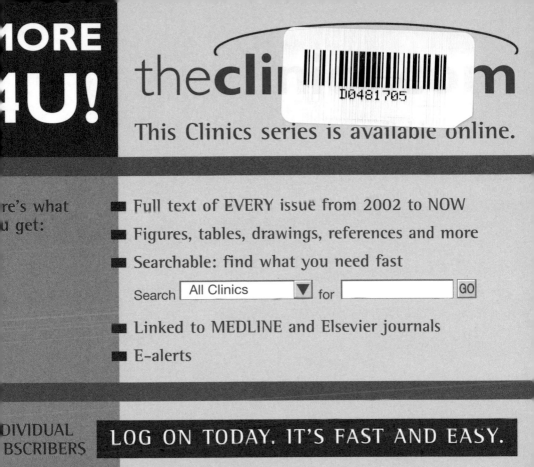
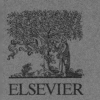

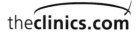

CHILD AND ADOLESCENT PSYCHIATRIC CLINICS OF NORTH AMERICA

Anxiety

GUEST EDITORS
Susan E. Swedo, MD, and
Daniel S. Pine, MD

CONSULTING EDITOR
Melvin Lewis, MBBS, FRCPsych, DCH

CONSULTING EDITOR (ACTING)
Andrés Martin, MD, MPH

October 2005 • Volume 14 • Number 4

SAUNDERS

An Imprint of Elsevier, Inc.
PHILADELPHIA   LONDON   TORONTO   MONTREAL   SYDNEY   TOKYO

W.B. SAUNDERS COMPANY
A Division of Elsevier Inc.

Elsevier, Inc. • 1600 John F. Kennedy Boulevard • Suite 1800 • Philadelphia, Pennsylvania 19103-2899

http://www.childpsych.theclinics.com

**CHILD AND ADOLESCENT PSYCHIATRIC CLINICS
OF NORTH AMERICA**   Volume 14, Number 4
October 2005   ISSN 1056-4993
Editor: Sarah E. Barth   ISBN 1-4160-2814-5

Reprints: For copies of 100 or more, of articles in this publication, please contact the Commercial Reprints Department, Elsevier Inc., 360 Park Avenue South, New York, New York 10010-1710. Tel. (212) 633-3813 Fax: (212) 462-1935 email: reprints@elsevier.com

The ideas and opinions expressed in *Child and Adolescent Psychiatric Clinics of North America* do not necessarily reflect those of the Publisher. The Publisher does not assume any responsibility for any injury and/or damage to persons or property arising out of or related to any use of the material contained in this periodical. The reader is advised to check the appropriate medical literature and the product information currently provided by the manufacturer of each drug to be administered to verify the dosage, the method and duration of administration, or contraindications. It is the responsibility of the treating physician or other health care professional, relying on independent experience and knowledge of the patient, to determine drug dosages and the best treatment for the patient. Mention of any product in this issue should not be construed as endorsement by the contributors, editors, or the Publisher of the product or manufacturers' claims.

Child and Adolescent Psychiatric Clinics of North America (ISSN 1056-4993) is published quarterly by W.B. Saunders Company. Corporate and editorial offices: Elsevier, Inc., 1600 John F. Kennedy Boulevard, Suite 1800, Philadelphia, PA 19103-2899. Accounting and circulation offices: 6277 Sea Harbor Drive, Orlando, FL 32887-4800. Periodicals postage paid at Orlando, FL 32862, and additional mailing offices. Subscription prices are $185.00 per year (US individuals), $280.00 per year (US institutions), $210.00 per year (Canadian individuals), $330.00 per year (Canadian institutions), $235.00 per year (foreign individuals), and $330.00 per year (foreign institutions). Foreign air speed delivery is included in all *Clinics* subscription prices. All prices are subject to change without notice. POSTMASTER: Send address changes to *Child and Adolescent Psychiatric Clinics of North America*, W.B. Saunders Company, Periodicals Fulfillment, Orlando, FL 32887-4800. **Customer Service: 1-800-654-2452 (US). From outside the US, call 1-407-345-4000. E-mail:** hhspcs@harcourt.com.

Child and Adolescent Psychiatric Clinics of North America is covered in *Index Medicus, ISI, SSCI, Research Alert, Social Search, Current Contents,* and *EMBASE/Excerpta Medica.*

Printed in the United States of America.

CONSULTING EDITOR

MELVIN LEWIS, MBBS, FRCPsych, DCH, Professor Emeritus, Senior Research Scientist, Yale Child Study Center, Yale University School of Medicine, New Haven, Connecticut; and Founding Consulting Editor, Emeritus

CONSULTING EDITOR (ACTING)

ANDRÉS MARTIN, MD, MPH, Associate Professor of Child Psychiatry and Psychiatry, Yale Child Study Center, Yale University School of Medicine; and Medical Director, Children's Psychiatric Inpatient Service, Yale-New Haven Children's Hospital, New Haven, Connecticut

GUEST EDITORS

DANIEL S. PINE, MD, Mood and Anxiety Disorders Program, Section on Development and Psychopathology, National Institute of Mental Health, Bethesda, Maryland

SUSAN E. SWEDO, MD, Behavioral Pediatric Section, Pediatrics and Developmental Neuropsychiatry Branch, National Institute of Mental Health, Bethesda, Maryland

CONTRIBUTORS

CHELSEA M. ALE, BA, The Pediatric Anxiety Research Clinic (PARC) at the Bradley Hasbro Research Center, Rhode Island Hospital, Providence, Rhode Island

ADRIAN ANGOLD, MRCPsych, Duke University Medical Center, Durham, North Carolina

SASHA G. ASCHENBRAND, MA, Doctoral Candidate in Clinical Psychology, Department of Psychology, Temple University, Philadelphia, Pennsylvania

DENISE A. CHAVIRA, PhD, Assistant Project Scientist, Anxiety and Traumatic Stress Disorders Clinic, Department of Psychiatry, University of California San Diego, La Jolla, California

E. JANE COSTELLO, PhD, Duke University Medical Center, Durham, North Carolina

RONALD E. DAHL, MD, Department of Psychiatry, University of Pittsburgh, School of Medicine/Medical Center, Western Psychiatric Institute and Clinic, Pittsburgh, Pennsylvania

MICHAEL D. DE BELLIS, MD, MPH, Professor of Psychiatry and Behavioral Sciences; and Director, Healthy Childhood Brain Development and Developmental Traumatology Research Program, Department of Psychiatry and Behavioral Sciences, Duke University Medical Center, Durham, North Carolina

HELEN L. EGGER, MD, Duke University Medical Center, Durham, North Carolina

ERIKA E. FORBES, PhD, Department of Psychiatry, University of Pittsburgh, School of Medicine/Medical Center, Western Psychiatric Institute and Clinic, Pittsburgh, Pennsylvania

NATHAN A. FOX, PhD, University of Maryland, College Park, Maryland

JENNIFER B. FREEMAN, PhD, The Pediatric Anxiety Research Clinic (PARC) at the Bradley Hasbro Research Center, Rhode Island Hospital, Providence, Rhode Island

ABBE M. GARCIA, PhD, The Pediatric Anxiety Research Clinic (PARC) at the Bradley Hasbro Research Center, Rhode Island Hospital, Providence, Rhode Island

PHILIP C. KENDALL, PhD, ABPP, Laura H. Carnell Professor of Psychology and Director, Child and Adolescent Anxiety Disorders Clinic, Department of Psychology, Temple University, Philadelphia, Pennsylvania

HENRIETTA L. LEONARD, MD, The Pediatric Anxiety Research Clinic (PARC) at the Bradley Hasbro Research Center, Rhode Island Hospital, Providence, Rhode Island

HEIDI J. LYNEHAM, PhD, Department of Psychology, Macquarie University, Sydney, New South Wales, Australia

KATHLEEN RIES MERIKANGAS, PhD, Senior Investigator, National Institute of Mental Health, Bethesda, Maryland

JACQUELINE MORENO, MS, Child Anxiety and Phobia Program, Child and Family Psychosocial Research Center, Department of Psychology, Florida International University, Miami, Florida

JANET S. NG, BA, The Pediatric Anxiety Research Clinic (PARC) at the Bradley Hasbro Research Center, Rhode Island Hospital, Providence, Rhode Island

KORALY PÉREZ-EDGAR, PhD, University of Maryland, College Park, Maryland

JOHN PIACENTINI, PhD, ABPP, Professor-in-Residence, Division of Child and Adolescent Psychiatry, Neuropsychiatric Institute; and Director, University of California Los Angeles Child OCD, Anxiety and Tic Disorders Program, University of California Los Angeles, Los Angeles, California

RONALD M. RAPEE, PhD, Department of Psychology, Macquarie University, Sydney, New South Wales, Australia

SHAUNA P. REINBLATT, MD, FRCPC, Postdoctoral Research Fellow, Division of Child and Adolescent Psychiatry, Johns Hopkins University School of Medicine, Baltimore, Maryland

TAMI ROBLEK, PhD, Postdoctoral Research Fellow in Child and Adolescent Psychiatry, Neuropsychiatric Institute; and School of Medicine, University of California Los Angeles, Los Angeles, California

NEAL D. RYAN, MD, Department of Psychiatry, University of Pittsburgh, School of Medicine/Medical Center, Western Psychiatric Institute and Clinic, Pittsburgh, Pennsylvania

WENDY K. SILVERMAN, PhD, ABPP, Professor of Psychology; and Director, Child Anxiety and Phobia Program, Child and Family Psychosocial Research Center, Department of Psychology, Florida International University, Miami, Florida

MURRAY B. STEIN, MD, MPH, FRCPC, Professor of Psychiatry, Anxiety and Traumatic Stress Disorders Clinic, Department of Psychiatry, University of California—San Diego, La Jolla, California

CYNTHIA SUVEG, PhD, Postdoctoral Research Fellow, Department of Psychology, Temple University, Philadelphia, Pennsylvania

THOMAS VAN DILLEN, PhD, Clinical Associate, Department of Psychiatry and Behavioral Sciences, Duke University Medical Center, Durham, North Carolina

JOHN T. WALKUP, MD, Associate Professor of Psychiatry, Division of Child and Adolescent Psychiatry, Johns Hopkins University School of Medicine, Baltimore, Maryland

DOUGLAS E. WILLIAMSON, PhD, Department of Psychiatry, University of Pittsburgh, School of Medicine/Medical Center, Western Psychiatric Institute and Clinic, Pittsburgh, Pennsylvania

CONTENTS

This article argues that the quality of diagnostic tools used to measure anxiety disorders in children and adolescents has improved enormously in the past few years. As a result, prevalence estimates are less erratic, understanding of comorbidity is increasing, and the role of impairment as a criterion for "caseness" is considered more carefully. Several of the instruments developed for epidemiologic research are now being used in clinical settings. Further integration of laboratory methods and clinical and epidemiologic ideas will benefit children with anxiety disorders and their families.

With the maturation of community studies of adults in the past decade, there has been growing awareness of the importance of the magnitude and impact of anxiety disorders in the general population. The convergence of findings from adult and child epidemiology reveals that the onset of anxiety disorders occurs in childhood, and a substantial proportion of youth with anxiety continues to manifest lifelong problems with anxiety and other mental disorders. In this article, the major risk factors for the development of anxiety disorders in childhood and adolescence are reviewed.

specific phobia, and presents assessment and treatment issues. Finally, a case study is offered that serves to illuminate the major topics outlined in the article.

Evaluation and Treatment of Anxiety Disorders in the General Pediatric Population: A Clinician's Guide

Heidi J. Lyneham and Ronald M. Rapee

This article provides an overview of research on the recognition, assessment, and treatment of children and adolescents who have anxiety disorders and emphasizes practical issues facing clinicians. Discussion includes an overview of the prevalence and consequences of anxiety and reviews assessment tools, maintenance factors, and evidence-based approaches to treatment. Topics also include developmental considerations, approaches to informant discrepancy, predictors of treatment outcome, and recent innovative approaches to treatment that may potentially improve dissemination to the general pediatric population.

Cognitive-Behavior Therapy for Childhood Anxiety Disorders

Tami Roblek and John Piacentini

Over the past decade, multiple controlled trials have demonstrated the efficacy of cognitive-behavior therapy (CBT) for the treatment of anxiety disorders in children and adolescents. Relying heavily on behavioral exposure, cognitive restructuring, and psychoeducation, CBT for child anxiety has been shown to be adaptable to a variety of implementation formats, including individual, family, and group treatment. This article describes the conceptual framework underlying CBT and the key elements of this treatment approach. Important developmental and family considerations in treatment are discussed, and the empirical literature is reviewed.

Psychopharmacologic Treatment of Pediatric Anxiety Disorders

Shauna P. Reinblatt and John T. Walkup

This article reviews the psychopharmacologic treatment of child and adolescent anxiety disorders and is divided into the following sections: historical background, general treatment principles, obsessive-compulsive disorder, other anxiety disorders, including separation anxiety disorders, generalized anxiety disorder, and social phobia, elective mutism, and post-traumatic stress disorder and specific phobia. Short-term and long-term psychopharmacologic treatment strategies are reviewed, as are approaches for managing comorbidity and treatment-refractory cases. This article is organized by diagnostic categories rather than by medication classes to emphasize the clinical perspective.

FORTHCOMING ISSUES

RECENT ISSUES

ELSEVIER
SAUNDERS

Child Adolesc Psychiatric Clin N Am
14 (2005) xiii–xiv

CHILD AND
ADOLESCENT
PSYCHIATRIC CLINICS
OF NORTH AMERICA

Foreword

Nervous Energy

Where did you come from, lamentable quality?
. . .
I hadn't any other experience of enemies from inside.
They were all from outside—big boys
Who cursed me and hit me; motorists; falling trees.
All these you were as bad as, yet inside.

—Kenneth Koch: To Stammering

All movement is precipitated by dissatisfaction with where you currently are.

—Blaise Pascal, Pensees

Anxiety is about more than fear and trembling. Beyond children's suffering, anxiety can, in reasonable doses, stimulate their adaptive growth. It may be argued that anxiety of some sort invariably precedes all mobilization. While the common parlance suggests that the spiritually enlightened eliminate all anxiety, those without any to speak of are more commonly found within our prisons: a little anxiety appears to be a good thing. As child psychiatrists, though, we see the excesses of the trait. Fears of contamination may spiral children into paralyzing washing rituals, and those of academic performance or social engagement may shut them out of classrooms or circles of friends. But the self-same fears that in full expression may become the OCD, school phobia, or PTSD so familiar to clinicians, may in smaller servings yield the meticulous cleanliness, attention to organization and detail, or apprehension of strangers so cherished and instilled by attentive parents everywhere. Perhaps no functional domain so clearly exemplifies the thin line between adaptive value and the burdens of excess as does anxiety.

And as this issue of the *Clinics* makes clear, children's anxiety has spurred the mobilization of more than cleanliness, good work habits, or stranger danger. Research on anxiety disorders has served as a guide and provided a model for other areas of pediatric mental health and developmental psychopathology. No

1056-4993/05/$ – see front matter © 2005 Elsevier Inc. All rights reserved.
doi:10.1016/j.chc.2005.07.002

less should be expected from a group of disorders with a penchant to collect first places: first in prevalence for sure (although that particular distinction is threatened once functional impairment is factored in seriously); first in novel mechanisms of etiologic understanding (be they immunologic, as in PANDAS, or in the unveiling of neural pathways through basic science and functional neuroimaging); a series of firsts in treatment (for example, acral lick disorder, that loaner from veterinary medicine, remains a compelling animal model for a human psychiatric disorder [OCD], and one of the more pharmacologically responsive ones at that [starting with clomipramine and heralding the ascendancy of the SSRIs]).

The contributors to this issue make clear how much we have advanced in our understanding of these disorders—and that there is much more still to know. It is a good thing, then, that anxiety precedes mobilization but precludes rest, for we have much left to do and can ill afford to remain inactive. This field of inquiry, just as our children and the federal dependency that stewards their mental well-being, are and will be the better for the combined wisdom and restless efforts of Guest Editors Sue Swedo and Danny Pine. May we all be kindled by a spark from their unique brand of nervous energy.

Andrés Martin, MD, MPH
Consulting Editor (Acting)
Yale Child Study Center
Yale University School of Medicine
230 South Frontage Road
New Haven, CT 06520-7900, USA
E-mail address: andres.martin@yale.edu

ELSEVIER
SAUNDERS

Child Adolesc Psychiatric Clin N Am
14 (2005) xv–xviii

CHILD AND
ADOLESCENT
PSYCHIATRIC CLINICS
OF NORTH AMERICA

Preface

Anxiety

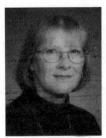 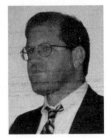

Susan E. Swedo, MD   Daniel S. Pine, MD
Guest Editors

This issue of the *Child and Adolescent Psychiatric Clinics of North America* reviews recent research findings on pediatric anxiety disorders. This provides an important opportunity to reflect on progress in various areas of research on developmental psychopathology during the past 10 to 15 years. Both the major breakthroughs and the major questions in research on pediatric anxiety parallel many of the broader advances and uncertainties in other areas of psychiatry and psychology. Thus, a review of work in this area is prescient both for considerations specifically on anxiety and for broader issues affecting the mental well being of children and adolescents. Findings and central questions in five major areas of research are summarized in this issue, each pertaining to pediatric anxiety disorders. In the current summary, we briefly outline the nature of these five areas.

First, considerable advances have emerged in psychiatric epidemiology, as applied to various forms of developmental psychopathology. These advances have stimulated a series of large-scale studies that document the prevalence of pediatric mental disorders and their distributions across various sectors of the population. Based on these studies, pediatric anxiety disorders are recognized as the most common form of developmental psychopathology. The high prevalence of pediatric anxiety disorders emphasizes the importance of work summarized in this issue. Nevertheless, this major finding has also led to many unanswered questions. In particular, prevalence estimates for pediatric anxiety disorders are highly sensitive to impairment thresholds, such that relatively minor alterations in algorithms for defining impairment in a structured assessment for anxiety lead to relatively marked changes in estimated prevalence. As in many other areas of psychiatric epidemiology, this finding has raised major questions concerning the nature of psychiatric diagnosis. Particularly pressing questions emerge concerning the degree to which psychiatric phenotypes, such as pediatric anxiety disorders, might be most appropriately characterized as continuously distributed traits, without clear boundaries separating health and disease, as opposed to categorical entities. These questions appear particularly pressing in research on anxiety, given the ubiquity of anxiety as a part of normal development and the effects on prevalence of minor alterations in diagnostic algorithms.

Second, longitudinal and family genetic research has revealed strong relationships between pediatric anxiety disorders and various forms of adult psychopathology. Thus, longitudinal studies demonstrate within-subject relationships across development, in that pediatric anxiety disorders confer a high risk for both adult anxiety and mood disorders. Similarly, family studies demonstrate across-subject relationships within families, in that both anxiety and depression in parents confers a high risk for pediatric anxiety disorders in offspring. Given the high prevalence of pediatric anxiety disorders, data linking pediatric anxiety disorders with adult psychopathology lends further emphasis to the importance of advancing understandings of pathophysiology and treatment. Nevertheless, major questions also remain in studies linking pediatric anxiety to adult psychopathology. In particular, while strong relationships do exist, early anxiety is by no means a fait accompli, in that the majority of children and adolescents with anxiety disorders will not suffer from a mood or anxiety disorder when assessed as adults. These findings raise major questions regarding factors that distinguish among children and adolescents with transient as opposed to more persistent forms of psychopathology that begin as pediatric anxiety disorders.

Third, this issue reviews data on multiple forms of anxiety currently classified as distinct conditions in the *Diagnostic and Statistical Manual of Mental Disorders* (DSM-IV). This includes separation anxiety disorder, social anxiety disorder, generalized anxiety disorder, phobias, obsessive-compulsive disorder, and a series of other related conditions. As reviewed in this issue, these conditions show certain shared features in that each represents a developmental condition characterized by high levels of fear and apprehension concerning various stimuli or situations. On the other hand, these conditions also can be distinguished from one another in that unique symptom profiles and associated features can also clearly be differentiated among the various pediatric anxiety disorders. The degree to which current categorizations in the DSM-IV genuinely achieve the goal of "carving nature at its joints" in capturing categories of syndromes that relate to genuine differences in pathophysiology remains unclear.

Fourth, efforts to validate current anxiety disorder diagnoses, and determine the accuracy of current classifications, will benefit from recent breakthroughs in neuroscience. Relative to other complex behaviors, research on the neural circuitry of fear and anxiety has progressed relatively far during the past two decades. Studies in rodents and non-human primates have delineated the neural circuitry that has evolved to facilitate the mammalian response to various forms of danger. Central to these responses are the key defining features of the anxiety disorders, including hypervigilance, avoidance, and defensive physiologic responses. Neuroscientific understandings have also led to some appreciation of specificity in response to divergent forms of danger. Thus, the neural circuitry mediating learned fears can be differentiated from that mediating innate fears. Similarly, circuitry engaged by toxins that pose a threat to safety when ingested can be differentiated from circuitry engaged by stimuli that threaten mammals by other routes. Advances in neuroimaging have set the stage for studies that will determine the degree to which these distinctions can be used to inform classification in pediatric anxiety. Thus, it may be that distinct forms of anxiety involve distinct forms of circuitry dysfunction. If confirmed, this finding might lead to a modification of psychiatric nosology based on understandings of brain function.

Finally, the past decade has also witnessed considerable advances in treatment. As a rule, advances during recent years have emerged largely by applying to children and adolescent treatments with a long history of use in adult anxiety disorders. Specifically, a series of studies have used cognitive behavioral therapy (CBT) in various forms of pediatric anxiety disorders. These studies have demonstrated clear benefits of this treatment over various control conditions, although the precise aspect of CBT that is most beneficial remains incompletely understood. Similarly, large-scale medication trials have been executed during the past decade. Although major questions have emerged concerning safety, large-scale randomized controlled trials leave little doubt that selective serotonin reuptake inhibitors (SSRIs) represent efficacious treatments for many forms of pediatric anxiety disorders. Despite these advances, major questions remain. For example, it is unclear which treatments are best suited for which patients with most anxiety disorders, given the dearth of head-to-head comparison randomized controlled trials using SSRIs and CBT. Similarly, while efficacy has been clearly established for SSRIs and CBT, these treatments remain far from panaceas. Even in ideal settings, many children and adolescents will exhibit only a modest symptomatic response to these treatments. Considerably more work is needed in the development of therapeutic modalities.

In closing, it is clear that major progress has been made in research on pediatric anxiety disorders. This progress has delineated many of the major questions that have yet to be answered, providing important guidelines for future research approaches. Perhaps most importantly, research in pediatric anxiety disorders has defined key issues confronting studies in many other areas of developmental psychopathology. As a result, the material in this issue might provide key insights relevant to pediatric anxiety disorders as well as other forms of psychopathology.

Susan E. Swedo, MD
Behavioral Pediatric Section
Pediatrics and Developmental Neuropsychiatry Branch
National Institute of Mental Health
10 Center Drive MSC 1255
Building 10, Room 4N208
Bethesda, MD 20892-1255, USA
E-mail address: swedos@irp.nimh.nih.gov

Daniel S. Pine, MD
Mood and Anxiety Disorders Program
Section on Development and Psychopathology
National Institute of Mental Health
15K North Drive
Room 110
Bethesda, MD 20892, USA
E-mail address: pined@mail.nih.gov

ELSEVIER
SAUNDERS

Child Adolesc Psychiatric Clin N Am
14 (2005) 631–648

CHILD AND
ADOLESCENT
PSYCHIATRIC CLINICS
OF NORTH AMERICA

The Developmental Epidemiology of Anxiety Disorders: Phenomenology, Prevalence, and Comorbidity

E. Jane Costello, PhD*, Helen L. Egger, MD,
Adrian Angold, MRCPsych

Duke University Medical Center, Box 3454 DUMC, Durham, NC 27710, USA

Anxiety has been one of the most difficult areas of child psychopathology to study in representative population samples. The main reasons for this are clinical uncertainty about the boundaries of the various anxiety disorders and the rarity of several of the disorders in population-based samples. Although the taxonomic problems are far from resolved, there has been considerable progress in the past decade.

First, longitudinal and laboratory-based studies have made it clear that different types of anxiety have different correlates, predictors, and courses across childhood and adolescence [1]. Second, although there are still many problems with assessment, the situation is improving. Direct assessment of young children is always difficult because they often lack the cognitive abilities needed to talk about worry, fear, and panic [2]. However, parents have been shown to be reliable reporters about their young children's anxieties (Angold, submitted for publication, 2005). In addition, most current assessment instruments incorporate measures of functioning so that researchers can decide what level of impairment is required to make a diagnosis. When functional impairment is required, the

This work is based in part on Costello EJ, Egger HL, Angold A. The developmental epidemiology of anxiety disorders. In: Ollendick T, March J, editors. Phobic and anxiety disorders in children and adolescents. New York: Oxford University Press; 2004. p. 61–91; copyright 2004, Oxford University Press; with permission.

* Corresponding author.
E-mail address: jcostell@psych.mc.duke.edu (E.J. Costello).

prevalence of some anxiety disorders such as simple phobias falls dramatically [3] and rates become much more consistent across studies [4].

A third issue for assessment is the overlap of depression and anxiety. The two types of disorders predict one another developmentally [5,6] and often respond to the same treatments [7], which has led some clinicians to treat them as part of the same syndrome [8]. However, a closer look suggests that the overlap of anxiety and depression applies only to some anxiety disorders [5]. It would be premature to change the taxonomy at this stage; we need to know a lot more about the developmental pathways of the various types of anxiety and depression, before that point is reached.

Prevalence and comorbidity

This article reviews the epidemiologic literature on anxiety disorder in general and, when they are specified, on separation anxiety disorder (SAD), generalized anxiety disorder (GAD), overanxious disorder (OAD), specific phobias, panic, agoraphobia, social phobia, post-traumatic stress disorder (PTSD), and obsessive-compulsive disorder (OCD). However, many epidemiologic studies have reported on "anxiety" in general, without distinguishing among the specific categories set out in, for example, the Diagnostic and Statistical Manual of Mental Disorders (DSM), Third Edition, Revised (III-R) or DSM-IV, and it is often unclear how many different diagnoses have been included in the research protocol.

Prevalence of anxiety disorders in preschool children

Most of the research on anxiety and fear in young children has been conducted from the perspective of temperament and normal development, not psychopathology. In these approaches, anxiety or fear in young children is seen either as a normative phase of development or, in a subset of children, a risk factor for anxiety disorders. Between the age of 7 and 12 months, most infants develop a fear of strangers and express distress when they are separated from their primary caregivers. These fears peak between 9 and 18 months of age and decrease for most children by age 2.5 [9]. Approximately 15% of young children display more intense and persistent fear, shyness, and social withdrawal in response to unfamiliar people, situations, or objects than other children do [10–12]. Behaviorally inhibited young children display characteristic patterns of physiology (high heart rate, low heart rate variability, high baseline levels of morning cortisol, and elevated startle responses) [13] and are more likely to develop an anxiety disorder later in childhood or adolescence or to have first-degree relatives with anxiety disorders [12,14–18]. Recent advances in the nosology and diagnosis of psychiatric symptoms and disorders in preschool children [19,20] have made it possible to begin to define the boundaries between normative anxiety, temperament variation, and clinically significant anxiety disorders in very young children.

Until 5 years ago, there were only three studies that could approximate community-based estimates of the prevalence of DSM anxiety disorders in preschool-aged children. The 1982 study by Earls [21] was ahead of its time, using questionnaires followed by clinical judgment, and applying DSM-III criteria to all of the 3-year-old children on Martha's Vineyard (Massachusetts). Fifteen years later, Keenan and colleagues [22] studied another small sample of children in poverty, who were assessed with a structured clinical interview. Lavigne and colleagues [23] used a combination of the Child Behavior Checklist [8], observational assessments, and measures of adaptive behaviors to make clinical consensus diagnoses of the preschoolers in a pediatric primary care setting. Recently, the Preschool Age Psychiatric Assessment (PAPA) [19,24] was developed for use with parents of children ages 2 through 5 years old. Table 1 [21–23,25] shows the prevalence of anxiety disorders from these four studies of preschoolers in nonpsychiatric settings, providing an approximation to expected general population rates.

The PAPA study, for which information was available by gender, found no significant gender differences for anxiety disorders overall or for specific anxiety disorders. Four- and 5-year-old children were significantly more likely than 2- and 3-year-old children were to have any anxiety disorder (11.9% versus 7.7%, respectively) or PTSD (1.3% versus 0.0%, respectively). African-American children were less likely to meet criteria for any anxiety disorder (6.4% versus 14.0%, respectively) or social phobia (0.6% versus 4.3%, respectively) than were non-African-American children. Comorbidity with other psychiatric disorder was common, ranging from 53% of cases of generalized anxiety disorder to 100% of cases of specific phobia. The most common type of comorbidity with nonanxiety disorders was with depression.

Prevalence of anxiety disorders in school-aged children and adolescents

Table 2 [3,26–50] summarizes information on prevalence from recent epidemiologic studies of older children and adolescents. It includes all published studies using DSM-III-R (the earliest published in 1992) or DSM-IV (1996 onward). Studies are listed in order of their period of reference (current, 3-, 6-, or 12-month and lifetime.)

Any anxiety disorder

Studies with a short assessment interval and a single data wave had the lowest prevalence; for example, the current prevalence of one or more anxiety disorders was 2.8% in the Oregon Adolescent Depression Project [26]. Three-month estimates ranged from 2.2% to 8.6%; 6-month estimates ranged from 5.5% to 17.7%; 12-month estimates ranged from 8.6% to 20.9%; and lifetime estimates ranged from 8.3% to 27.0%. Not surprisingly, using a lifetime criterion on the oldest samples generated the highest estimates.

Table 1
Prevalence of anxiety disorders in community studies of preschoolers

Study [reference]	Diagnostic criteria	Age (y)	N	Any anxiety disorder (%)	SAD (%)	GAD (%)	OAD (%)	Specific phobia (%)	Social phobia (%)	Selective mutism (%)
Earls et al, 1982 [21]	Questionnaire and clinical interview DSM-III	3	100	NR	5.0	NR	NR	0.0	2.0	NR
Keenan et al, 1997 [22]	Modified K-SADS DSM-III-R	5	104	NR	11.5	NR	NR	4.6	2.3	NR
Lavigne et al, 1996 [23]	Clinical consensus DSM-III-R	2–5	510	NR	0.5	NR	NR	0.6	0.7	NR
Briggs-Gowan et al, 2000 [25]	DISC DSM-III-R	4–6	516[a]	6.1	3.6	NR	0.5	3.7	NR	NR
Angold et al, submitted for publication, 2005	PAPA DSM-IV	2–5	307[b]	9.5	2.4	6.5	0.0	2.3	2.2	0.6

Abbreviations: DISC, Diagnostic Interview Schedule for Children; K-SADS, Kiddie-Schedule for Affective Disorders and Schizophrenia; NR, not reported.
[a] Total sample of 1060.
[b] Data weighted back to screening population of 1073.

Specific anxiety disorders

Recent studies have provided new information about the prevalence of specific anxiety disorders. They show that DSM-III-R OAD and DSM-IV GAD are the most common anxiety diagnoses and that panic disorder and agoraphobia (separately or together) are the least common. In the first prevalence studies, the reported rates of specific phobias ("simple phobias" in DSM-III-R) were extremely high, but most diagnostic instruments for children have now resolved this problem by taking disability into account in making the diagnosis. Two studies using adult instruments (the Diagnostic Interview Schedule [DIS] and the Composite International Diagnostic Interview [CIDI]) continued to report high rates of specific and social phobias and agoraphobia. This suggests that attention needs to be paid to the use of adult measures when assessing phobias in children. In contrast, the Bremen study of adolescents [51], which also used the CIDI, reported rates of specific and social phobia well within the range found in other studies of children and adolescents.

Anxiety and disability

One of the most hotly debated areas in the past few years has been the relationship between psychiatric diagnosis and the level of functioning. When the first versions of the DIS for Children (DISC) were introduced in the 1980s, they were found to generate extremely high prevalence rates for some disorders, among which were some anxiety disorders [3,52]; for example, according to data from the four-site Methods for the Epidemiology of Child and Adolescent (MECA) mental disorders study, 39.5% of the children had at least one anxiety diagnosis in the previous 12 months [3]. At the same time, health maintenance organization (HMO) insurance companies and governmental agencies were concerned about whether all these children "really needed" treatment [53,54].

One solution to both problems was to require that, to receive a diagnosis, a child should show a significant degree of functional impairment or disability (to use the World Health Organization's preferred term). In 1993, the Federal Register defined a new class of psychiatric disorders, called Serious Emotional Disturbance (SED), which required "significantly impaired functioning" or disability in addition to a diagnosis [55]. SED was to be used as the criterion for assessing the prevalence of child psychiatric disorder in each state for the purpose of allocating federal block grants, and disability criteria were added to psychiatric diagnoses.

Disability can be measured at several different levels. Each symptom can require impaired functioning; disability can be evaluated at the level of the syndrome or diagnosis or in the presence of any diagnosis, irrespective of which one causes impaired functioning; the interviewer could rate the child's level of functioning without making a diagnosis, using a separate measure [55,56]; or, of course, more than one method can be used.

Table 2
Summary of Diagnostic and Statistical Manual of Mental Disorders (III-R and IV) and International Classification of Diseases (Tenth Revision) studies of anxiety disorder prevalence

Study [reference]	Diagnostic criteria	Age of child/adolescent (y)	N	Period of reference	SAD (%)	Panic disorder (%)	OCD (%)	Specific phobia (%)	Agoraphobia with or without panic (%)	Social phobia (%)	PTSD (%)	Avoidant disorder (%)	OAD (%)	GAD (%)	Any anxiety disorder (%)
Oregon Adolescent Depression [26,27]	DSM-III-R, K-SADS	14–18	1709	Current	0.2	0.3	—	1.3	0.1	0.9	—	—	0.5	—	2.8
				Lifetime											8.3
				Lifetime by age 19											27.0
Virginia Twin Study of Adolescent Behavioral Development [28]	DSM-III-R, CAPA	8–17	2824	3 mo	1.2	—	—	4.4	1.1	2.5	—	—	4.4	—	8.6
Caring for Children in the Community [29]	DSM-III-R, DSM-IV, CAPA	9–12	388	3 mo	3.6	0.2	0.1	0.3	0.4	0.8	2.6	0.0	1.5	1.4	5.0
Great Smoky Mountains [30]	DSM-III-R, DSM-IV, CAPA	9–12	2709	3 mo	2.1	0.1	0.1	0.1	0.2	0.3	0.5	0.0	0.6	1.4	2.9
Caring for Children in the Community [29]	DSM-III-R, DSM-IV, CAPA	13–17	532	3 mo	2.6	1.8	0.3	0.5	0.6	1.7	4.0	0.1	3.6	3.9	5.9

Study	Diagnostic criteria	Age	N	Time frame											
Great Smoky Mountains [30]	DSM-III-R, DSM-IV, CAPA	13–16	3895	3 mo	0.4	0.3	0.2	0.3	0.3	0.7	1.0	0.1	1.5	2.3	2.2
Quebec Child Mental Health Survey [31]	DSM-III-R, DISC 2.25	6–14	2400	6 mo	2.6 (child) 1.6 (parent)	—	—	4.9 (child) 11.5 (parent)	—	—	—	—	3.1 (child) 3.8 (parent)	—	9.1 (child) 14.7 (parent)
Methods for the Epidemiology of Child and Adolescent Mental Disorders [3]	DSM-III-R, DISC 2.3 (Dx + CGAS <71)	9–17	1285	6 mo	3.9	—	—	2.6	3.3	5.4	—	—	5.7	—	13.0
Health Maintenance Organization [32]	DSM-III-R, DISC 2.3	12–18	278	6 mo	3.2	1.1	—	3.6	2.2	5.1	—	1.8	7.1	4.6	17.7
Random sample (The Netherlands) [33]	DSM-III-R, DISC 2.3	13–18	274	6 mo	1.8	0.4	1.0	12.7	2.6	9.2	—	4.0	3.1	1.3	23.5 / 9.7 with CGAS <71 / 5.3 without CGAS <61
Northern Plains (child only) [34]	DSM-III-R, DISC 2.1C	14–16	109	6 mo	1.9	—	—	2.9	—	2.0	—	—	1.9	—	5.5

(continued on next page)

Table 2 (continued)

Study [reference]	Diagnostic criteria	Age of child/adolescent (y)	N	Period of reference	SAD (%)	Panic disorder (%)	OCD (%)	Specific phobia (%)	Agoraphobia with or without panic (%)	Social phobia (%)	PTSD (%)	Avoidant disorder (%)	OAD (%)	GAD (%)	Any anxiety disorder (%)
Christchurch Longitudinal [35]	DSM-III-R, DISC 2.3	15	1000	6 mo	—	—	—	—	—	—	—	—	—	—	12.8
Early Developmental Stages of Psychopathology [36]	DSM-IV, CIDI	14–24	3021	12 mo	—	1.2	0.6	1.8	1.6 (without panic)	2.6	0.7	—	—	0.5	9.3
				Lifetime	—	1.6	0.7	2.3	2.6 (without panic)	3.5	1.3	—	—	0.8	14.4
National Comorbidity Survey [37,38]	DSM-III-R, CIDI	15–17	479	12 mo	—	3.0	—	11.8	4.0	12.4	—	—	—	0.3	20.9
				Lifetime	—	3.1	—	12.2	9.1	13.1	—	—	—	0.6	24.7
Dunedin Longitudinal [39,40]	DSM-III-R, DIS, DISC	18	993	12 mo (DIS)	—	—	4.0	—	—	11.1	—	—	—	—	12.4

Study	Instrument	Age	N	Timeframe												
Dunedin Longitudinal [41]	DSM-III-R, DIS, DISC	21	960	12 mo (DIS, DISC)	—	0.6	7.1	8.4	3.8	9.7	—	—	—	—	1.9	20.3
Puerto Rico [42]	DSM-IV, DISC	4–17	1897	12 mo	3.1	0.7	—	—	—	2.8	0.8	—	—	—	2.4	9.5
Iowa Family [43]	DSM-III-R, UM-CIDI	Any onsets during 15–19	303	—	—	1.3 (attack)	—	2.6	1.7	5.0	—	—	—	—	—	8.6
Essau Bremen [44–47]	DSM-IV, CIDI	12–17	1035	Lifetime	—	0.5	—	3.5	—	1.6	1.6	—	—	—	—	—
Minnesota Parent-Child Project [48]	K-SADS, DSM-III-R	17.5	172	Lifetime	4.6	1.7	1.7	—	—	5.8	—	1.7	4.6	—	—	15.1
New York State Longitudinal [49]	DSM-III-R, DISC	Any onsets by 18	551	—	—	—	—	—	—	—	—	—	—	—	—	15.1
Boston Longitudinal [50]	DSM-III-R	21	384	Lifetime	—	—	—	—	—	—	6.0	—	—	—	—	—

Abbreviations: CAPA, Child and Adolescent Psychiatric Assessment; CGAS, Children's Global Assessment Scale; CIDI, Composite International Diagnostic Interview; DIS, Diagnostic Interview Schedule; DISC, Diagnostic Interview Schedule for Children; Dx, diagnosis; K-SADS, Kiddie-Schedule for Affective Disorders and Schizophrenia; UM-CIDI, University of Michigan Composite International Diagnostic Interview.

The effects on the prevalence of anxiety disorders of assessing disability in different ways can be seen in the four-site MECA study using the DISC version 2.3. The study used two kinds of disability assessment: one type attached to each symptom cluster such that the interviewer asked about disability if the child or parent endorsed "half plus one" symptoms (ie, one more than half the symptoms needed for the diagnosis) and one that required the interviewer to rate the child on a scale of 0 to 100 on a level of functioning using the Children's Global Assessment Scale (CGAS) [56] after the interview was ended. Adding either diagnosis-specific impairment or "mild impairment" (70 or less) on the CGAS halved the prevalence rate; adding both reduced it by two-thirds. A requirement of both diagnosis-specific impairment and "severe" (50 or below) impairment on the CGAS reduced it by almost 90% [3]. Anxiety was of all diagnoses the area most severely affected by requiring impairment, and among the anxiety disorders, simple phobia was the most affected; the prevalence estimate fell from 21.6% (no impairment requirements) to 0.7% (diagnosis-specific plus CGAS ≤ 50).

Requiring disability as a criterion for making the diagnosis brings the rates down to levels that certainly make provider institutions more comfortable. However, there is growing evidence that disability can be associated with anxiety symptoms that do not reach the threshold for a diagnosis [57] and that even controlling for comorbidity with other psychiatric disorders anxiety disorders are associated with a high degree of disability [58]. The true burden to children, families, and society associated with these conditions is still unclear and needs further longitudinal research.

Sex and age differences in the prevalence of anxiety disorders

Girls are somewhat more likely than boys are to report an anxiety disorder of some sort. However, at the level of individual diagnoses, few of the gender differences are large. If we assume that the difference is likely to be clinically and statistically meaningful if twice as many girls as boys reported a diagnosis, then only the eight studies cited in Table 2 reported any meaningful gender differences. Three studies reported more specific phobias in girls; two studies reported more panic disorder; two studies reported more agoraphobia; and one study reported more separation anxiety disorder and OAD. Lewinsohn and colleagues [26], in one of the few studies to examine the effects of potentially confounding factors associated with both gender and anxiety, found that controlling for 15 such factors did not eliminate the excess of anxiety disorders in girls.

It is difficult to draw conclusions about age trends from this review because, in many cases, the age of subjects was confounded with the time frame of the interview. Thus, the 3-month studies had both the lowest prevalence rates and the youngest subjects, whereas the 12-month studies tended to have the highest prevalence as well as the oldest subjects. It is worth noting that Lewinsohn and

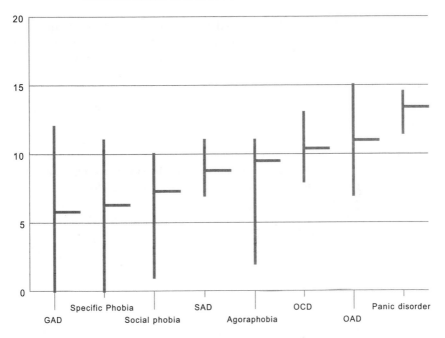

Fig. 1. Mean age of onset by age 16, and interquartile range, anxiety disorders. (*From* Phobic and anxiety disorders in children and adolescents: a clinician's guide to effective psychosocial and pharmacological interventions by Thomas Ollendick, edited by John S. March, copyright Oxford University Press, Inc.; with permission.)

colleagues [26], using retrospective data, identified the female preponderance in anxiety disorders as emerging by age 6 years.

Fig. 1 summarizes the ages of onset of different anxiety disorders. It represents the range and median ages for the studies from Table 2 for which this information is available. It shows that GAD began earliest, with a median age of around 6 years, whereas panic disorders rarely began before midadolescence. It is important to note that the range of estimates is very wide for some anxiety disorders.

Comorbidity among anxiety disorders

Comorbidity among anxiety disorders has historically been a problem, not only for nosology and epidemiology but also for diagnosis and treatment. This is an area in which the high level of comorbidity found in clinical samples is mirrored in community samples. A review of published studies yields inconclusive results because (1) not all diagnoses were included in every study, and the number of anxiety disorders included in the analyses of comorbidity varies from study to study; (2) there is a lack of consensus about whether to control for comorbidity with other anxiety disorders or with other diagnoses when examining the strength of a particular association; and (3) concurrent and sequential comorbidity are not always distinguished clearly. The two published studies that have explored the issue of comorbidity among anxiety disorders [27,28] used bivariate analyses (corrected for gender and age in the latter case), so it is hard to interpret the finding that the majority of comparisons yielded a significant odds ratio.

The present authors attempted to conduct a meta-analysis of the available data sets along the lines of work on psychiatric comorbidity that we have published previously [59]. However, for many of the diagnostic comparisons, there were too few data sets for such analyses to be feasible. Therefore, we can only draw some very tentative conclusions based mainly on studies for which we had direct access to the data: the Great Smoky Mountains Study (GSMS) [30], the Caring for Children in the Community (CCC) study [29], the Virginia Twin Study of Adolescent Behavioral Development [28], the HMO study [32], and the National Comorbidity Survey [37,38] (see Table 2).

Generalized anxiety disorder and overanxious disorder

A question of nosologic interest is the extent to which the older overanxious disorder category overlaps with the DSM-IV generalized anxiety diagnosis. The intention was that children who would formerly have received a diagnosis of overanxious disorder of childhood would be subsumed into the new GAD category. The criteria for GAD were loosened for children, who could receive the diagnosis if they had only one of the six symptoms of criterion C (restlessness, fatigue, difficulty concentrating, irritability, muscle tension, and sleep disturbance). However, with one exception, these symptom classes are very different from those defined for overanxious disorder (worries about the past or future, concerns about one's competence, need for reassurance, somatic symptoms, self-consciousness, and muscle tension). Although it is mentioned briefly in the description of criterion A (excessive anxiety or worry), the latter symptoms are not set out in the new formal diagnostic criteria. On the other hand, five of the six new criterion C symptoms are very similar to symptoms of major depressive episode; it is very difficult to write diagnostic questions that reliably capture the subtle differences between, for example, the fatigue associated with depression and that associated with GAD. Thus, any examination of the overlap between OAD and GAD should take into account the possibility of their overlap with depression.

Only three data sets (GSMS, CCC, and HMO) permitted a comparison of GAD, OAD, and depression in the same children. Here we use GSMS data to examine concurrent comorbidity among OAD using DSM-III-R criteria, GAD, using DSM-IV criteria, and DSM-IV depression. Over the course of the study, 182 children (11.6% of the sample) had one or more of the three diagnoses by the age of 16 years. Of those who were comorbid (5.4% of the sample or 47% of those with any of the three diagnoses) more than half (52%) had all three disorders. Because GAD was supposed to subsume OAD, one might expect this combination to be quite common. In fact, only 12 children (weighted 16% of those with either GAD or OAD) had both disorders without depression over the course of the study. Of the children with OAD without GAD, 36 of 88 (weighted 42%) also had a depressive disorder, not far from the 135 of 296 (weighted 34%) children with GAD but not OAD. There is a great deal of similarity between many of the symptoms of depression and GAD in DSM-IV. Therefore, one might have expected more comorbidity between depression and GAD than between depression and OAD, but this did not occur. In summary, although there is evidence for considerable comorbidity among GAD, OAD, and depression, tracing the extent to which this degree of comorbidity is "real" rather than methodological will require detailed longitudinal investigation.

Comorbidity among the phobias and separation and anxiety disorders

Almost all the studies confirmed significant comorbidities among the phobias: specific, social, and agoraphobia. The concurrent association between panic disorder and separation anxiety was nonsignificant in three out of the four studies that measured it.

Absence of comorbidity

Evidence for the lack of comorbidity among disorders generally lumped together under the label "anxiety" is as interesting as evidence for comorbidity. Little connection was found between separation anxiety and the group of phobias or between separation anxiety and overanxious disorder. GAD and OAD were unrelated to simple or specific phobias. There was, however, a consistent pattern of significant association between OAD and social phobia. Interestingly, in light of the clinical data suggesting a developmental link, there was no evidence of a cross-sectional association between separation anxiety and panic disorder. However, it must be emphasized that the evidence is often patchy: some associations could only be examined in two or three studies. Also, most studies examined were cross-sectional and could not test for possible sequential or developmental relationships.

Comorbidity with other disorders

A review of comorbidity with anxiety disorders published in 1999 [59] showed that, controlling for other comorbid conditions, the highest level of anxious comorbidity was with depression, with a median odds ratio of 8.2 (95% CI, 5.8–12.0). This means that across all available studies, depression was 8.2 times as likely in children with anxiety disorders as in children without anxiety disorders and that 95 of 100 times the increase in likelihood of depression in the presence of anxiety would lie between 5.8 and 12 times. The odds ratio for comorbidity with conduct disorder or oppositional defiant disorder (ODD) was 3.1 (95% CI, 2.2–4.6) and that with attention deficit-hyperactivity disorder (ADHD) was 3.0 (95% CI, 2.1–4.3). These confidence intervals all exclude 1, indicating a statistically and substantively significant degree of comorbidity. In the case of substance use or abuse, although the bivariate odds ratios were significant in some studies, the association disappeared once comorbidity between anxiety and other psychiatric disorders was controlled [60].

There are few published reports that permit a review of comorbidity between specific anxiety disorders and other psychiatric diagnoses. Comorbidity analyses of the Oregon Adolescent Depression Study data set [27] looking at lifetime diagnoses showed that depression was significantly associated with each of the anxiety disorders except OCD, controlling for other disorders. Other lifetime associations found were ADHD with simple phobia, ODD with OCD, bipolar disorder with separation anxiety (in males), and alcohol abuse or dependence with OAD. The importance of a more detailed approach is shown by Kaplow and colleagues' [61] reanalysis of the data from GSMS. This found that different anxiety disorders had different relationships to the risk of beginning substance use. Children with separation anxiety symptoms were less likely than other children to begin drinking alcohol and did so later than others, whereas those with generalized anxiety symptoms were more likely than other children to begin drinking and did so earlier.

Homotypic and heterotypic continuity

An important question for clinicians is whether children with anxiety disorders can be expected to have further episodes of the same disorder (homotypic continuity) or to develop other psychiatric conditions (heterotypic continuity). There are few studies that deal thoughtfully with issues of concurrent versus sequential comorbidity [62]. Some studies have suggested that childhood anxiety predicts adolescent depression [5], but there also is evidence that early depression predicts anxiety [6]. Study of GSMS subjects [61] has demonstrated that the relationships among OAD, SAD, and alcohol use changed across development. The confused temporal relationship between anxiety and depression also may need more fine-grained analysis before we understand it properly.

There are few epidemiologic studies that provide information about continuity among the anxiety disorders. The clinical literature suggests that separation anxiety is a predictor of later panic disorder [31,63–65], for which there is some support in the GSMS (Bittner, submitted for publication, 2005). Controlling for concurrent comorbidity among the anxiety disorders, the GSMS showed a high degree of homotypic continuity of separation anxiety and social phobia. DSM-III-R overanxious disorder also showed significant continuity. There was relatively little heterotypic continuity, which suggests a level of predictive validity in the diagnostic categories for the anxiety disorders across childhood and adolescence.

Summary

This article argues that the quality (accuracy, reliability, validity) of measures used to measure anxiety disorders in the child and adolescent population have improved enormously in the past few years. As a result, prevalence estimates are less erratic, our understanding of comorbidity is increasing, and the role of impairment as a criterion for "caseness" is more carefully considered. Several of the instruments developed for epidemiologic research are now being used in clinical settings. The further integration of research methods can be expected in the next few years as, for example, laboratory methods for testing stress response become available for use in the field. The integration of laboratory, clinical, and epidemiologic ideas and methods can only benefit children with anxiety disorders and their families.

References

[1] Ollendick T, March JS, editors. Phobic and anxiety disorders in children and adolescents: a clinician's guide to effective psychosocial and pharmacological interventions. New York: Oxford University Press; 2004.

[2] Dadds MR, James RC, Barrett PM, et al. Diagnostic issues. In: Ollendick TH, March JS, editors. Phobic and anxiety disorders in children and adolescents: a clinician's guide to effective psychosocial and pharmacological interventions. New York: Oxford University Press; 2004. p. 3–33.

[3] Shaffer D, Fisher PW, Dulcan M, et al. The NIMH diagnostic interview schedule for children (DISC 2.3): description, acceptability, prevalences, and performance in the MECA study. J Am Acad Child Adolesc Psychiatry 1996;35:865–77.

[4] Costello EJ, Egger HL, Angold A. The developmental epidemiology of anxiety disorders. In: Ollendick T, March J, editors. Phobic and anxiety disorders in children and adolescents: a clinician's guide to effective psychosocial and pharmacological interventions. New York: Oxford University Press; 2004. p. 61–91.

[5] Costello EJ, Mustillo S, Keeler G, et al. Prevalence of psychiatric disorders in childhood and adolescence. In: Lubotsky Levin B, Petrila J, Hennessey K, editors. Mental health services: a public health perspective. New York: Oxford University Press; 2004. p. 111–28.

[6] Silberg J, Rutter M, Eaves L. Genetic and environmental influences on the temporal association between earlier anxiety and later depression in girls. Biol Psychiatry 2001;49:1040–9.

[7] Ferdinand R, Barrett J, Dadds MR. Anxiety and depression in childhood: prevention and intervention. In: Ollendick TH, March JS, editors. Phobic and anxiety disorders in children and adolescents: a clinician's guide to effective psychosocial and pharmacological interventions. New York: Oxford University Press; 2004. p. 459–75.

[8] Achenbach TM. Manual for the child behavior checklist 4–18 and 1991 profile. Burlington (VT): University of Vermont, Department of Psychiatry; 1991.

[9] Warren SL, Sroufe LA. Developmental issues. In: Ollendick TH, March JS, editors. Phobic and anxiety disorders in children and adolescents: a clinician's guide to effective psychosocial and pharmacological interventions. New York: Oxford University Press; 2004. p. 92–115.

[10] Kagan J, Snidman N. Infant predictors of inhibited and uninhibited profiles. Psychol Sci 1991;2:40–4.

[11] Biederman J, Rosenbaum JF, Hirshfeld DR, et al. Psychiatric correlates of behavioral inhibition in young children of parents with and without psychiatric disorders. Arch Gen Psychiatry 1990;47:21–6.

[12] Hirshfeld DR, Rosenbaum JF, Biederman J, et al. Stable behavioral inhibition and its association with anxiety disorder. J Am Acad Child Adolesc Psychiatry 1992;31:103–11.

[13] Kagan J, Reznick JS, Snidman N. The physiology and psychology of behavioral inhibition in young children. Child Dev 1987;58:1459–73.

[14] Biederman J, Rosenbaum JF, Bolduc-Murphy EA, et al. A 3-year follow-up of children with and without behavioral inhibition. J Am Acad Child Adolesc Psychiatry 1993;32:814–21.

[15] Kagan J, Snidman N. Early childhood predictors of adult anxiety disorders. Biol Psychiatry 1999;46:1536–41.

[16] Rosenbaum JF, Biederman J, Hirshfeld DR, et al. Further evidence of an association between behavioral inhibition and anxiety disorders: results from a family study of children from a non-clinical sample. J Psychiatr Res 1991;25:49–65.

[17] Rosenbaum JF, Biederman J, Hirshfeld DR, et al. Behavioral inhibition in children: a possible precursor to panic disorder or social phobia. J Clin Psychiatry 1991;52:5–9.

[18] Rosenbaum JF, Biederman J, Bolduc EA, et al. Comorbidity of parental anxiety disorders as risk for childhood-onset anxiety in inhibited children. Am J Psychiatry 1992;149:475–81.

[19] Egger HL, Angold A. The preschool age psychiatric assessment (PAPA): a structured parent interview for diagnosing psychiatric disorders in preschool children. In: DelCarmen-Wiggins R, Carter A, editors. Handbook of infant, toddler, and preschool mental assessment. New York: Oxford University Press; 2004. p. 223–43.

[20] Angold A, Egger HL. Psychiatric diagnosis in preschool children. In: DelCarmen-Wiggins R, Carter A, editors. Handbook of infant, toddler, and preschool mental health assessment. New York: Oxford University Press; 2004. p. 123–39.

[21] Earls F. Application of DSM-III in an epidemiological study of preschool children. Am J Psychiatry 1982;139:242–3.

[22] Keenan K, Shaw DS, Walsh B, et al. DSM-III-R disorders in preschool children from low-income families. J Am Acad Child Adolesc Psychiatry 1997;36:620–7.

[23] Lavigne JV, Gibbons RD, Christoffel KK, et al. Prevalence rates and correlates of psychiatric disorders among preschool children. J Am Acad Child Adolesc Psychiatry 1996;35:204–14.

[24] Egger HL, Ascher BH, Angold A. The preschool age psychiatric assessment: version 1.1. Durham (NC): Center for Developmental Epidemiology, Department of Psychiatry and Behavioral Sciences, Duke University Medical Center; 1999.

[25] Briggs-Gowan MJ, Horwitz SM, Schwab-Stone ME, et al. Mental health in pediatric settings: distributions of disorders and factors related to service juse. J Am Acad Child Adolesc Psychiatry 2000;39:841–9.

[26] Lewinsohn PM, Lewinsohn M, Gotlib IH, et al. Gender differences in anxiety disorders and anxiety symptoms in adolescents. J Abnorm Psychol 1998;107:109–17.

[27] Lewinsohn P, Zinbarg J, Lewinsohn M, et al. Lifetime comorbidity among anxiety disorders and between anxiety disorders and other mental disorders in adolescents. J Anxiety Disord 1997; 11:377–94.

[28] Simonoff E, Pickles A, Meyer JM, et al. The Virginia twin study of adolescent behavioral development: influences of age, sex and impairment on rates of disorder. Arch Gen Psychiatry 1997;54:801–8.

[29] Angold A, Erkanli A, Farmer EMZ, et al. Psychiatric disorder, impairment, and service use in rural African American and white youth. Arch Gen Psychiatry 2002;59:893–901.

[30] Costello EJ, Angold A, Burns BJ, et al. The Great Smoky Mountains Study Of Youth: goals, designs, methods, and the prevalence of DSM-III-R disorders. Arch Gen Psychiatry 1996; 53:1129–36.

[31] Silove D, Manicavasagar V, Curtis J, et al. Is early separation anxiety a risk factor for adult panic disorder? A critical review. Compr Psychiatry 1996;37:167–79.

[32] Costello EJ, Angold A, Keeler GP. Adolescent outcomes of childhood disorders: the consequences of severity and impairment. J Am Acad Child Adolesc Psychiatry 1999;38: 121–8.

[33] Verhulst FC, van der Ende J, Ferdinand RF, et al. The prevalence of DSM-III-R diagnoses in a national sample of Dutch adolescents. Arch Gen Psychiatry 1997;54:329–36.

[34] Beals J, Piasecki J, Nelson S, et al. Psychiatric disorder among American Indian adolescents: prevalence in northern plains youth. J Am Acad Child Adolesc Psychiatry 1997;36:1252–9.
[35] Fergusson DM, Horwood LJ, Lynskey MT. Prevalence and comorbidity of DSM-III-R diagnoses in a birth cohort of 15 year olds. J Am Acad Child Adolesc Psychiatry 1993;32:1127–34.
[36] Wittchen H-U, Nelson CB, Lachner G. Prevalence of mental disorders and psychosocial impairments in adolescents and young adults. Psychol Med 1998;28:109–26.
[37] Kessler RC. The national comorbidity survey of the united states. Int Rev Psychiatry 1994; 6:365–76.
[38] Brady KT, Killeen TK, Brewerton T, et al. Comorbidity of psychiatric disorders and post-traumatic stress disorder. J Clin Psychiatry 2000;61(Suppl 7):S22–32.
[39] Feehan M, McGee R, Williams SM. Mental health disorders from age 15 to age 18 years. J Am Acad Child Adolesc Psychiatry 1993;32:1118–26.
[40] Douglass HM, Moffitt TE, Dar R, et al. Obsessive-compulsive disorder in a birth cohort of 18-year-olds: prevalence and predictors. J Am Acad Child Adolesc Psychiatry 1995;34:1424–31.
[41] Newman DL, Moffitt TE, Caspi A, et al. Comorbid mental disorders: implications for treatment and sample selection. J Abnorm Psychol 1998;107:305–11.
[42] Canino G, Shrout P, Rubio-Stipec M, et al. The DSM-IV rates of child and adolescent disorders in Puerto Rico. Arch Gen Psychiatry 2004;61:85–93.
[43] Rueter MA, Scaramella L, Wallace LE, et al. First onset of depressive or anxiety disorders predicted by the longitudinal course of internalizing symptoms and parent-adolescent disagreements. Arch Gen Psychiatry 1999;56:726–32.
[44] Essau CA, Karpinski NA, Petermann F, et al. Frequency and comorbidity of psychological disorders in adolescents: results of the Bremen adolescent study. Z Klin Psychol Psychopathol Psychother 1998;46:105–24.
[45] Essau CA, Conradt J, Petermann F. Frequency and comorbidity of social phobia and social fears in adolescents. Behav Res Ther 1999;37:8321–843.
[46] Essau CA, Conradt J, Petermann F. Incidence of post-traumatic stress disorder in adolescents: results of the Bremen adolescent study. Z Kinder Jugenpsychiatr 1999;27:37–45.
[47] Essau CA, Conradt J, Petermann F. Frequency of panic attacks and panic disorder in adolescents. Depress Anxiety 1999;9:19–26.
[48] Warren SL, Huston L, Egeland B, et al. Child and adolescent anxiety disorders and early attachment. J Am Acad Child Adolesc Psychiatry 1997;36:637–44.
[49] Kasen S, Cohen P, Skodol AE, et al. Influence of child and adolescent psychiatric disorders on young adult personality disorder. Am J Psychiatry 1999;156:1529–35.
[50] Giaconia RM, Reinherz HZ, Silverman AB, et al. Traumas and posttraumatic stress disorder in a community population of older adolescents. J Am Acad Child Adolesc Psychiatry 1995; 34:1369–80.
[51] Essau CA, Conradt J, Petermann F. Frequency and comorbidity of social anxiety and social phobia in adolescents: Results of a Bremen adolescent study. Fortschr Neurol Psychiatr 1998; 66:524–30.
[52] Costello AJ, Edelbrock CS, Dulcan MK, et al. Development and testing of the NIMH diagnostic interview schedule for children in a clinic population: final report. Contract no. Rfp-db-81-0027. Rockville (MD): NIMH Center for Epidemiologic Studies; 1984.
[53] Costello EJ, Burns BJ, Angold A, et al. How can epidemiology improve mental health services for children and adolescents? J Am Acad Child Adolesc Psychiatry 1993;32:1106–13.
[54] US Government. Fed Regist 1993;58:29425.
[55] Hodges K, Doucette-Gates A, Liao Q. The relationship between the child and adolescent functional assessment scale (CAFAS) and indicators of functioning. J Child Fam Stud 1999;8: 109–22.
[56] Bird HR, Andrews H, Schwab-Stone M, et al. Global measures of impairment for epidemiologic and clinical use with children and adolescents. Int J Psych Res 1996;6:295–307.
[57] Angold A, Costello EJ, Farmer EMZ, et al. Impaired but undiagnosed. J Am Acad Child Adolesc Psychiatry 1999;38:129–37.

[58] Ezpeleta L, Keeler G, Erkanli A, et al. Epidemiology of psychiatric disability in childhood and adolescence. J Child Psychol Psychiatry 2001;42:901–14.

[59] Angold A, Costello EJ, Erkanli A. Comorbidity. J Child Psychol Psychiatry 1999;40:57–87.

[60] Armstrong TD, Costello EJ. Community studies on adolescent substance use, abuse, or dependence and psychiatric comorbidity. J Consult Clin Psychol 2002;70:1224–39.

[61] Kaplow JB, Curran PJ, Angold A, et al. The prospective relation between dimensions of anxiety and the initiation of adolescent alcohol use. J Clin Child Psychol 2001;30:316–26.

[62] Orvaschel H, Lewinsohn PM, Seeley JR. Continuity of psychopathology in a community sample of adolescents. J Am Acad Child Adolesc Psychiatry 1995;34:1525–35.

[63] Perwien AR, Bernstein GA. Separation anxiety disorder. Phobic and Anxiety Disorders in Children and Adolescents 2004;10:272–305.

[64] Klein RG. Is panic disorder associated with childhood separation anxiety disorder? Clin Neuropharmacol 1995;18:S7–14.

[65] Breton J-J, Bergeron L, Valla J-P, et al. Quebec child mental health survey: prevalence of DSM-III-R mental health disorders. J Child Psychol Psychiatry 1999;40:375–84.

CHILD AND
ADOLESCENT
PSYCHIATRIC CLINICS
OF NORTH AMERICA

ELSEVIER
SAUNDERS

Child Adolesc Psychiatric Clin N Am
14 (2005) 649–679

Vulnerability Factors for Anxiety Disorders in Children and Adolescents

Kathleen Ries Merikangas, PhD

National Institute of Mental Health, 35 Convent Drive, MSC 3720, Bethesda, MD 20892, USA

With the maturation of community studies of adults in the past decade, there has been growing awareness of the importance of the magnitude and impact of anxiety disorders in the general population [1]. The convergence of findings from adult and child epidemiology reveals that the onset of anxiety disorders occurs in childhood, and a substantial proportion of youth with anxiety continue to manifest lifelong problems with anxiety and other mental disorders.

In evaluating the rates and risk factors for the development of anxiety disorders, several issues require consideration. First, there is substantial overlap between the anxiety disorders and other psychiatric disorders, both concomitantly and longitudinally. Second, manifestations of anxiety change substantially across the life course, particularly during childhood and adolescence. A developmental perspective is essential in evaluating links between risk factors and anxiety disorders. Third, the assessment of anxiety requires evaluation of the context in which an individual experiences anxiety and the subjective response to anxiety-inducing situations. As such, anxiety becomes a disorder when there is a mismatch between the inherent threat posed by a particular stimulus or situation and the cognitive or somatic response. In this article, the major risk factors for the development of anxiety disorders in childhood and adolescence are reviewed. The magnitude and risk factors for the development of the major Diagnostic and Statistical Manual (DSM-III-R) and DSM-IV anxiety disorders are evaluated [2,3], as are the specific anxiety disorders of childhood, including separation anxiety disorder and overanxious disorder. Although overanxious disorder was omitted and subsumed under generalized anxiety disorder in the DSM-IV, there is a substantial amount of information regarding the prevalence and prognostic

E-mail address: merikank@mail.nih.gov

significance of this disorder on the subsequent course and development of anxiety disorders in adulthood.

To tap the diagnostic criteria for specific anxiety disorders, several structured and semi-structured diagnostic interviews have been developed. Community studies generally ascertain diagnostic criteria in highly structured interviews, such as the Diagnostic Interview Schedule for Children and Adolescents, which can be administered by nonclinicians to ascertain diagnostic criteria for all of the major mental disorders experienced by children and adolescents [4]. Some semi-structured diagnostic interviews require interviewers with clinical experience. The Kiddie-Schedule for Affective Disorders and Schizophrenia [5] is the most widely used semi-structured diagnostic interview for children and adolescents. Other semi-structured diagnostic interviews for children include the Child and Adolescent Psychiatric Assessment [6] and the Anxiety Disorders Interview Schedule, Revised, which collects extensive information on childhood anxiety disorders, including separation anxiety, overanxious disorder, and phobic states [7].

Numerous symptom scales also assess anxiety symptoms on a continuum. Some of the most widely used dimensional assessments of childhood anxiety are the Fear Survey Schedule, the Revised Child Manifest Anxiety Scale, the State Trait Anxiety Inventory for Children, the Multidimensional Anxiety Scale for Children [8], and the Screen for Childhood Anxiety Related Emotional Disorders [9]. A review of these measures is provided by Schniering and colleagues [10].

Several psychophysiologic indicators of anxiety also have been used in adults and children. Experimental models that induce stress and measure autonomic output to test the human "fight or flight" response to threat have been used to study the range of triggers, correlates, and responses to fear-provoking situations. Behavioral tasks, such as giving a speech or response to novelty, have been used to experimentally induce anxiety states in normal subjects and persons with anxiety disorders. Measures of changes in pulse, galvanic skin response, heart rate, and temperature regulation and observations of facial expression, blushing, and other overt signs of anxiety are presumed to provide a more accurate depiction of the disorder than self-reports or interviews about typical response patterns to stress.

Magnitude and demographic risk factors

Community studies of anxiety disorders

There are an increasing number of community studies of children and adolescents. It is difficult to draw conclusions across the aggregate data because of differences in diagnostic criteria and instruments, and variations in the source, and age and sex composition of the sample. Table 1 presents the methods of contemporary large-scale community studies of children and adolescents [4,11–32]. Anxiety disorders are the most common mental disorder in the general population of children and adolescents. Table 2 presents the magnitude of anxiety disorders in community surveys for children and adolescents [4,11–32]. In general, approximately 20% of youth suffer from one of the anxiety disorders, and half as many have impairment in functioning that results from anxiety or phobias. The most common disorders are overanxious disorder and separation anxiety disorder, which are specific anxiety disorders of childhood. Estimates of the lifetime prevalence of overanxious disorder range from 1.3% to 2.9%, with a median of 1.7%. Estimates of separation anxiety disorder are consistent across all studies, with a median of 3.5%.

The phobic disorders are even more frequent in children than childhood anxiety disorders. The rates of specific phobias range from 0.3% to 2.4%, with a median of 2.3%. The rates of social phobia in children were fairly consistent across studies, with a range of 0.6% to 3.5% and a median of approximately 1.3%.

Panic, generalized anxiety disorder (GAD), and obsessive-compulsive disorder are infrequent among children and youth. Rates of panic disorder range from 0.03% to 1.6%, with a median of 0.8%. Likewise, rates of generalized anxiety and obsessive-compulsive disorder are low, with ranges of rates of 0.08% to 2.4% and 0.2% to 0.7%, respectively.

Sex differences in anxiety disorders

Similar to the sex ratio for adults, girls tend to have more of all subtypes of anxiety disorders across all developmental phases [20,30,31,33]. The rates of anxiety disorders in community or school-based surveys of children and adolescents as defined by contemporary diagnostic criteria range from 0.1% to 13.3% in boys and 0.4% to 28.6% in girls. There is an approximately equal male-to-female ratio for obsessive-compulsive disorder [34].

Evidence regarding the evolution of sex differences in anxiety disorders in community samples of children and adolescents is sparse. One prospective longitudinal study of adolescents aged 14 to 18 years from the general community examined sex differences in the prevalence, course, risk factors, onset, and co-morbidity of anxiety disorders [35]. As compared with boys, girls had greater rates of current anxiety disorders (ie, 12.2% versus 8.5%), past anxiety disorders (5.2% versus 2.7%), and anxiety symptom scores on a dimensional rating $(M = 1.9$ versus 0.9) [36].

Explanations that may elevate falsely the sex ratio for anxiety disorders include sampling bias, reporting differences, artifacts of the classification system, and confounds with other clinical or demographic correlates. Possible mechanisms for the sex difference in anxiety, such as historical (evolutionary), demographic, developmental, genetic, biologic, and psychosocial risk factors, have been reviewed by Merikangas and Pollack [37] and Pollack and colleagues [38].

Age-specific patterns of expression of anxiety disorders

Retrospective reports of adults with anxiety disorders suggest that the onset of anxiety disorders generally occurs in childhood or adolescence. Fig. 1 shows

Table 1
Community studies of child and adolescent mood and anxiety disorders

Study [reference]	Location	Wave	N	Age (y)	Diagnostic criteria	Diagnostic interview	Period
United States							
Bird et al, 1988 [12]	Puerto Rico		386[a]	4–16	DSM-III	DISC	
Cohen et al, 1993 [16]	New York	T1	776	9–18	DSM-III-R	DISC	PT, 12 mo
Velez et al, 1989 [29]		T2	760	11–20			
Pine et al, 1998 [27]		T3	716	17–26			
Costello, 1988 [17]	Pittsburgh (Pennsylvania)		300[a]	7–11	DSM-III	DISC	12 mo
Costello et al, 1996 [18]	North Carolina		1015	9, 11, 13	DSM-III-R	CAPA	12 mo
Kashani et al, 1987 [21]	Missouri		150	14–16	DSM-III (+treatment)	DICA	3 mo
Kashani et al, 1989 [22]	Missouri		210	8, 12, 17	DSM-III	CAS	PT
Lewinsohn et al, 1994 [23]	Oregon	T1	1709	14–18	DSM-III-R	K-SADS-E	PT, LT
		T2	1507	15–19			PT, LT
		T3	893[a]	24	DSM-IV		PT, LT
Shaffer et al, 1996 [4]	Atlanta (Georgia), New Haven (Connecticut), New York, Puerto Rico		1285	9–17	DSM-III-R	DISC	6 mo
Simonoff et al, 1997 [28]	Virginia		2762 twins	8–16	DSM-III-R	CAPA	3 mo
Whitaker et al, 1990 [31]	New Jersey		356[a]	13–18	DSM-III	Clinical interview	LT

International

Study	Location		n	Age	Criteria	Instrument	Time frame
Anderson et al, 1987 [11]	Dunedin (New Zealand)	T1	792	11	DSM-III	DISC	12 mo
McGee et al, 1990 [24]		T3	943	15	DSM-III	DISC short	PT
Feehan et al, 1994 [19]		T4	930	18	DSM-III-R	DIS-III-R	PT, 12 mo
Newman et al, 1996 [25]		T5	961	21	DSM-III-R	DIS	12 mo
Bowen et al, 1990 [13]	Ontario (Canada)		2852	6-16	DSM-III	SDI	6 mo
Offord et al, 1989 [26]							
Canals et al, 1995 [15]	Spain	T1	500	10-11	DSM-III-R		
Canals et al, 1997 [14]		T2	290	18 (follow-up)	DSM-III-R	SCAN	PT
Fergusson et al, 1993 [20]	Christchurch (New Zealand)		1265	15	DSM-III-R	DISC	PT, 12 mo
Verhulst et al, 1997 [30]	The Netherlands		780[a]	13-18	DSM-III-R	DISC	6 mo
Wittchen et al, 1998 [32]	Munich (Germany)		3021	14-24	DSM-IV	CIDI	12 mo, LT

Abbreviations: CAPA, Child and Adolescent Psychiatric Assessment; CAS, Child Assessment Schedule; CIDI, Composite International Diagnostic Interview; DICA, Diagnostic Interview for Children and Adolescents; DIS, Diagnostic Interview Schedule; DISC, Diagnostic Interview Schedule for Children; K-SADS, Schedule for Affective Disorders & Schizophrenia for School-Aged Children; LT, lifetime; PT, point; SCAN, Schedules for Clinical Assessment in Neuropsychiatry; SDI, Survey Diagnostic Instrument.

[a] Screened from larger population.

Data from Merikangas KR, Avenevoli S. Epidemiology of mood and anxiety disorders in children and adolescents. In: Tsaung MT, Tohen M, editors. Textbook in psychiatric epidemiology. 2nd edition. New York: Wiley-Liss; 2002. p. 657–704.

Table 2
Rates of anxiety disorders in community samples of children and adolescents

Study [reference]	Age (y)	Anxiety			Phobias				Total (%)
		Separation anxiety (%)	Overanxiety (%)	General anxiety (%)	Panic (%)	Specific (%)	Social (%)	Agoraphobia (%)	
United States									
Bird et al, 1988 [12]	4–16	4.7				2.6			
Cohen et al, 1993 [16]	9–18	M: 7.7 F: 9.5	M: 3.6 F: 18.0		M: 0 F: 0	M: 7.7 F: 17.8	M: 6.7 F: 10.1		
Velez et al, 1989 [29]	11–20	M: 3.7 F: 3.7	M: 5.8 F: 10.3		M: 0 F: 0	M: 3.7 F: 8.2	M: 6.8 F: 12.6		
Pine et al, 1998 [27]	17–26			M: 2.2 F: 7.8	M: 0.3 F: 1.7	M: 12.0 F: 32.1	M: 1.7 F: 9.5		
Costello, 1988 [17]	7–11	4.1	4.6		0	9.2	1.0	1.2	15.4
Costello et al, 1996 [18]	9, 11, 13	3.5	1.4	1.7	0	0.3	0.6	0	5.7
Kashani et al, 1987 [21]	14–16	4.1				9.1			8.7
Kashani et al, 1989 [22]	8, 12, 17								25.7, 15.7, 21.4
Lewinsohn et al, 1993 [22a]	14–18 15–19	0.2 (PT) 0.1 (PT) 4.3 (LT)	0.5 (PT) 0.1 (PT) 1.2 (LT)		0.4 (PT) 0.3 (PT) 1.2 (LT)	1.4 (PT) 0.5 (PT) 2.1 (LT)	0.9 (PT) 0.2 (PT) 1.5 (LT)	0.4 (PT) 0.1 (PT) 0.6 (LT)	3.2 1.3 (PT) 9.2 (LT)

Study	Age								
Shaffer et al, 1996 [4]		6.5 (I) 5.8 (noI) 1.5 (I) 7.2 (noI)	11.4 (I) 7.7 (noI) 4.4 (I) 10.8 (noI)		— —	21.6 (I) 3.3 (noI) 4.4 (I) 21.2 (noI)	15.1 (I) 7.6 (noI) 2.5 (I) 8.4 (noI)	6.5 (I) 4.8 (noI) 1.1 (I) 2.7 (noI)	39.5 (I) 20.5 (noI)
Simonoff et al, 1997 [28]	8–16								
Whitaker et al, 1990 [31]	13–18			3.7	0.6				
International									
Anderson et al, 1987	11	3.5	2.9			2.4	0.9		7.4
McGee et al, 1990	15	2.0	5.9			3.6	1.1		10.7
Feehan et al, 1994	18			1.8	0.8	6.1	11.1	4.0	
Newman et al, 1996	21			1.9	0.6	8.4	9.7	3.8	
Bowen et al, 1990	12–16	3.6	2.4	3.7	0.6				
Offord et al, 1989	14–17				0.6				
Canals et al, 1995	10–11			0	0.3	1.7		0.7	2.7
Canals et al, 1997	18			1.7		1.3	0.7		12.8
Fergusson et al, 1993	15	0.5	2.1	1.3	0.4	12.7	9.2	2.6	23.5
Verhulst et al, 1997	13–18	1.8	3.1	4.3 (12 mo)	1.2 (12 mo)	1.8 (12 mo)	2.6 (12 mo)	1.6 (12 mo)	9.3 (12 mo)
Wittchen et al, 1998	14–24	—	—	0.8 (LT)	1.6 (LT)	2.3 (LT)	3.5 (LT)	2.6 (LT)	14.4 (LT)

Abbreviations: F, female; I, with impairment; LT, lifetime; M, male; noI, without impairment; PT, point.

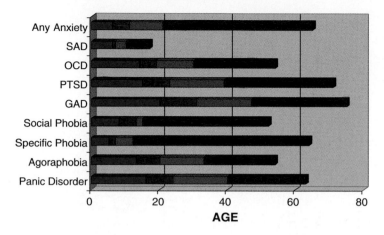

Fig. 1. Median age at onset of anxiety disorders in United States general population. N = 9282. Blue, 25th percentile; green, 50th percentile; yellow, 75th percentile; red, 99th percentile. (*From* Kessler RC, Berglund P, Demler O, et al. Lifetime prevalence and age-of-onset distributions of DSM-IV disorders in the National Comorbidity Survey Replication. Arch Gen Psychiatry 2005;62:597; with permission.)

the median age of onset of specific anxiety disorders reported by adults in a population-based survey of the United States [1]. Although there is substantial variation across studies, the results of prospective community-based research reveal differential peak periods of onset of specific subtypes of anxiety: separation anxiety and specific phobias in middle childhood (ie, ages 7–9), overanxious disorder in late childhood (ie, ages 10–13), social phobia in middle adolescence (ie, ages 15–16), and panic in late adolescence (ie, ages 17–18) [16,27,39–41]. The median age of onset of all of the anxiety disorders is approximately 10 to 12 years. Specific phobias have the earliest onset (median age, 6 years), followed by social phobia (median age, 12 years) and agoraphobia, obsessive-compulsive disorder, post-traumatic stress disorder, panic, and GAD, which had the latest age at onset (median age, 28 years).

Inspection of incidence curves reveals a sharp increase in girls beginning as early as age 5 with a continuously increasing slope throughout adolescence. Although rates of anxiety among boys also increase throughout childhood and adolescence, the rise is far more gradual than that of girls, and they begin to level off in late adolescence. By age 6, girls have significantly greater rates of anxiety than boys. Lewinsohn and colleagues [42] also showed that there was no sex difference in the duration of anxiety. Examining the age at which the sex difference in anxiety become apparent and concomitant changes in the risk factors and correlates of anxiety across the period of risk for onset may inform etiologic pathways to anxiety disorders.

Anxiety disorders, particularly the phobias, tend to persist across the life course. There are major differences among the anxiety subtypes in terms of specificity and chronicity, however. Although the phobic states tend to be fairly stable and nonprogressive, generalized anxiety and panic tend to be less specific and less stable over time [27,43,44].

Several follow-up studies of children and adolescents have shown that anxiety symptoms and disorders in general tend to exhibit some stability, but with substantial switching across categories of anxiety disorders over time [45]. A recent 8-year follow-up study of a community sample of youth aged 9 to 18 at study entry provides compelling evidence for the stability of specific and social phobias and yields some interesting sex differences in the stability of anxiety over time [42].

Social class and ethnicity

Rates of anxiety disorders in general are greater among persons at lower levels of socioeconomic status [46]. Several community studies have yielded greater rates of anxiety disorders, particularly phobic disorders, among African Americans [47]. With respect to children, Compton and colleagues [41] found that white children were more likely to report symptoms of social phobia, whereas African-American children had more separation anxiety symptoms. Pine and colleagues [48] reported that phobias were greater among persons at lower levels of social class. The reasons for ethnic and social class differences have not yet been evaluated systematically; however, methodologic factors and differences in exposure to stressors have been advanced as possible explanations.

Familial factors

The familial aggregation of all of the major subtypes of anxiety disorders has been well established [49,50]. The results of more than a dozen controlled family studies of probands with specific subtypes of anxiety disorders converge in demonstrating a three- to five-fold increased risk of anxiety disorders among first-degree relatives of affected probands compared with controls.

Of the subtypes of anxiety, panic disorder is the anxiety syndrome that has been shown to have the strongest degree of familial aggregation. A recent review of family studies of panic disorder by Gorwood and colleagues [51] cited 13 studies that included 3700 relatives of 780 probands with panic disorder compared with 3400 relatives of 720 controls. The lifetime prevalence of panic was 10.7% among relatives of panic probands compared with 1.4% among relatives of controls, which yielded a relative risk of 6.8. Early-onset panic has been shown to have a higher familial loading than later onset panic disorder [52].

Although there has been some inconsistency reported by twin studies of panic disorder [53], two studies that applied modern diagnostic criteria demonstrated considerably higher rates for monozygotic compared with dizygotic twins [54,55]. Current estimates derived from the Virginia Twin Registry show that panic disorder has the highest heritability of all anxiety disorders at 44% [56].

Although there are far fewer controlled family and twin studies of the other anxiety subtypes, all of the phobic states (ie, specific phobia, agoraphobia) have been shown to be familial [43,57–62]. The average relative risk of phobic disorders in the relatives of phobia is 3.1. Stein and colleagues [60] found that the familial aggregation of social phobia could be attributed to the generalized subtype of social phobia. Data from the Virginia Twin Study reported the estimated total heritability for phobias to be 35% [63]. Twin studies of children and adolescents have yielded similar findings to those of adults [64,65].

Evidence also exists for the familial aggregation and heritability of generalized anxiety disorder in a limited number of studies. The average familial odds ratio is approximately five [66,67], and the heritability was 0.32 among female twin pairs [68]. Few controlled family studies have been conducted on obsessive-compulsive disorder. Two of the three studies [69,70] reported familial relative risks of three to four, whereas Black and colleagues [71] found no evidence for familial aggregation. Nestadt and colleagues [70] found that the early age of onset and obsessional symptoms were associated with greater familiality. Twin studies have yielded weak evidence for heritability of obsessive-compulsive disorder [72–74].

The importance of the role of genetic factors in the familial clustering of anxiety has been demonstrated by numerous twin studies of anxiety symptoms and disorders. The relatively moderate magnitude of heritability also strongly implicates environmental etiologic factors, however.

Genetic factors

Based on indirect evidence implicating the adrenergic system in panic disorder [75], several linkage studies have investigated the role of mutations in adrenergic receptor loci on chromosomes 4, 5, or 10 [76], but without success. Other work similarly has excluded linkage with GABA- A receptor genes [77]. Reports from a genomic survey of panic disorder using 600 markers have not yielded evidence of linkage [78].

The lack of success in identifying specific genes for anxiety disorders to date is not surprising given their complexity. Similar to several other psychiatric disorders, the anxiety disorders are complicated by etiologic and phenotypic heterogeneity, a lack of valid diagnostic thresholds, unclear boundaries between discrete anxiety subtypes, and comorbidity with other forms of psychopathology. In a comprehensive consideration of what may be inherited, a review of the components of anxiety that have been investigated in human and animal studies has been compiled. Evidence from twin studies has indicated that somatic manifestations of anxiety may lie under some degree of genetic control. These studies demonstrate that physiologic responses, such as pulse, respiration rate, and galvanic skin response, are more alike in monozygotic than dizygotic twin pairs. Twin studies of personality factors have shown high heritability of anxiety reaction. Finally, the results of animal studies have suggested that anxiety or emotionality is under genetic control. Selective breeding experiments with mammals have demonstrated that emotional activity analogous to anxiety is controlled by multiple genes. These findings suggest that anxiety and fear states are highly heterogeneous and that future studies must investigate the extent to which the components of anxiety result from common versus unique genetic factors and the role of environmental factors, either biologic or social, in either potentiating or suppressing their expression.

High-risk studies of anxiety disorders

Studies of children of parents with anxiety have become an increasingly important source of information on the premorbid risk factors and early forms of expression of anxiety. Numerous studies have shown that there are increased rates of anxiety symptoms and disorders among offspring of parents with anxiety disorders [79–88]. Table 3 presents a summary of the controlled studies of offspring of parents with anxiety disorders. Derivation of an aggregate estimate of the risk for anxiety disorders based on parental anxiety is precluded by the lack of comparability of the selection of parental anxiety disorders across studies. In general, the results reveal an increased relative risk in anxiety disorders among offspring of parents with anxiety disorders compared with offspring of controls with a range of 1.3 to 13.3 [79,81,84–86,88–92].

Similar to studies of adults, which show common familial and genetic risk factors for anxiety and depression [93–95], these studies also have revealed that there is a lack of specificity with respect to depression. Studies that used a

Table 3
Controlled high-risk studies of anxiety

Study [reference]	Parent probands		Spouse	Offspring		
	Anxiety	Other		N	Age (y)	Relative risk
Sylvester et al, 1987 [90]	Panic	MDD	No disorder	91	7–17	13.3
Turner et al, 1987 [79]	Agoraphobia/ obsessive-compulsive disorder	Dysthymia	Not evaluated	43	7–12	4.8
Capps et al, 1996 [86]	Agoraphobia	Agoraphobia/ panic	Not evaluated	43	8–24	—
Warner et al, 1995 [84]	Panic/MDD	Panic	Disorder	145	6–29	1.3
Beidel et al, 1997 [85]	Anxiety + depression	Anxiety	No disorder	129	7–12	4.0
Merikangas et al, 1998 [87]	Panic/social phobia	Alcohol or drugs	Disorder	192	7–17	2.0
Unnewehr et al, 1998 [88]	Panic	Simple	Not evaluated	87	5–15	9.2
Biederman et al, 2001 [81]	Panic + MDD	Panic only	Not evaluated	312	5–18	5.9
Lieb et al, 2003	Social phobia	MDD	History	1047	14–17	4.7 (social phobia)
Pine et al, 2005 [92]	Panic	MDD	Not evaluated	142	9–19	3.8 (panic)

Abbreviation: MDD, major depressive disorder.

comparison group of parent probands with depressive disorders have shown that rates of anxiety disorders also increase among the offspring of these parents [79,84,91,92,96,97]. Conversely, offspring of parents with anxiety disorders and depression have elevated rates of depression when compared with offspring of controls [82] or offspring of anxiety-disordered parents without depression [80]. Similar findings emerged from the family study by Last and colleagues [83], who found an increase in rates of major depression among the adult relatives of children with anxiety. These findings are often interpreted as providing evidence for age-specific expression of common risk factors for anxiety in childhood and depression with or without comorbid anxiety in adulthood.

The links between anxiety and depression in parents and youth may be sex specific. For example, Beidel and Turner [85] reported no sex difference in the rates of anxiety disorders among offspring of parents with anxiety compared with offspring of parents with depression or anxiety plus depression. Whereas the magnitude of the association between parental and child anxiety was stable across childhood for girls, there was a large increase with increasing age among male offspring.

The high rates of anxiety disorders among offspring of parents with anxiety suggest that there may be underlying psychological or biologic vulnerability factors for anxiety disorders in general, which may already manifest in children before puberty. Previous research has shown that children at risk for anxiety disorders are characterized by behavioral inhibition [98], autonomic reactivity [99,100], somatic symptoms [79,100,101], social fears [79,82], enhanced startle reflex [100], and respiratory sensitivity [102]. Rosenbaum and colleagues [103] also found that the parents of children with behavioral inhibition are more likely to have anxiety disorders than parents of uninhibited children. Empirical research on each of these domains of risk is reviewed in the next section.

Vulnerability factors

A summary of individual and contextual risk factors for the development of anxiety disorders is presented in Box 1. The following section summarizes the current knowledge base for each of these vulnerability factors. It is likely, however, that combinations of individual and environmental factors play a more important role in influencing children who develop anxiety disorders in adulthood.

Temperament and personality

Behavioral inhibition

One of the earliest indicators of vulnerability to the development of anxiety is behavioral inhibition, which is characterized by increased physiologic reactivity or behavioral withdrawal in the face of novel stimuli or challenging situations [104]. In a summary of the evidence regarding behavioral inhibition as a precursor to the development of anxiety disorders, Hirshfeld-Becker and colleagues

---

Box 1. Vulnerability factors for anxiety disorders

Individual

Genetic factors
Temperament

- Behavioral inhibition
- Anxiety sensitivity
- Vigilance to threat

Pre-existing psychiatric or medical disorder
Autonomic reactivity
Respiratory sensitivity
Neurobiologic factors
Neuroendocrine factors

Exogenous

Exposure to stress/life events
Drug use
Parenting

- Modeling
- Sensitization

---

[105] found a strong association between childhood behavioral inhibition and social anxiety disorder in high-risk and prospective studies. There is an increased frequency of behavioral inhibition among children of parents with anxiety disorders compared with children of normal controls [98,103,105–108]. Behavioral inhibition may be a manifestation of a biologic predisposition characterized by overt behavioral (eg, cessation of play, latency to interact in the presence of unfamiliar objects and people) and physiologic indicators (eg, low heart rate variability, accelerated heart rate, increased salivary cortisol level, pupillary dilation, increased cortisol level).

The expression of behavioral inhibition studied prospectively may reveal patterns of anxiety symptomatology similar to those endorsed in adult populations. Some studies suggest that behavioral inhibition is moderately stable over time [109–111]. In a prospective study of a large community cohort of subjects aged 3 months to 13 years, Prior and colleagues [112] found that maternal ratings of persistent shyness and shyness in late childhood were associated with the development of anxiety disorders in adolescence. Most children with anxiety disorders in adolescence were not shy in childhood, however, nor do most shy children develop anxiety disorders.

Finally, there is also some evidence that social problems and aggressive behavior in childhood are associated with the development of anxiety disorders in adolescence and early adulthood [113].

Anxiety sensitivity

Anxiety sensitivity is another potential trait marker for the development of anxiety disorders [114]. Anxiety sensitivity is characterized by beliefs that anxiety sensations indicate harmful physiologic, psychological, or social consequences (eg, fainting or an impending heart attack). The misinterpretation of bodily cues that characterize anxiety sensitivity may lead to a self-perpetuating "fear of fear" cycle. The fear of benign arousal sensations produces anxiety, which in turn increases the frequency and intensity of physiologic sensations and subsequently fuels apprehension regarding the significance of these sensations. This process ultimately may result in a full-blown panic attack.

Anxiety sensitivity is believed to represent a stable trait-like factor that is qualitatively different from general fear and anxiety [115]. It has been proposed that anxiety sensitivity may interact with environmental experiences (eg, hearing misinformation about the negative outcome of certain bodily sensations) to shape beliefs about the dangers of anxiety sensations. Anxiety sensitivity may be involved in the development of certain anxiety disorders, particularly panic disorder [116,117]. Of particular interest is the finding of the specificity of anxiety sensitivity with respect to development of anxiety disorders but not depression in a nonclinical sample [118]. Likewise, Pollock and colleagues [38] reported that anxiety sensitivity seems to be specific to anxiety, because it did not contribute unique variance above self-rated anxiety symptoms in the prediction of depressive symptoms.

Anxiety sensitivity has been shown to be under genetic and familial influence [119]; anxiety sensitivity was found to constitute a potential premorbid marker for the development of anxiety disorders in high-risk but not low-risk youth [38,120,121]. Prospective studies of youth also have demonstrated the prognostic significance of anxiety sensitivity in predicting the development of anxiety disorders. Based on the results of a 5-year prospective study of adolescents, Hayward and colleagues [122] concluded that anxiety sensitivity seemed to be a specific risk factor for the development of panic attacks in adolescents. These findings from prospective research, particularly the specificity with respect to anxiety, together with the importance of genetic and familial liability, suggest that anxiety sensitivity is an important vulnerability factor that should be examined in future studies.

Other temperamental factors

The results of several prospective studies of children suggest that negative affectivity may presage the development of anxiety disorders [123]. The results of prospective longitudinal studies are particularly informative in linking childhood temperament and the subsequent manifestation of emotional disorders in adolescence and adulthood. For example, Craske and colleagues [124] found that emotional reactivity at age 3 predicted panic/agoraphobia in early adulthood, but only in male subjects. Lonigan and colleagues [125] proposed that attentional bias toward threat-relevant information may combine with negative affect and other temperamental processes to lead to the development of anxiety disorders. Few studies have investigated the joint influence of these temperamental factors for the development of anxiety disorders. For example, Stewart and colleagues [126] found that negative affectivity and anxiety sensitivity significantly predicted the development of panic attacks in adolescents. Most studies have not examined sex differences in the association between profiles of risk factors and the development of anxiety disorders in adulthood. In general, the childhood risk factors for the development of adult anxiety disorders tend to be far more common in girls than boys. Finally, the developmental aspects of the childhood precursors and early cognitive and somatic manifestations of anxiety in childhood require more intensive evaluation to identify youths in whom the increased interpersonal social demands or biologic maturation lead to the expression of the full diagnostic entity.

Comorbid disorders

Psychiatric

The magnitude of comorbidity in adults and adolescents with anxiety suggests that investigation of the role of other disorders in enhancing the risk for the development of anxiety disorders may be fruitful. The difficulty in dating onset of specific disorders, particularly from retrospective data, diminishes our ability to determine the temporal relations between disorders. Some prospective studies have examined the links between anxiety disorders and earlier expression of other forms of psychopathology [127].

The association between specific subtypes of anxiety disorders in childhood and those manifested later in life reveal that most adults with a major anxiety disorder have a history of one of the childhood anxiety disorders, including separation anxiety, overanxious disorder, or phobic disorder. Few adults manifest only one anxiety disorder either concomitantly or across their lifetime [43,128]. There does not seem to be much specificity in the extent to which childhood anxiety disorders predict the development of specific anxiety disorders in adulthood. For example, Aschenbrand and colleagues [129] found that separation anxiety in childhood was not specifically associated with agoraphobia and panic disorder in adolescence.

Depression is the disorder that is most frequently associated with anxiety disorders in youth. A review of comorbidity of anxiety and depression by Brady and Kendall [130] suggested that anxiety and depression may be part of a developmental sequence in which anxiety is expressed earlier in life than depression. The association between anxiety and depression may be bilateral, however, as demonstrated by the results of a large prospective study, which suggested a bilateral temporal association between panic attacks and depression [122]. Substance use disorders also have been found to increase the risk for the development of anxiety disorders. The potential mechanisms through which anxiety may be associated with smoking in adolescents were examined by Patton and colleagues [131], who found that anxiety and depression were associated with smoking initiation through increased susceptibility to peer influences. In older adolescents, anxiety disorders are more strongly associated with regular substance use, including cigarettes, alcohol, and illicit substances, in girls than in boys. In a clinical sample, Rao and colleagues [132] found that anxiety disorders may comprise a mediator of the link between depression and the subsequent development of substance use disorders.

Conversely, some research suggests that substance use may trigger anxiety disorders in susceptible youth. For example, a prospective study of a community sample revealed that post-traumatic stress disorder may be triggered by substance abuse in approximately 50% of the cases [133]. Similarly, Johnson and colleagues [134] found that adolescent smoking predicted adult onset of panic attacks, panic disorder, and agoraphobia. Although comorbidity between anxiety and substance problems is common in children and adolescents, further research on the mechanisms for links between specific disorders across and within genders is necessary. One of the most intriguing associations that may have preventive implications is the association between anxiety disorders and substance use and abuse in youth [135]. Kendall and colleagues [136] showed that treatment responders had a greater decrease in substance use than individuals who did not respond to treatment.

Medical symptoms and disorders

Several studies also have suggested an association between childhood medical conditions and the subsequent development of anxiety. In a retrospective review of pre- and perinatal and early childhood risk factors for different forms of psychiatric disorders in adolescence and early adulthood, Allen and colleagues [137] found that anxiety disorders in adolescents were associated specifically with illness during the first year of life, particularly high fever. Taylor and colleagues [138] reported that immunologic diseases and infections were specifically associated with emotional disorders because children with developmental or behavioral disorders had no elevation in infections or allergic diseases. Kagan and colleagues [139] found an association between allergic symptoms, particularly hay fever, and inhibited temperament in young children. An association between allergy and atopic disorders and panic disorder also has been found [140,141]. These findings suggest that it may be fruitful to examine links between immunologic function and the development of anxiety disorders.

Allen and Matthews [142] also found that adolescents and young adults with anxiety disorders were more likely to have suffered from infections during early childhood than others. Likewise, the prevalence of high fevers in childhood along with diseases associated with the immune system was elevated among offspring of parents with anxiety disorders in the Yale High Risk Study [100]. Cohen and colleagues [143] found that immunologic illnesses in adolescents showed stronger associations with depressive as opposed to anxiety disorders.

Taken together, these findings suggest future inquiry into the possible role of the immune system in anxiety states.

Allergies and atopic disorders.   The link between childhood allergies and eczema and behavioral inhibition was discussed by Kagan [144], who proposed that the high levels of cortisol associated with anxiety may lead to immunologic sensitivity to environmental stimuli. Slattery and colleagues [141] found increased rates of atopic disorders in offspring of parents with panic disorder. Children with separation anxiety disorder also had increased rates of atopic disorders. Kovalenko and colleagues [140] found that the strongest association between allergy and psychiatric disorders was between allergy and panic disorder. Respiratory ill health at age 3 also was a predictor of panic disorder and agoraphobia more than 15 years later in a cohort study from New Zealand [124].

Migraine.   Migraine has been shown to have a strong association with anxiety disorders and depression in adulthood, but limited data are available on the developmental patterns of evolution of these conditions in childhood. Several studies have shown that anxiety disorders tend to onset before migraine, whereas the age of onset of depression tends to occur after that of migraine [145]. Premorbid phobic disorders are particularly strongly associated with migraine [145,146]. In a prospective longitudinal study, Waldie and Poulton [147] found that migraine was related to anxiety symptoms in childhood, anxiety disorders in adolescence and young adulthood, and stress reactivity personality trait at the age of 18. The results of family studies and prospective cohort studies suggest that there may be a subtype of migraine with shared liability for anxiety and depression [145].

Cardiovascular.   Prospective studies have revealed that the anxiety disorders may comprise risk factors for the development of some cardiovascular and neurologic diseases. Haines and colleagues [148] reported that phobic anxiety was associated with ischemic heart disease, particularly fatal ischemic events. Bovasso and Eaton [149] used cardiac and respiratory symptoms and illness to subtype panic attacks and their association with depression in a large community-based sample. They found that respiratory panic attacks were associated with the subsequent risk of myocardial infarction.

Head injury and anxiety.   Vasa and colleagues [150] found an increase in anxiety symptoms after head injury, with the most frequent symptoms being obsessive-compulsive disorder, separation anxiety, and simple phobia. Luis and Mittenberg [151] reported new-onset mood or anxiety disorders after brain injury, with the likelihood of developing one or both of these disorders positively corresponding with stress after the injury and the severity of the injury.

Neurologic signs.   Neurologic soft signs in childhood, particularly motor impairment, also have been associated with the subsequent development of anxiety disorders. Shaffer and colleagues [152] reported that neurologic soft signs in childhood predicted anxiety symptoms in late adolescence. In the 1958 UK Birth Cohort and the National Child Development Study, Sigurdsson and colleagues [153] found that motor impairment at ages 7 and 11 was associated with a more than threefold increased odds of developing anxiety at the age of 16 among boys but not girls.

Autonomic reactivity

Reactions to threatening stimuli among various organisms, including primates and lower mammals, involve changes in the autonomic nervous system. These changes can be detected through an analysis of time-series for heart rate, heart period variability, blood pressure, and catecholamine levels. There is a long history of research in this area, and much of the initial work concerned the assessment of physiologic changes associated with acute anxiety states. Acute episodes of anxiety, in the laboratory and in natural settings, are typically characterized by acute changes in heart rate, blood pressure, and heart period variability [154]. These changes result from coordinated changes in the parasympathetic and sympathetic innervation of the cardiovascular system.

More recent work on physiologic changes during acute anxiety states has attempted to identify specific physiologic patterns associated with one or another emotion. The identification of emotion-specific patterns may provide insights on emotion-specific patterns of brain activity. For example, some forms of anxiety, such as acute panic, may be characterized by marked parasympathetic withdrawal in the face of sympathetic enhancement. Other emotions, such as anger, may be characterized by a physiologic "finger print," which reflects the involvement of distinct brain systems across emotions [155–157]. In general, consistent associations are found across development between acute anxiety states and changes in peripheral autonomic indices, including heart rate, blood pressure, and heart period variability. As a result, some researchers suggest that perturbations in autonomic regulation may index an underlying vulnerability to develop anxiety disorders. This underlying vulnerability is believed to relate to the functioning of particular neural circuits within the brain that exert effects on subjective internal states and physiologic activity. Potentially relevant neural circuits have been identified through basic science studies on the neural basis of fear and anxiety, as described in the following section.

Despite consistent evidence of an association between acute anxiety states and changes in autonomic physiology, the degree to which such changes index vulnerability for anxiety, as opposed to the acute state of anxiety, remains unclear. Autonomic indices might index vulnerability in a fashion that is more sensitive than indices derived through self-report measures.

Autonomic physiologic profiles have been studied among individuals who face high risk for anxiety disorders. Physiologic profiles have been linked to other indicators of risk, including behavioral inhibition [158], a parental history of panic disorder [159], and a history of traumatic life events in childhood [160].

Psychophysiologic function

Research on fear conditioning and physiologic reactions to innate and learned fears has shown that children at risk for anxiety disorders have elevated psychophysiologic reactivity to fear. Recent studies that have used the startle reflex to evaluate vulnerability to anxiety have found abnormalities in children at high risk for anxiety disorders and among children with behavioral inhibition born to adults with an array of anxiety disorders. Startle was found to discriminate between children at high and low risk for anxiety disorders and discriminate between children at risk for anxiety compared with children at risk for alcoholism [161,162].

A sex difference in anxiety vulnerability is suggested by the finding that the startle amplitude was elevated among high-risk girls, whereas high-risk boys exhibited greater magnitude of startle potentiation during aversive anticipation. Two possible explanations for the gender differences in the high-risk groups were suggested by the authors: (1) differential sensitivity among boys and girls to explicit threat versus the broader contextual stimuli that are mediated by different neurobiologic pathways and (2) different developmental levels in boys and girls in which the vulnerability to anxiety may be physiologically expressed earlier in girls. A subsequent study of startle among youth at risk for depression based on parental depression yielded similar findings to those that emerged for offspring of parents with anxiety disorders [163]. This finding suggests that there may be common pathways underlying the development of depression and anxiety disorders through increased vigilance to stressful stimuli.

Respiratory function

As in the area of autonomic physiology, a wealth of research delineates associations between respiratory perturbation and acute anxiety. This association has been most convincingly demonstrated in panic disorder, in which various forms of respiratory stimulation consistently produce high degrees of anxiety and more pronounced perturbations in respiratory physiologic parameters. Of note, these associations extend beyond the specific diagnosis of panic disorder, because enhanced sensitivity to respiratory perturbation is also found in conditions that exhibit strong familial or phenomenologic associations with panic disorder. These conditions include limited symptom panic attacks, certain forms of situational phobias, childhood anxiety disorders, particularly separation anxiety disorder, and high ratings of anxiety sensitivity scales.

The link between respiratory indices and panic disorder is strongly heritable, which suggests potential shared genetic vulnerability for panic attacks and respiratory dysregulation. Pine and colleagues [164] reported increased carbon dioxide sensitivity in children with anxiety disorders. Such data are also consistent with work on respiratory disease [165] and smoking [166], which suggest that abnormalities in respiration predispose individuals to later anxiety. Pine and colleagues [92] found that children at high risk for panic disorder did not have greater sensitivity to carbon dioxide than their low risk counterparts, however, which suggests that respiratory dysfunction could be a correlate rather than a vulnerability factor for panic disorder and other anxiety disorders.

Neural pathways

Integration of preclinical and clinical research on anxiety has advanced our understanding of the neural pathways underlying anxiety disorders in humans. The three areas of research that have informed the pathophysiologic models include neural circuits involved in fear conditioning, behaviors and physiologic perturbations that distinguish pathologic anxiety from normal fear, and neural effects of environmental perturbations that may disrupt reaction to stress [166a]. The results of fear conditioning studies suggest that the amygdala translates perception of threat and initiates a biochemical reaction in response to acute threats [167]. Human studies suggest that people with anxiety disorders may be more attuned to threat stimuli than warranted by the nature of the stimulus [168]. Similar to depression, dysfunction of the hypothalamic pituitary adrenal axis also has been related to vulnerability to anxiety. Integration of preclinical fear studies and research on human anxiety suggests that the neuroendocrine cascade provoked by fear acts through induction of corticotropin releasing factor on activity of the amygdala. Research in the third area, alteration of fear circuits through environmental stressors, particularly early in development, also has identified the neural circuits underlying the threat response and human anxiety [169].

Vigilance and attention

Studies of the association between attention regulation and anxiety have revealed that adults with anxiety disorders exhibit enhanced vigilance for threat cues, as indexed by effects of fear-related words or pictures on reaction times. These effects have been attributed to amygdala influences on attention allocation [125]. Enhanced attentional bias in acute anxiety represents a particularly robust finding, noted in numerous studies using various paradigms across virtually all anxiety disorders. Lonigan and colleagues [125] posit a model indicating that reactive and effortful temperamental processes, possibly mediated by an attentional bias toward threat-relevant information, interact to produce problems of dysregulated negative affect and elevated levels of pathologic anxiety.

Environmental exposures

Perinatal exposures

There is no evidence that either prenatal factors or delivery complications enhance the risk for the development of anxiety disorders. The results of three studies that retrospectively assessed perinatal events converged in linking such exposures to behavioral outcomes but not to subsequent anxiety. For example, Allen and colleagues [137] found that children who suffered from various exposures, which ranged from prenatal substance use to postnatal injuries, were more likely to develop behavioral disorders, particularly attention deficit disorder and conduct problems, but not anxiety disorders. Likewise, the results of the Yale High Risk Study yielded no association between pre- and perinatal risk factors and the subsequent development of anxiety disorders [100].

Life events and stressors

The role of life experiences in the etiology of anxiety states, particularly phobias and panic disorder, has been studied widely [170–173]. Life events often have been designated a causal role in the onset of phobias, which are linked inherently to particular events or objects. More broadly, life experiences that to some extent threaten one's notion of safety and security in the world are often at least retrospectively perceived to trigger or precipitate the onset of anxiety disorders. In evaluating the evidence on the causal role of life experiences, it is critical to consider separately the subtypes of anxiety disorders. Although it is likely that life stress may exacerbate phobic and generalized anxiety states, Marks [174] concluded that phobic states that result from exposure are rarer than conditions that emerge with no apparent exposure. In contrast, post-traumatic stress disorder is defined as a sequela of a catastrophic life event.

The major impediment to evaluation of the causal role of life events in anxiety (or depression) is the retrospective nature of most research that addresses this issue. For example, Lteif and Mavissakalian [175] found that patients with panic or agoraphobia exhibited an increased tendency to report life events in general. This finding suggests that studies that limit assessment of life events to events preceding onset of a disorder may be misleading because they fail to provide comparison for the time period of onset. Stressful life events may interact with other risk factors, such as a family history of depression, in precipitating episodes of panic [176].

In terms of specific environmental risk factors, there has been abundant literature on the role of parenting in enhancing vulnerability to anxiety disorders. Based on Bowlby's [177] theory that anxiety is a response to disruption in the mother-child relationship, researchers have postulated that maternal overprotection is related to anxiety, particularly separation anxiety. Using the Parental Bonding Instrument of Parker and colleagues [178], several studies of clinical samples have found that adult patients with anxiety disorders recall their parents as less caring and more overprotective than did controls [179]. These findings also have been supported in nonclinical samples [91,180]. All of these studies caution that a causal link cannot be established because of the lack of independence of assessment of parent behaviors and offspring anxiety.

Another parental behavior that may enhance risk of anxiety in offspring is parental sensitization of anxiety through enhancing cognitive awareness of a child to specific events and situations, such as bodily functions, social disapproval, the importance of routines, and necessity for personal safety [180]. Bennet and Stirling [180] found that subjects with anxiety disorders and individuals with high trait anxiety reported increased maternal sensitization to anxiety stimuli than controls.

Another feature of the parental relationship that has received widespread attention in recent research has been exposure to severe childhood trauma through either separation or abuse [177,181]. There is increasing animal research on the impact of early adverse experiences on brain systems and subsequent development [182,183]. Pynoos and colleagues [184] presented a comprehensive developmental life-trajectory model for evaluating the effects of childhood traumatic stress and anxiety disorders. They proposed different avenues by which dangerous circumstances, childhood traumatic experiences, and post-traumatic stress disorder can intersect with other anxiety disorders across the life span. The developmental perspective is critical in light of different levels of neural response to experience at different stages of development [185].

Summary

Anxiety disorders are the most common mental disorder in the general population of children and adolescents. In general, approximately 20% of youth suffer from one of the anxiety disorders, and half as many have impairment in functioning that results from anxiety or phobias. The most common anxiety disorder is specific phobia, followed by social phobia and overanxious disorder. Similar to the sex ratio for adults, girls tend to have more of all subtypes of anxiety disorders across all developmental phases [20,30,31,33]. The prevalence of panic disorder is rare in community surveys of youth. Retrospective reports of adults with anxiety disorders suggest that the onset of anxiety disorders generally occurs in childhood or adolescence.

The key vulnerability factors for the development of anxiety disorders are female gender, inhibited or anxious temperament, anxiety sensitivity, parental anxiety or mood disorder, increased startle reflex, and increased autonomic reactivity. Future prospective studies that integrate the temperamental and biologic factors underlying anxiety with environmental exposures that may lead to the development of anxiety disorders may inform etiology and lead to more informed interventions [186].

Acknowledgments

The author appreciates the editorial assistance of Erin Knight, BA.

References

[1] Kessler RC, Berglund P, Demler O, et al. Lifetime prevalence and age-of-onset distributions of DSM-IV disorders in the National Comorbidity Survey Replication. Arch Gen Psychiatry 2005;62:593–602.

[2] American Psychiatric Association. Diagnostic and statistical manual of mental disorders (DSM-III-R). 3rd edition, revised. Washington (DC): American Psychiatric Press; 1987.

[3] American Psychiatric Association. Diagnostic and statistical manual of mental disorders (DSM-IV). 4th edition. Washington (DC): American Psychiatric Press; 1994.

[4] Shaffer D, Fisher P, Dulcan MK, et al. The NIMH Diagnostic Interview Schedule for Children Version 2.3 (DISC-2.3): description, acceptability, prevalence rates, and performance in the MECA study. J Am Acad Child Adolesc Psychiatry 1996;35:865–77.

[5] Orvaschel H, Puig-Antich J, Chambers LW, et al. Retrospective assessment of prepubertal major depression with the Kiddie-SADS-E. J Am Acad Child Adolesc Psychiatry 1982;21: 392–7.

[6] Angold A, Costello EJ. A test-retest reliability study of child-reported psychiatric symptoms and diagnoses using the child and adolescent psychiatric assessment (CAPA-C). Psychol Med 1995;25:755–62.

[7] Di Nardo PA, Barlow DH. Anxiety Disorders Interview Schedule–Revised (ADIS-R). Albany (NY): Phobia and Anxiety Disorders Clinic; 1988.

[8] March JS, Parker JD, Sullivan K, et al. The Multidimensional Anxiety Scale for Children (MASC): factor structure, reliability, and validity. J Am Acad Child Adolesc Psychiatry 1997; 36:554–65.

[9] Birmaher B, Khetarpal S, Brent D, et al. The Screen for Child Anxiety Related Emotional Disorders (SCARED): scale construction and psychometric characteristics. J Am Acad Child Adolesc Psychiatry 1997;36:545–53.

[10] Schniering CA, Hudson JL, Rapee RM. Issues in the diagnosis and assessment of anxiety disorders in children and adolescents. Clin Psychol Rev 2000;20:453–78.

[11] Anderson JC, Williams S, McGee R, et al. DSM-III disorders in preadolescent children: prevalence in a large sample from the general population. Arch Gen Psychiatry 1987;44:69–76.

[12] Bird HR, Canino G, Rubino-Stipec M, et al. Estimates of the prevalence of childhood maladjustment in a community survey in Puerto Rico: the use of combined measures. Arch Gen Psychiatry 1988;45:1120–6.

[13] Bowen RC, Offord DR, Boyle MH. The prevalence of overanxious disorder and separation anxiety disorder: results from the Ontario Child Health Study. J Am Acad Child Adolesc Psychiatry 1990;29:753–8.

[14] Canals J, Domenech E, Carbajo G, et al. Prevalence of DSM-III-R and ICD-10 psychiatric disorders in a Spanish population of 18-year olds. Acta Psychiatr Scand 1997;96:287–94.

[15] Canals J, Marti-Henneberg C, Fernandez-Ballart J, et al. A longitudinal study of depression in an urban Spanish pubertal population. Eur Child Adolesc Psychiatry 1995;4:102–11.

[16] Cohen P, Cohen J, Kasen S, et al. An epidemiological study of disorders in late childhood and adolescence. I. Age and gender-specific prevalence. J Child Psychol Psychiatry 1993;34: 851–67.

[17] Costello EJ, Edelbrock C, Costello AJ, et al. Psychopathology in pediatric primary care: the new hidden morbidity [abstract]. Pediatrics 1988;82(3):415–24.

[18] Costello J, Angold A, Burns BJ, et al. The Great Smoky Mountains study of youths: goals, design, methods, and the prevalence of DSM-III-R disorders. Arch Gen Psychiatry 1996;53: 1129–36.

[19] Feehan M, McGee R, Raja SN, et al. DSM-III-R disorders in New Zealand 18-year-olds. Aust N Z J Psychiatry 1994;28:87–99.

[20] Fergusson DM, Horwood LJ, Lynskey MT. Prevalence and comorbidity of DSM-III-R diagnoses in a birth cohort of 15 year olds. J Am Acad Child Adolesc Psychiatry 1993;32: 1127–34.

[21] Kashani J, Beck N, Hoeper E, et al. Psychiatric disorders in a community sample of adolescents. Am J Psychiatry 1987;144:584–9.

[22] Kashani J, Orvaschel H, Rosenberg T, et al. Psychopathology in a community sample of children and adolescents: a developmental perspective. J Am Acad Child Adolesc Psychiatry 1989;28:701–6.

[22a] Lewinsohn PM, Hops H, Roberts RE, et al. Adolescent psychopathology: I. Prevalence and incidence of depression and other DSM-III-R disorders in high school students. J Abnorm Psychol 1993;102:133–44.

[23] Lewinsohn PM, Roberts RE, Seeley JR, et al. Adolescent psychopathology: II. Psychosocial risk factors for depression. J Abnorm Psychol 1994;103:302–15.

[24] McGee R, Feehan M, Williams S, et al. DSM-III disorders in a large sample of adolescents. J Am Acad Child Adolesc Psychiatry 1990;29:611–9.

[25] Newman DL, Moffitt TE, Caspi A, et al. Psychiatric disorder in a birth cohort of young adults: prevalence, comorbidity, clinical significance, and new case incidence from ages 11–21. J Consult Clin Psychol 1996;64:552–62.

[26] Offord DR, Boyle MH, Fleming JE, et al. Ontario Child Health Study: summary of selected results. Can J Psychiatry 1989;34:483–91.

[27] Pine DS, Cohen P, Gurley D, et al. The risk for early adulthood anxiety and depressive disorders in adolescents with anxiety and depressive disorders. Arch Gen Psychiatry 1998;55:56–64.

[28] Simonoff E, Pickles A, Meyer J, et al. The Virginia twin study of adolescent behavioral development: influences of age, sex, and inpairment on rates of disorders. Arch Gen Psychiatry 1997;47:487–96.

[29] Velez C, Johnson J, Cohen P. A longitudinal analysis of selected risk factors for childhood psychopathology. J Am Acad Child Adolesc Psychiatry 1989;28:861–4.

[30] Verhulst FC, van der Ende J, Ferdinand RF, et al. The prevalence of DSM-III-R diagnoses in a national sample of Dutch adolescents. Arch Gen Psychiatry 1997;54:329–36.

[31] Whitaker A, Johnson J, Shaffer D, et al. Uncommon troubles in young people: prevalence estimates of selected psychiatric disorders in a nonreferred population. Arch Gen Psychiatry 1990;47:487–96.

[32] Wittchen H-U, Nelson CB, Lachner G. Prevalence of mental disorders and psychosocial impairments in adolescents and young adults. Psychol Med 1998;28:109–26.

[33] Feehan M, McGee R, Williams SM. Mental health disorders from age 15 to 18 years. J Am Acad Child Adolesc Psychiatry 1993;32:1118–26.

[34] Douglass HM, Moffitt TE, Dar R, et al. Obsessive-compulsive disorder in a birth cohort of 18 year-olds: prevalence and predictors. J Am Acad Child Adolesc Psychiatry 1995;34:1424–31.

[35] Lewinsohn PM, Rohde P, Seeley JR. Major depressive disorder in older adolescents: prevalence, risk factors, and clinical implications. Clin Psychol Rev 1998;18:765–94.

[36] Lewinsohn PM, Rhode P, Klein DN, et al. Natural course of adolescent major depressive disorder: I. Continuity into young adulthood. J Am Acad Child Adolesc Psychiatry 1999;38:56–63.

[37] Merikangas KR, Pollock R. Anxiety disorders in women. In: Goldman M, Hatch M, editors. Women and health. San Diego (CA): Academic Press; 2000. p. 1010–23.

[38] Pollock RA, Carter AS, Dierker L, et al. Anxiety sensitivity in adolescents at risk for psychopathology. J Child Clinical Psychology 2002;31:343–53.

[39] Last CG, Perrin S, Hersen M, et al. DSM-III-R anxiety disorders in children: sociodemographic and clinical characteristics. J Am Acad Child Adolesc Psychiatry 1992;31:1070–6.

[40] Costello EJ, Messer SC, Bird HR, et al. The prevalence of serious emotional disturbance: a reanalysis of community studies. J Child Fam Stud 1998;7:411–32.

[41] Compton SN, Nelson AH, March JS. Social phobia and separation anxiety symptoms in community and clinical samples of children and adolescents. J Am Acad Child Adolesc Psychiatry 2000;39:1040–6.

[42] Lewinsohn PM, Lewinsohn M, Gotlib IH, et al. Gender differences in anxiety disorders and anxiety symptoms in adolescents. J Abnorm Psychol 1998;107:109–17.

[43] Merikangas KR, Angst J. Comorbidity and social phobia: evidence from clinical, epidemiologic and genetic studies. Eur Arch Psychiatry Clin Neurosci 1995;244:297–303.

[44] Last CG, Perrin S, Hersen M, et al. A prospective study of childhood anxiety disorders. J Am Acad Child Adolesc Psychiatry 1996;35:1502–10.

[45] Ialongo N, Edelsohn G, Werthamer-Larsson L, et al. The significance of self-reported anxious symptoms in first grade children: prediction to anxious symptoms and adaptive functioning in fifth grade. J Child Psychol Psychiatry 1995;36:427–37.

[46] Horwath E, Weissman MM. Epidemiology of depression and anxiety disorder. In: Tsuang MT, Tohen M, Zahner GEP, editors. Textbook in psychiatric epidemiology. New York: Wiley-Liss, Inc.; 1995. p. 389–426.

[47] Eaton WW, Dryman A, Weissman MM. Panic and phobia. In: Robins LN, Regier DA, editors. Psychiatric disorders in America: the epidemiological catchment area study. New York: Free Press; 1991. p. 155–79.

[48] Pine DS, Cohen P, Gurley D, et al. The risk for early-adulthood anxiety and depressive disorders in adolescents with anxiety and depressive disorders. Arch Gen Psychiatry 1998;55: 56–64.

[49] Merikangas KR, Swendsen J. Genetic epidemiology of psychiatric disorders. Epidemiol Rev 1997;19:144–55.

[50] Smoller JW, Finn C, White C. The genetics of anxiety disorders: an overview. Psychiatr Ann 2000;30:745–53.

[51] Gorwood P, Feingold J, Ades J. Epidemiologie genetique et psychiatrie(I): portees et limites des etudes de concentration familiale exemple du trouble panique. Encephale 1999;10:21–9.

[52] Goldstein RB, Wickramaratne PJ, Horwath E, et al. Familial aggregation and phenomenology of early-onset (at or before age 20 years) panic disorder. Arch Gen Psychiatry 1997;54:271–8.

[53] McGuffin P, Asherson P, Owen M, et al. The strength of the genetic effect. Is there room for an environmental influence in the aetiology of schizophrenia? Br J Psychiatry 1994;164:593–9.

[54] Kendler KS, Neale MC, Kessler RC. Panic disorder in women: a population-based twin study. Psychol Med 1993;23:397–406.

[55] Skre I, Onstad S, Torgersen S, et al. A twin study of DSM-III-R anxiety disorders. Acta Psychiatr Scand 1993;88:85–92.

[56] Kendler KS, Walters EE, Neale MC, et al. The structure of the genetic and environmental risk factors for six major psychiatric disorders in women: phobia, generalized anxiety disorder, panic disorder, bulimia, major depression, and alcoholism. Arch Gen Psychiatry 1995;52: 374–83.

[57] Fyer AJ, Mannuzza S, Chapman TF, et al. A direct interview family study of social phobia. Arch Gen Psychiatry 1993;50:286–93.

[58] Fyer AJ, Mannuzza S, Chapman TF, et al. Specificity in familial aggregation of phobic disorders. Arch Gen Psychiatry 1995;52:564–73.

[59] Noyes Jr R, Clarkson C, Crowe RR. A family study of generalized anxiety disorder. Am J Psychol 1987;144:1019–24.

[60] Stein MB, Chartier MJ, Hazen AL, et al. A direct-interview family study of generalized social phobia. Am J Psychiatry 1998;155:90–7.

[61] Woodman C, Crowe R. The genetics of the anxiety disorders. Bailliere's Clinical Psychiatry 1996;2:47–57.

[62] Smoller JW, Tsuang MT. Panic and phobic anxiety: defining phenotypes for genetic studies. Am J Psychiatry 1998;155:1152–62.

[63] Kendler KS, Karkowski LM, Prescott CA. Fears and phobias: reliability and heritability. Psychol Med 1999;29:539–53.

[64] Silberg J, Rutter M, Neale M, et al. Genetic moderation of environmental risk for depression and anxiety in adolescent girls. Br J Psychiatry 2001;179:116–21.

[65] Lichtenstein P, Annas P. Heritability and prevalence of specific fears and phobias in childhood. J Child Psychol Psychiatry 2000;41:927–37.

[66] Noyes R, Woodman C, Garvey MJ, et al. Generalized anxiety disorder vs. panic disorder: distinguishing characteristics and patterns of comorbidity. J Nerv Ment Dis 1992;180:369–79.

[67] Mendlewicz J, Papdimitriou G, Wilmotte J. Family study of panic disorder: comparison with generalized anxiety disorder, major depression and normal subjects. Psychiatr Genet 1993;3:73–8.

[68] Kendler KS, Neale MC, Kessler RC, et al. Generalized anxiety disorder in women: a population-based twin study. Arch Gen Psychiatry 1992;49:267–72.

[69] Pauls DL, Alsobrook JP, Goodman W, et al. A family study of obsessive-compulsive disorder. Am J Psychiatry 1995;152:76–84.

[70] Nestadt G, Samuels J, Riddle M, et al. A family study of obsessive-compulsive disorder. Arch Gen Psychiatry 2000;57:358–63.

[71] Black DW, Noyes RJ, Goldstein RB, et al. A family study of obsessive-compulsive disorder. Arch Gen Psychiatry 1992;49:362–8.

[72] Carey G, Gottesman II. Twin and family studies of anxiety, phobic, and obsessive disorders. New York: Raven Press; 1981.

[73] Lenane MC, Swedo SE, Leonard H, et al. Psychiatric disorders in first-degree relatives of children and adolescents with obsessive-compulsive disorder. J Am Acad Child Adolesc Psychiatry 1990;29:766–72.

[74] Bellodi L, Battaglia M, Diaferia G, et al. Lifetime prevalence of depression and family history of patients with panic disorder and social phobia. Eur Psychiatry 1993;8:147–52.

[75] Goddard AW, Woods SC, Charney DS. A critical review of the role of norepinephrine in panic disorder: focus on its interaction with serotonin. In: Westenberg HGM, Den Boer JA, Murphy DL, editors. Advances in the neurobiology of anxiety disorders. New York: John Wiley and Sons; 1996. p. 107–37.

[76] Wang ZW, Crowe RR, Noyes RJ. Adrenergic receptor genes as candidate genes for panic disorder: a linkage study. Am J Psychiatry 1992;149:470–4.

[77] Schmidt SM, Zoega T, Crowe RR. Excluding linkage between panic disorder and the gamma-aminobutynic acid beta I reactor locus in five Icelandic pedigrees. Acta Psychiatr Scand 1993;88:225–8.

[78] Nurnberger J, Byerley WF. Molecular genetics of anxiety disorders. Psychiatr Genet 1995;5:5–7.

[79] Turner SM, Beidel DC, Costello A. Psychopathology in the offspring of anxiety disorders patients. J Consult Clin Psychol 1987;55:229–35.

[80] Biederman J, Rosenbaum JF, Bolduc EA, et al. A high risk study of young children of parents with panic disorders and agoraphobia with and without comorbid major depression. Psychiatry Res 1991;37:333–48.

[81] Biederman J, Faraone SV, Hirshfeld-Becker DR, et al. Patterns of psychopathology and dysfunction in high-risk children of parents with panic disorder and major depression. Am J Psychiatry 2001;158:49–57.

[82] Sylvester CE, Hyde TS, Reichler RJ. Clinical psychopathology among children of adults with panic disorder. In: Dunner DL, Gershon ES, Barrett JE, editors. Relatives at risk for mental disorder. New York: Raven Press; 1988. p. 87–102.

[83] Last C, Hersen M, Kazdin A, et al. Anxiety disorders in children and their families. Arch Gen Psychiatry 1991;48:928–34.

[84] Warner V, Mufson L, Weissman M. Offspring at high risk for depression and anxiety: mechanisms of psychiatric disorder. J Am Acad Child Adolesc Psychiatry 1995;34:786–97.

[85] Beidel DC, Turner SM. At risk for anxiety: I. Psychopathology in the offspring of anxious parents. J Am Acad Child Adolesc Psychiatry 1997;36:918–24.

[86] Capps L, Sigman M, Sena R, et al. Fear, anxiety and perceived control in children of agoraphobic parents. J Child Psychol Psychiatry 1996;37:445–52.

[87] Merikangas KR, Mehta RL, Molnar BE, et al. Comorbidity of substance use disorders with mood and anxiety disorders: results of the international consortium in psychiatric epidemiology. Addict Behav 1998;23:893–907.

[88] Unnewehr S, Schneider S, Florin I, et al. Psychopathology in children of patients with panic disorder or animal phobia. Psychopathology 1998;31:69–84.

[89] Merikangas KR, Dierker LC, Szatmari P. Psychopathology among offspring of parents with substance abuse and/or anxiety: a high risk study. J Child Psychol Psychiatry 1998;39: 711–20.

[90] Sylvester CE, Hyde TS, Reichler RJ. The diagnostic interview for children and personality inventory for children in studies of children at risk for anxiety disorders or depression. J Am Acad Child Adolesc Psychiatry 1987;26:668–75.

[91] Lieb R, Wittchen H-U, Hofler M, et al. Parental psychopathology, parenting styles and the risk of social phobia in offspring: a prospective-longitudinal community study. Arch Gen Psychiatry 2000;57:859–66.

[92] Pine DS, Klein RG, Roberson-Nay R, et al. Response to 5% carbon dioxide in children and adolescents: relationship to panic disorder in parents and anxiety disorders in subjects. Arch Gen Psychiatry 2005;62:73–80.

[93] Kendler K, Neale M, Kessler R, et al. Major depression and phobias: the genetic and environmental sources of comorbidity. Psychol Med 1993;23:361–71.

[94] Merikangas K. Comorbidity for anxiety and depression: a review of family and genetic studies. In: Maser J, Cloninger C, editors. Comorbidity of mood and anxiety disorders. Washington (DC): American Psychiatric Press; 1990. p. 331–48.

[95] Stavrakaki C, Vargo B, The relationship of anxiety and depression: a review of literature. Br J Psychiatry 1986;149:7–16.

[96] Foley DL, Pickles A, Simonoff E, et al. Parental concordance and comorbidity for psychiatric disorder and associate risks for current psychiatric symptoms and disorders in a community sample of juvenile twins. J Child Psychol Psychiatry 2001;42:381–94.

[97] Weissman MM, Wickramaratne P, Nomura Y, et al. Families at high and low risk for depression: a 3-generation study. Arch Gen Psychiatry 2005;62:29–36.

[98] Rosenbaum JF, Biederman J, Gersten M. Behavioral inhibition in children of parents with panic disorder and agoraphobia: a controlled study. Arch Gen Psychiatry 1988;45:463–70.

[99] Beidel DC. Psychophysiological assessment of anxious emotional states in children. J Abnorm Psychol 1988;97:80–2.

[100] Merikangas KR, Avenevoli S, Dierker L, et al. Vulnerability factors among children at risk for anxiety disorders. Biol Psychiatry 1999;46:1523–35.

[101] Reichler RJ, Sylvester CE, Hyde TS. Biological studies on offspring of panic disorder probands. In: Dunner DL, Gershon ES, Barrett JE, editors. Relatives at risk for mental disorders. New York: Raven Press; 1988. p. 103–26.

[102] Pine DS, Cohen E, Cohen P, et al. Social phobia and the persistence of conduct problems. J Child Psychol Psychiatry 2000;41:657–65.

[103] Rosenbaum JF, Biederman J, Hirshfeld DR, et al. Further evidence of an association between behavioral inhibition and anxiety disorders: results from a family study of children from a non-clinical sample. J Psychiatr Res 1991;25:49–65.

[104] Hirshfeld DR, Rosenbaum JF, Biederman J, et al. Stable behavioral inhibition and its association with anxiety disorder. J Am Acad Child Adolesc Psychiatry 1992;31:103–11.

[105] Hirshfeld-Becker DR, Biederman J, Calltharp S, et al. Behavioral inhibition and disinhibition as hypothesized precursors to psychopathology: implications for pediatric bipolar disorder. Biol Psychiatry 2003;53:985–99.

[106] Battaglia M, Bajo S, Strambi LF, et al. Physiological and behavioral responses to minor stressors in offspring of patients with panic disorder. J Psychiatr Res 1997;31:365–76.

[107] Manassis K, Bradley S, Goldberg S, et al. Behavioral inhibition, attachment and anxiety in children of mothers with anxiety disorders. Can J Psychiatry 1995;40:87–92.

[108] Rosenbaum JF, Biederman J, Hirshfeld-Becker DR, et al. A controlled study of behavioral inhibition in children of parents with panic disorder and depression. Am J Psychiatry 2000; 157:2002–10.

[109] Asendorpf J. Development of inhibition during childhood: evidence for situation specificity and a two-factor model. Dev Psychol 1990;26:721–30.

[110] Scarpa A, Raine A, Venables PH, et al. The stability of inhibited/uninhibited temperament from ages 3 to 11 years in Mauritian children. J Abnorm Child Psychol 1995;23:607–18.

[111] Stevenson-Hinde J, Shouldice A. 4.5 to 7 years: fearful behaviour, fears and worries. J Child Psychol Psychiatry 1995;36:1027–38.

[112] Prior M, Smart D, Sanson A, et al. Does shy-inhibited temperament in childhood lead to anxiety problems in adolescence? J Am Acad Child Adolesc Psychiatry 2000;39:461–8.

[113] Roza SJ, Hofstra MB, van der Ende J, et al. Stable prediction of mood and anxiety disorders based on behavioral and emotional problems in childhood: a 14-year follow-up during childhood, adolescence, and young adulthood. Am J Psychiatry 2003;160:2116–21.

[114] Reiss S, Peterson RA, Gursky DM, et al. Anxiety sensitivity, anxiety frequency and the prediction of fearfulness. Behav Res Ther 1986;24:1–8.

[115] McNally RJ. Panic disorder: a critical analysis. New York: Guilford Press; 1994.

[116] McNally RJ. Psychological approaches to panic disorder: a review. Psychol Bull 1990;108: 403–19.

[117] Schmidt N, Lerew D, Jackson R. The role of anxiety sensitivity in the pathogenesis of panic: prospective evaluation of spontaneous panic attacks during acute stress. J Abnorm Psychol 1997;106:355–64.

[118] Schmidt NB, Lerew DR, Joiner Jr TE. Anxiety sensitivity and the pathogenesis of anxiety and depression: evidence for symptom specificity. Behav Res Ther 1998;36:165–77.

[119] Stein MB, Jang KL, Livesley WJ. Heritability of anxiety sensitivity: a twin study. Am J Psychiatry 1999;156:246–51.

[120] Pollock RA, Carter AS, Dierker L, et al. Anxiety sensitivity in adolescents at risk for psychopathology. J Child Clinical Psychology 2002;31:343–53.

[121] Calamari JE, Hale LR, Heffelfinger SK, et al. Relations between anxiety sensitivity and panic symptoms in nonreferred children and adolescents. J Behav Ther Exp Psychiatry 2001; 32:117–36.

[122] Hayward C, Killen JD, Kraemer HC, et al. Predictors of panic attacks in adolescents. J Am Acad Child Adolesc Psychiatry 2000;39:207–14.

[123] Hayward C, Wilson KA, Lagle K, et al. Parent-reported predictors of adolescent panic attacks. J Am Acad Child Adolesc Psychiatry 2004;43:613–20.

[124] Craske MG, Poulton R, Tsao JC, et al. Paths to panic disorder/agoraphobia: an exploratory analysis from age 3 to 21 in an unselected birth cohort. J Am Acad Child Adolesc Psychiatry 2001;40:556–63.

[125] Lonigan CJ, Vasey MW, Phillips BM, et al. Temperament, anxiety, and the processing of threat-relevant stimuli. J Clin Child Adolesc Psychol 2004;33:8–20.

[126] Stewart SH, Taylor S, Jang KL, et al. Causal modeling of relations among learning history, anxiety sensitivity, and panic attacks. Behav Res Ther 2001;39:443–56.

[127] Kessler KC. The epidemiology of pure and comorbid generalized anxiety disorder: a review and evaluation of recent research. Acta Psychiatr Scand 2000;102:7–13.

[128] Kessler RC. Agoraphobia, simple phobia, and social phobia in the National Community Survey. Arch Gen Psychiatry 1996;53:159–68.

[129] Aschenbrand SG, Kendall PC, Webb A, et al. Is childhood separation anxiety disorder a predictor of adult panic disorder and agoraphobia? A seven-year longitudinal study. J Am Acad Child Adolesc Psychiatry 2003;42:1478–85.

[130] Brady EU, Kendall PC. Comorbidity of anxiety and depression in children and adolescents. Psychol Bull 1992;111:244–55.

[131] Patton GC, Carlin JB, Coffey C, et al. Depression, anxiety, and smoking initiation: a prospective study over 3 years. Am J Public Health 1998;88:1518–22.

[132] Rao U, Ryan ND, Dahl RE, et al. Factors associated with the development of substance use disorder in depressed adolescents. J Am Acad Child Adolesc Psychiatry 1999;38:1109–17.

[133] Giaconia RM, Reinherz HZ, Hauf A, et al. Comorbidity of substance use and post-traumatic stress disorders in a community sample of adolescents. Am J Orthopsychiatry 2000;70:253–62.

[134] Johnson JG, Cohen P, Pine DS, et al. Association between cigarette smoking and anxiety disorders during adolescence and early adulthood. JAMA 2000;284:2348–51.

[135] Merikangas KR, Dierker LC, Fenton B. Familial factors and substance abuse: implications for prevention. In: Ashery RS, Robertson EB, Kumpfer KL, editors. Drug abuse prevention through family interventions. NIDA Research Monograph 177. Bethesda (MD): NIH Publications; 1998. p. 511.

[136] Kendall PC, Safford S, Flannery-Schroeder E, et al. Child anxiety treatment: outcomes in adolescence and impact on substance use and depression at 7.4-year follow-up. J Consult Clin Psychol 2004;72:276–87.

[137] Allen NB, Lewinsohn PM, Seeley JR. Prenatal and perinatal influences on risk for psychopathology in childhood and adolescence. Dev Psychopathol 1998;10:513–29.

[138] Taylor EA, Sandberg SJ, Thorley G, et al. The epidemiology of childhood hyperactivity. Oxford (UK): Oxford University Press/Maudsley Monographs; 1991.

[139] Kagan J, Reznick SJ, Clarke C, et al. Behavioral inhibition to the unfamiliar. Child Dev 1984; 55:2212–25.

[140] Kovalenko PA, Hoven CW, Wu P, et al. Association between allergy and anxiety disorders in youth. Aust N Z J Psychiatry 2001;35:815–21.

[141] Slattery MJ, Klein DF, Mannuzza S, et al. Relationship between separation anxiety disorder, parental panic disorder, and atopic disorders in children: a controlled high-risk study. J Am Acad Child Adolesc Psychiatry 2002;41:947–54.

[142] Allen M, Matthews K. Hemodynamic responses to laboratory stressors in children and adolescents: the influences of age, race, and gender. Psychophysiology 1997;34:329–39.

[143] Cohen P, Brook JS, Cohen J, et al. Common and uncommon pathways to adolescent psychopathology and problem behavior. In: Robins L, Rutter M, editors. Straight and devious pathways from childhood to adulthood. London: Cambridge University Press; 1990. p. 242–58.

[144] Kagan J. Galen's prophecy: temperament in human nature. New York: Basic Books; 1994.

[145] Merikangas KR, Stevens DE, Merikangas JR. Migraine and other psychiatric disorders. In: Robinson RG, Yates WR, editors. Psychiatric treatment of the medically ill. New York: Marcel Dekker; 1999. p. 425–42.

[146] Swartz KL, Pratt LA, Armenian HK, et al. Mental disorders and the incidence of migraine headaches in a community sample. Arch Gen Psychiatry 2000;57:945–50.

[147] Waldie KE, Poulton R. Physical and psychological correlates of primary headache in young adulthood: a 26 year longitudinal study. J Neurol Neurosurg Psychiatry 2002;72:86–92.

[148] Haines AP, Imeson JD, Meade TW. Phobic anxiety and ischaemic heart disease. BMJ 1987; 295:297–9.

[149] Bovasso G, Eaton W. Types of panic attacks and their association with psychiatric disorder and physical illness. Compr Psychiatry 1999;40:469–77.

[150] Vasa RA, Gerring JP, Grados M, et al. Anxiety after severe pediatric closed head injury. J Am Acad Child Adolesc Psychiatry 2002;41:148–56.

[151] Luis CA, Mittenberg W. Mood and anxiety disorders following pediatric traumatic brain injury: a prospective study. J Clin Exp Neuropsychol 2002;24:270–9.

[152] Shaffer D, Schonfeld I, O'Connor PA, et al. Neurological soft signs: their relationship to psychiatric disorder and intelligence in childhood and adolescence. Arch Gen Psychiatry 1985;42:342–51.

[153] Sigurdsson E, Van Os J, Fombonne E. Are impaired childhood motor skills a risk factor for adolescent anxiety? Results from the 1958 UK birth cohort and the National Child Development Study. Am J Psychiatry 2002;159:1044–6.

[154] Freedman RR, Ianni P, Ettedgui E, et al. Psychophysiological factors in panic disorder. Psychopathy 1984;17:66–73.

[155] Davidson RJ, Abercrombie H, Nitschke JB, et al. Regional brain function, emotion and disorders of emotion. Curr Opin Neurobiol 1999;9:228–34.

[156] Lang PL, Bradley MM, Cuthbert BN. Emotion, motivation and anxiety: brain mechanisms and psychophysiology. Biol Psychiatry 1998;44:1248–63.

[157] Levenson RW, Ekman P, Heider K, et al. Emotion and autonomic nervous system activity in the Minangkabau of west Sumatra. J Pers Soc Psychol 1992;62:972–88.

[158] Kagan J, Snidman N, Arcus D. The role of temperament in social development. In: Chrousos GP, McCarty R, editors. Stress: basic mechanisms and clinical implications. New York: New York Academy of Sciences; 1995. p. 485–90.

[159] Bellodi L, Perna G, Caldirola D, et al. CO_2-induced panic attacks: a twin study. Am J Psychiatry 1998;155:1184–8.

[160] Shalev A, Bloch M, Peri T, et al. Alprazolam reduces response to loud tones in panic disorder but not in posttraumatic stress disorder. Biol Psychiatry 1998;44:64–8.

[161] Grillon C, Dierker L, Merikangas KR. Startle modulation in children at risk for anxiety disorders and/or alcoholism. J Am Acad Child Adolesc Psychiatry 1997;36:925–32.

[162] Grillon C, Dierker L, Merikangas KR. Fear-potentiated startle in adolescent offspring of parents with anxiety disorders. Biol Psychiatry 1998;44:990–7.

[163] Grillon C, Warner V, Hille J, et al. Families at high and low risk for depression: a three-generation startle study. Biol Psychiatry 2005;57:953–60.

[164] Pine DS, Klein RG, Coplan JD, et al. Differential carbon dioxide sensitivity in childhood anxiety disorders and non-ill comparison group. Arch Gen Psychiatry 2000;57:960–7.

[165] Pine DS, Weese-Mayer D, Silvestri JM, et al. Anxiety and congenital central hypoventilation syndrome. Am J Psychiatry 1994;151:864–70.

[166] Breslau N, Klein DF. Smoking and panic attacks: an epidemiologic investigation. Arch Gen Psychiatry 1999;56:1141–7.

[166a] Monk CS, Nelson EE, Woldehawariat G, et al. Related articles, links experience-dependent plasticity for attention to threat: behavioral and neurophysiological evidence in humans. Biol Psychiatry 2004;56(8):607–10.

[167] Gewirtz JC, McNish KA, Davis M. Lesions of the bed nucleus of the stria terminalis block sensitization of acoustic startle reflex produced by repeated stress, but not fear-potentiated startle. Prog Neuropsychopharmacol Biol Psychiatry 1998;22:625–48.

[168] LeDoux J. Emotion, memory and the brain. Sci Am 1994;270:50–7.

[169] Coplan JD, Andrews MW, Rosenblum LA, et al. Persistent elevations of cerebrospinal fluid concentrations of corticotropin-releasing factor in adult nonhuman primates exposed to early-life stressors: implications for the pathophysiology of mood and anxiety disorders. Proc Natl Acad Sci U S A 1996;93:1619–23.

[170] Faravelli C, Guerrini Degl'Innocenti B, Giardnelli L. Epidemiology of anxiety disorders in Florence. Acta Psychiatr Scand 1989;79:308–12.

[171] Roy-Bryne P, Geraci M, Uhde T. Life events and the onset of panic disorder. Am J Psychiatry 1986;143:1424–7.

[172] De Loof C, Zandbergen J, Lousberg H, et al. The role of life events in the onset of panic disorder. Behav Res Ther 1989;27:461–3.

[173] Last C, Barlow D, O'Brien G. Precipitants of agoraphobia: role of stressful life events. Psychol Rep 1984;54:567–70.

[174] Marks IM. Genetics of fear and anxiety disorders. Br J Psychiatry 1986;149:406–18.

[175] Lteif GN, Mavissakalian MR. Life events and panic disorder/agoraphobia: a comparison at two time periods. Compr Psychiatry 1996;37:241–4.

[176] Manfro GG, Otto MW, McArdle ET, et al. Relationship of antecedent stressful life events to childhood and family history of anxiety and the course of panic disorder. J Affect Disord 1996;41:135–9.

[177] Bowlby J. The making and breaking of affectional bonds. Br J Psychiatry 1960;130:201–10.

[178] Parker G, Tupling H, Brown LB. A parental bonding instrument. Br J Med Psychol 1979;52:1–10.

[179] Silove D, Parker G, Hadzipavlovic D, et al. Parental representations of patients with panic disorder and generalised anxiety disorder. Br J Psychiatry 1991;159:835–41.

[180] Bennet A, Stirling J. Vulnerability factors in the anxiety disorders. Br J Med Psychol 1998;71:311–21.

[181] Stein MB, Walker JR, Anderson G, et al. Childhood physical and sexual abuse in patients with anxiety disorders and in a community sample. Am J Psychiatry 1996;153:275–6.

[182] Lewis MH, Gluck JP, Petitto JM, et al. Early social deprivation in nonhuman primates: long-term effects on survival and cell-mediated immunity. Biol Psychiatry 2000;47:119–26.

[183] Heim C, Newport DJ, Miller AH, et al. Long-term neuroendocrine effects of childhood maltreatment. JAMA 2000;284:2321.

[184] Pynoos RS, Steinberg AM, Piacentini JC. A developmental psychopathology model of childhood traumatic stress and intersection with anxiety disorders. Biol Psychiatry 1999;1999: 1542–54.

[185] Spear LP. The adolescent brain and age-related behavioral manifestations. Neurosci Biobehav Rev 2000;24:417–63.

[186] Robaey P, Breton F, Duga M, et al. An event-related potential study of controlled and automatic processes in 6–8 year old boys with attention deficit hyperactivity disorder. Electroencephalogr Clin Neurophysiol 1992;82:330–40.

ELSEVIER
SAUNDERS

Child Adolesc Psychiatric Clin N Am
14 (2005) 681–706

CHILD AND
ADOLESCENT
PSYCHIATRIC CLINICS
OF NORTH AMERICA

Temperament and Anxiety Disorders

Koraly Pérez-Edgar, PhD*, Nathan A. Fox, PhD

University of Maryland, 3304 Benjamin Building, College Park, MD 20742, USA

As a relatively new contributor to the world of empirical science, the field of psychology has spent the last century working first to prove its scientific underpinnings and then to generate an understanding of human behavior that truthfully portrays the present and accurately predicts the future. This has at times proven quite difficult because the object of study is much less orderly and rule-bound than the target of other disciplines, such as the atom or the cell. However, a consensus has arisen in the last decade that much of this empirical frustration may have been self-inflicted. By subdividing the field into parsimonious and atomic subdisciplines, researchers have created units that are almost by definition ill suited to capturing the complexity and multidimensionality of human behavior. Leaders in the field are attempting to bridge these gaps by forming multidisciplinary research groups that can bring together disparate literatures and methodologies to create a more three-dimensional view of the phenomenon of interest.

This article focuses on the attempt to link early appearing temperamental traits to the later emergence of psychopathology, particularly in the form of anxiety disorders. The discussion defines and characterizes the current understanding of temperament and anxiety as separate constructs; reviews the evidence to date linking temperament and anxiety; and explores the environmental, cognitive, and neural mechanisms that have been suggested as potential mediators for this effect. The article also highlights the strength of bringing together converging data from multiple sources and levels of analysis.

Anxiety and anxiety disorders can have a large affect on the daily functioning of an individual, coloring interactions with both the environment and personal assessments of internal states. The affect can be particularly damaging if anxiety

---

* Corresponding author.
E-mail address: kpe@umd.edu (K. Pérez-Edgar).

1056-4993/05/$ – see front matter © 2005 Elsevier Inc. All rights reserved.
doi:10.1016/j.chc.2005.05.008

first emerges in childhood and adolescence because this has been linked to increases in both the severity and longevity of the disorder [1]. As such, researchers and clinicians have been keen on identifying factors that may predict the emergence of anxiety. In this regard, differentiating the symptoms or characteristics of the disorder may help researchers delineate the multiple pathways to disease [2].

A number of reviews [3–5] have noted a variety of behavioral similarities between shy or inhibited temperament groups and anxious individuals. Both groups are marked by social awkwardness and withdrawal, an avoidant coping style, and a constellation of psychophysiologic markers (Table 1). Because temperament is early appearing, the construct may help outline early risk factors, even before a disorder is visibly manifested.

There are, however, a number of limitations to the potential bridge between temperament and anxiety that should be kept in mind when reviewing the discussion. First, our definition of temperament must be further refined and solidified. As Vasey and Dadds [4] have noted, many of the measures of temperament in infancy and early childhood have been rationally rather than empirically derived. This has led to some confusion within the temperament literature regarding the core characteristics of a particular temperament trait, the observed behavioral phenotype, its developmental concomitants, and its impact on socioemotional development.

Table 1
Defining characteristics shared by anxiety and behavioral inhibition

Behavior	Characteristics
Overly sensitive danger detection systems	Anxious and behaviorally inhibited individuals show a tendency to feel frightened by objects or situations that most individuals experience as nonthreatening.
Attentional bias to threat	Individuals monitor the environment for potential threat. In addition, anxious or inhibited individuals detect and respond to "threat" cues at lower thresholds. This may lead the individual to find the environment more subjectively threatening.
Avoidant coping style	Having detected an environmental threat, anxious and behaviorally inhibited individuals often respond by withdrawing from the situation and avoiding the trigger both at that moment in time and in future encounters.
Psychophysiologic patterns	Electroencephalographic asymmetry: likely to show greater activation in the right frontal lobe Startle responses: greater potentiated startle to threat cues Heart rate and heart rate variability: show high heart rate and low heart rate variability at rest Pupil dilation: show greater dilation during cognitive tasks Salivary cortisol: tend to show higher levels of stress hormone at rest and after provocation
Over-reactive amygdala	The preliminary definition of behavioral inhibition was based on behaviors linked to amygdalar activity. Recent functional MRI studies have documented increased amygdala activation to threatening and salient stimuli for both clinical and temperament groups.

Second, even with a better-defined construct, it is unlikely that research will reveal a clear linear relationship between early emerging traits and later anxiety. Developmental changes often occur as a result of reciprocal interactions between an active child and his or her environmental context, making the child both the producer and product of the environment [6]. As such, attempts to draw a link from early temperament to the later emergence of psychopathology must contend with the fact that a difficult temperament may push a child in the direction of any number of developmental outcomes (multifinality), and the targeted outcome can result from a host of predisposing pathways (equifinality). Research must therefore account for a number of potential moderating factors that can come into play at various points throughout development.

Third, just as temperament must be rigorously defined, our understanding of anxiety and psychopathology in childhood also must be better delineated. Currently, it is unclear whether these disorders can be viewed as equivalent to the adult template, simply shifted down to younger individuals. Alternatively, anxiety may be a truly developmental phenomenon that takes on a unique form and course in the young child. Beyond outlining the link between early temperament and childhood anxiety, we must therefore also examine the relationships between childhood anxiety and anxiety in adulthood.

Anxiety disorders in childhood

Anxiety is marked by a "sense of uncontrollability focused on possible future threat, danger, or other upcoming, potentially negative events" [7]. There is a sense of fear and helplessness in anxiety that is coupled with a somatically aroused central nervous system [8]. This leads the danger detection system to be maladaptively engaged [8], making it difficult to regulate emotional responses to potentially threatening stimuli. Unlike the symptoms of severe psychopathology (ie, delusions), anxiety is a normal state of functioning that has been experienced at one point by all children and adults and can often serve an adaptive purpose. Therefore, researchers must delineate the extent and depth of the anxiety state and distinguish between normative and pathologic anxiety.

In doing so, researchers often make the distinction between state anxiety, trait anxiety, and anxiety disorders. State anxiety is defined normally as a measure of the acute or immediate level of anxiety. Trait anxiety, in contrast, is the long-term tendency of an individual to show an anxiety response to environmental events. Across the clinical divide are a cluster of related disorders, which include generalized anxiety disorder, social phobia, simple phobia, panic disorder, post-traumatic stress disorder (PTSD), and obsessive-compulsive disorder. Together, these disorders affect over 20% of the adult population at one point in life and can exact an annual estimated cost of $44 billion in the United States alone [9]. Anxiety also produces a large individual burden, limiting a person's ability to freely navigate his or her environment free of excess worry and fear. Indeed, perhaps the most important distinction between state or trait anxiety and anxiety disorders is the degree of impairment that occurs as a result of the state (or trait).

Although they are heterogeneous in behavioral profile, the anxiety disorders are believed to share common physiologic or biologic characteristics, in part because they respond to a similar spectrum of drug treatments [10]. For example, the drugs most commonly used work to increase the potency of the main inhibitory neurotransmitter, γ-aminobutyric acid (GABA), or the serotonin (5-hydroxytryptamine$_3$ [5HT]) neurotransmitters. Recent work also has pointed to a shared genetic component. Approximately 30% to 40% of the variance in anxiety can be attributed to genetic variation [11], although the specificity of the genetic predisposition is unclear [12,13]. Overall, the magnitude of the genetic contribution is relatively moderate and is less than for more heritable disorders such as schizophrenia [14], indicating that gene–environment interactions and correlations are most likely particularly important in the emergence of anxiety.

Much of the work to date has focused exclusively on adult populations. Yet, many cases of anxiety (eg, social phobia) first develop during early to mid-adolescence [15], and anxiety is one of the most common psychiatric conditions afflicting adolescents [16,17]. The prevalence of anxiety disorders is between 5% and 10%, and rates of social phobia, particularly, vary from 1.6% to 8.5% [18–21].

Although many childhood anxiety disorders remit within 3 to 4 years [22], they are likely to carry or signal significant risk for further psychopathology, particularly for other anxiety disorders and depression [23,24]. Indeed, adolescent anxiety (or depression) predicts an approximate 2- to 3-fold increase in risk for anxiety in adulthood [1]. Among children there is a high degree of comorbidity between anxiety disorder and depression (approximately 28%), and comorbidity has been linked to more severe anxiety symptoms [15]. There also may be a developmental progression in which anxiety precedes depression, leading to more detrimental outcomes [25].

As such, there is a need for targeted interventions that may help ameliorate early appearing anxiety disorders. This effort would be helped if researchers and clinicians could accurately predict the emergence of anxiety. Recent work has focused on outlining behavioral, environmental, and biologic markers of risk. One of the most promising lines of research has examined early temperamental traits as a predisposing factor for later psychopathology.

Temperament in childhood

Temperament research in both its ancient (eg, Galen) and modern (eg, Thomas and Chess [26]) forms has attempted to account for core behavioral and psychologic traits that appear to shape mood and behavior for an individual across contexts. The idealized definition of temperament points to a stable psychologic profile with a presumed physiologic foundation that creates an enduring pattern of behaviors that are early appearing and consistent across time and place [27]. Borrowing from Cairns' [28] notion of behavioral epigenesis, Lahey [29] suggests that temperament can be viewed as the simple (basic or nonspecific) form of socioemotional behavior that appears early in development and provides the elemental materials for later, more complex, forms of behavior.

Much of the current work on temperament has focused on early appearing signs of negative affect and its subsequent link to inhibition, shyness, or social withdrawal. This research can be roughly categorized into one of three different approaches: the use of the adult "Big Five" personality traits as a template for childhood temperament; a continuous model of the dynamic relationship between reactivity and self-regulation; and a categorical approach that identifies children based on a discrete cluster of behavioral and psychophysiologic traits. Common to each approach is a focus on "difficult" or "negative" temperament, which is characterized by the presence of negative emotionality coupled with reports that the child's behavior is hard to manage [30].

The first strategy has attempted to map early temperament onto the adult Big Five model of personality. From this view, temperament is the "nonintellectual component or developmental precursor of personality" [4]. In trying to map onto the Big Five, Lonigan and Dyer conducted a large-scale principal component analysis using the Child Behavior Questionnaire [31] (Lonigan and Dyer, manuscript in preparation, 2000), the Emotion, Activity, Sociability, and Impulsivity (EASI) temperament scales [32], and the Positive and Negative Affective Schedule [33]. They found three factors, positive affect (PA), negative affect (NA), and effortful control, which roughly correspond with the adult constructs of surgency and extraversion, emotional stability/neuroticism, and conscientiousness [4]. Similar three-factor constellations have been found in additional independent samples [34,35].

Preliminary work has begun to link individual differences in PA or NA to childhood behavioral difficulties and psychopathology. For example, anxiety and depression show differing relationships with the temperament constructs. That is, although both anxious and depressed children show high levels of negative affect, only depressed children also show low levels of positive affect [36]. Findings such as these may allow researchers to tease apart the multiple mechanisms that can lead to behavioral profiles that appear similar at the surface.

There are a number of issues that remain to be addressed in this model. First, Vasey and Dadds [4] point out that scales that measure putatively the same dimension often have different patterns of association with other temperament dimensions, suggesting a lack of discriminant validity across the questionnaire-based constructs. This is particularly troubling given that little of this work has sought to reinforce the questionnaire data with either direct behavioral observations or psychophysiologic measures. Second, although the model includes effortful control as a third, more executive component of temperament, much of the work has focused on the PA or NA dimensions, hence the notion that temperament is a "nonintellectual" construct. This characterization would seem to limit the applicability of the model as children mature into late childhood and adolescence, the very point at which psychopathology often begins to emerge.

Third, there are little longitudinal data to help reinforce the initial similarities seen in developmental studies. On this point, Roberts and DelVecchio [37] have suggested that the available data on stability [38,39] indicate that temperament becomes more differentiated and hierarchically integrated with age, allowing for more stable temperamental profiles into adolescence and adulthood.

The second strategic approach has looked at the interaction between physical and emotional reactivity and higher order self-regulatory mechanisms in shaping behavior. The relationships between reactivity and self-regulation mechanisms are both genetically inherited and shaped by experience [40]. Reactivity is the individual's responsivity to changes in stimulation, shown at multiple levels of measurement, behavioral, autonomic, and neuroendocrine. Often, this response is seen in individual differences in the latency, rise time, peak intensity, recovery, and time of reaction when the child is confronted with emotionally evocative events. In contrast, self-regulation involves the processes modulating reactivity, including differences in the tendency to approach or avoid evocative people and events, inhibition in the face of stress, and attentional self-regulation. Generally, children are expected to become increasingly regulated over time, as attention and effortful control develop and can modulate initial reactive tendencies.

Although differences in reactivity appear quite early, it is difficult to judge the long-term impact on socioemotional development until the emergence of self-regulatory skills. This will help determine if underlying reactive tendencies are controlled successfully or are manifested in nonadaptive patterns of behavior. Generally, a child's inability to regulate negative affect can be expressed across three realms: behavior (eg, anxious withdrawal), cognition (eg, low self-worth), and psychophysiology (eg, elevated cortisol levels) [41]. The observed outcomes will depend on the strength and persistence of the underlying reactivity relative to the child's ability to draw on personal self-regulatory skills and environmental supports. High levels of negative affectivity have been linked to increased levels of internalizing problems, anxiety, and depression [2], while simultaneously acting as a protective factor against the development of externalizing disorders [42,43].

In measuring these relationships, it is important to note that stability in a temperamental profile across time appears to center on the high-order levels of temperament, rather than on the level of individual behaviors [4]. With development, the triggers for inhibited behavior change, and, similarly, the form of the behavioral response also changes. As such, the dynamic balance between reactivity and regulation must always be approached with the context of the developmental trajectory of the child. However, the assumption is that below the surface changes the underlying trait, at the biologic level, remains stable [41].

The third research approach has focused on behavioral inhibition as one of a number of discrete temperament categories that are evident in nature. Behavioral inhibition is found in approximately 15% of the population and is defined as the tendency to display signs of fear and wariness in response to unfamiliar stimuli [44–46]. As infants, behaviorally inhibited children show high levels of negative reactivity. That is, they respond with negative affect and vigorous activity when confronted with novelty. Later in life, behaviorally inhibited children are often "slow to warm up" in new social situations [47] and display unregulated social behavior that is characterized by social withdrawal to unfamiliar peers [48]. They are unlikely to initiate interaction, and they often do not respond positively when social initiations are made toward them [49].

Unlike the previous models, behavioral inhibition is defined by a constellation of traits at both the behavioral and psychophysiologic level. Specifically, inhibited children show a high- and low-heart rate variability [50,51], pupillary dilation during cognitive tasks [45], elevated salivary cortisol levels [46,52], an increased startle response [45,47,53], and right frontal electroencephalographic (EEG) asymmetry [50,54–57]. This profile is believed to be at least partially genetically mediated. For example, a recent study [58] found a strong link between behavioral inhibition and an allele of the corticotropin-releasing hormone, which is a key mediator of the stress response as it acts on the hypothalamic-pituitary-adrenal axis and the limbic system.

Long-term studies have noted moderate stability of behavioral inhibition from toddlerhood through middle childhood [59], from preschool age to middle and late childhood [60], and into early adulthood [39]. Among children selected for behavioral inhibition, Pearson correlations between repeated testing sessions, beginning in toddlerhood and ranging over 1 to 6 years, have been between $r = 0.24$ and $r = 0.64$ [60–63]. The correlations are higher among the extremely inhibited children [47]. In unselected samples, inhibition is shown to be moderately stable ($r = 0.33–0.42$) among preschoolers over the course of 2 years [64]. Again, extreme groups show much higher levels of stability, even over the course of 4 years [65].

In defining behavioral inhibition, Kagan [66] proposed that the observed physiologic and behavioral traits were linked to variations in amygdalar responses. In doing so, he drew on a line of research linking the amygdala to the acquisition of conditioned fear [67], the induction of vigorous limb movements [68], and the modulation of distress cries [69]. Behaviorally inhibited children appear to have an over-reactive amygdala, triggering a highly responsive sympathetic nervous system when confronted with stressful stimuli [46,70,71]. The role of the amygdala in behavioral inhibition and anxiety will be discussed in greater detail below.

Link between early temperament and childhood anxiety

Although research has generated a strong set of findings that help to characterize the form and function of temperamental traits, work linking early temperament to later risk for psychopathology is relatively new, limiting the conclusions that can be drawn concerning this relationship [72]. Frick [73] points out that the primary focus of research on temperament has been on its manifestations in infancy and early childhood. In contrast, research on psychopathology has understandably focused on its emergence in late childhood and adolescence [74]. As such, progress in the field will need to bridge developmental and clinical psychology, merging different theoretical constructs, research goals, research populations, and experimental methods [73,75].

Some investigators [4] argue that the low base rate of psychopathology makes studying the link between temperament and disorder difficult. However, a growing number of studies have found a persistent link between temperament-based negative affect in early childhood (variously defined) and the emergence of anxiety in mid to late adolescence [76–78]. Indeed, emerging data [77,79] suggest that the rate of psychopathology may be quite high at the temperamental extremes.

This section reviews the current descriptive findings concerning this relationship. The discussion will then turn to the mechanisms that may account for the findings to date.

The presence of behavioral inhibition in early childhood has been shown to be a risk factor for anxiety in childhood [80,81] and adolescence [77,82], particularly with regard to social phobia [77,83]. The link is strongest among adolescents who display consistent signs of inhibition across multiple testing points in childhood [84,85].

For example, a recent report [86] has found that 15% of young adults identified previously as behaviorally inhibited toddlers were diagnosed with generalized social phobia. Schwartz and colleagues [77] have found that adolescents who were inhibited at the age of 2 are more likely than their uninhibited peers to show symptoms of social anxiety as assessed by a semistructured diagnostic interview (ie, diagnostic interview schedule for children [DISC]). Indeed, 61% of the adolescents had current symptoms, and 80% had shown symptoms of anxiety at one point in their lifetime.

Using a Big Five perspective, Lonigan and colleagues [87] have found similarly that across 7 months fourth and 11th graders who were high in negative affect were likely to show increased levels of anxiety. Coupled with low levels of positive affect, negative affect also was predictive of increases in depression. Masi and colleagues [88] have found that the diagnosis of anxiety or anxiety comorbid with depression in adolescence is significantly linked to parental reports of emotionality and shyness, using Buss and Plomin's [89] EASI scale. The other two factors, activity and sociability, did not distinguish between the diagnostic groups and the controls. With regard to the emotionality and shyness scales, Buss and Plomin [89] suggest that these two factors in combination can be considered grossly equivalent to Kagan and colleagues' [70] construct of behavioral inhibition. Although direct comparisons of the two measures will be needed to confirm this relationship, it does suggest a stable core trait imparting risk in these children.

A study by Kagan and colleagues [90] has argued that because the relationships between temperament and socioemotional outcomes are nonlinear, it is important to examine subjects who have extreme scores. This will allow a clear differentiation across temperament groups because, in Kagan's formulation, individuals with extreme scores constitute discrete populations who have unique properties and developmental trajectories. In line with this admonition, Hayward and colleagues [91] have found that adolescents rated in the top 15% of self-reported behavioral inhibition had a 5-fold increase in developing social anxiety, relative to peers without an extreme temperamental profile.

Also in line with the notion that the relationship is clearer in extreme or discreet populations, a number of studies have found a clear link between temperament and anxiety in children of parents with panic disorder. Biederman and colleagues [83] have found that the rate of social anxiety disorder was significantly higher in inhibited children relative to children without behavioral inhibition. Although the interaction with parental diagnosis was not significant, the main effect of the behavioral inhibition group held only for those children who had a diagnosed parent. In addition, parallel studies have found that children of parents with anxiety disorders are more likely to show extreme behavioral inhibition [92]. A summary of these and other findings can be found in tabular form in Hirshfeld-Becker and colleagues' [93] review of the studies linking behavioral inhibition to vulnerability to psychopathology.

These initial results were not surprising given that researchers have long noted the surface similarities between negative affect and anxiety in both their operational definition and observed behavioral patterns (see Table 1). First, for example, Rapee [94] has suggested that a major component of withdrawn temperament is an avoidant style of coping. In turn, an avoidant coping style also is a central characteristic of children with clinical anxiety disorders [95].

Avoidance may help distinguish the shy child from other temperament or personality groups. For example, when they are given ambiguous social scenarios [96], withdrawn and oppositional children are highly likely to indicate a perceived threat. However, when asked to characterize their response to the threat, only the withdrawn children outlined an avoidant style. There are additional data indicating that mothers of withdrawn children may actively promote avoidance in their children [97].

Second, both anxiety and behavioral inhibition have been linked to difficulties in the deployment of the danger-detection system [8]. The tendency to feel frightened by objects or situations that most individuals experience as non-threatening represents a cardinal feature of most clinical anxiety disorders. This increased tendency to experience the subjective state of fear is associated with a variety of cognitive correlates, including thinking about feared objects or situations when they are not present, scanning the environment for signs of danger, and neglecting other nonfrightening aspects of the environment.

In particular, two studies using positive and negative facial expressions have found an explicit memory bias for negative or critical faces in social phobics [97,98]. Social phobics also have been found to display an attentional bias to words conveying a social threat [99,100]. Similarly, negative reactivity to novelty early in the first year of life is linked to a negative bias in information processing and social cognition.

Questions remain concerning the functional and structural relationships between temperament and anxiety. Temperament can either place a child at risk for developing certain forms of psychopathology or influence the stability or severity of the disorder [101]. This conceptualizes temperament as a separate construct from psychopathology [73]. Alternately, psychopathology could be construed as the extreme endpoint along a single temperamental spectrum [101]. The cut off between individual variation and psychologic disorder would be drawn when the child experiences psychosocial impairments [73]. Indeed, Lahey [29] argues that there is no inherent distinction between temperament and psychopathology in nature. Distinctions are simply imposed by experts in the field, taking into account the data revealing interconnections between basic temperamental traits (eg, irritability and anger) and specific psychopathologies (eg, oppositional defiant disorder). Along these lines, Akiskal [102] sees temperament as a subclinical variant of psychiatric disorders. This would be particularly the case among the extreme temperament types or spectrum.

Potential explanatory mechanisms

To date, the explanatory research has focused on three broad areas: environmental and parenting factors, cognitive or attentional mechanisms, and variations in neural functioning (particularly the amygdala and the orbital frontal cortex [OFC]).

Animal model for parenting

The literature in both the animal and human models suggests that parents and parenting style can influence the presence of negative temperament and the eventual emergence of anxiety. In doing so, the link appears to rely on both heritable traits passed along across generations and the parenting styles that color day-to-day interactions.

For example, in rat models, maternal licking of pups is believed to reflect the "conscientiousness" of the mother and is used as a marker for maternal effectiveness. Pups raised by mothers with impaired licking and grooming skills have higher levels of anxiety-related behavior than pups raised by high licking-and-grooming mothers [103]. Cross-fostering to a high-licking mother after birth will decrease anxiety-related behavior developing in the offspring of low-licking mothers [104]. However, the offspring of high-licking mothers will not take on the high-anxiety behaviors of their low-licking foster-mother. Francis and colleagues [105] have also shown that experimentally conferred high licking-and-grooming behavior can be passed on across generations. Females raised by high-licking mothers go on to become high-licking mothers themselves and have low-anxiety offspring, regardless of their genetic lineage.

These data suggest that although anxiety-related behaviors are amenable to environmental change, the buffering factors that protect an individual from disorder may be difficult to overcome, crumbling only in the face of multiple or severe insults. To examine the extent of the gene–environment dynamic, Francis and colleagues [105] transplanted embryos from a high-licking strain of mothers into a low-licking strain of surrogate mothers shortly after conception. The authors found that to confer low-licking behavior on the offspring of high-licking rats, the offspring must have exposure to a low-licking mother both in utero and after birth. No other combination of gestational and infant care produced low-licking rats. These data suggest that maternal characteristics that appear to shape behavioral outcomes begin to act long before birth. Although gestation may set the stage for later risk, this vulnerability must be reinforced early in life to have long-term consequences. Many of these issues are being explored in the human literature. Here, two factors have emerged as particularly important: parental intrusiveness or insensitivity and a parental history of anxiety disorders.

Parenting style

Thomas and Chess [26] were the first to introduce the concept of "goodness-of-fit" in arguing that the link between temperament and later adjustment cannot be understood without accounting for the dynamic characteristics of the child's environment, both in isolation and in direct response to the child's temperamental traits. Since then, a long line of research has argued that parenting styles, such as overprotective and controlling behavior and criticism and lack of warmth, are linked to the emergence of anxiety in children [106,107]. Sensitive parenting encourages mutual regulation between parent and child and contributes to the child mastering his or her own behavior [108]. In contrast, intrusive parenting may disrupt mutual regulation and interfere with the development of self-regulation [109]. A lack of strong self-regulatory skills would leave the child more vulnerable to underlying reactive tendencies.

Rubin and colleagues [110] have investigated whether the interaction of parenting behaviors and behavioral inhibition at 2 years of age explained child characteristics at 4 years of age, either directly or through the moderation of earlier inhibition. A maternal parenting style consisting of overly warm, intrusive, unresponsive, and derisive behavior moderated the concurrent association between shyness and behavioral inhibition at 2 years [111]. These associations remained 2 years later when children were reassessed at 4 years of age [110]. Inhibition at 2 years only predicted reticence with unfamiliar peers at 4 years when mothers behaved in a psychologically controlling or derisive manner.

Also affecting this relationship is the use of nonparental care. Fox and colleagues [56] have found that infants who show high negative emotionality at 4 months of age are more likely to change their behavior and become less inhibited over toddlerhood when they are placed in nonparental caregiving environments for at least 10 hours per week. Children who stay at home may be more likely to receive parenting that is more overcontrolling and oversolicitous, whereas children who go to daycare may be more likely to receive parenting that fosters independence [112]. In addition, children in out-of-home care have much more experience interacting with unfamiliar adults and peers, further ameliorating underlying reactive traits. Future work will need to determine if parenting style and care environment are risk factors independent of temperament or are directly associated with temperament [94].

Parental psychopathology

Parental behaviors, particularly when colored by the presence of mood or anxiety disorders, may mitigate or exacerbate the onset or maintenance of behavioral inhibition [113,114]. Several previous studies have reported higher risks of behavioral inhibition in children of adults with anxiety disorders [80,115] or major depression [116,117] as well as increased rates of parental anxiety disorders in children with inhibited behavior.

In examining this link, a number of potential moderating factors have been tested. Hirshfeld-Becker and colleagues [118] have found no relationships among behavioral inhibition and any of the following measures of psychosocial adversity: family conflict, low socioeconomic status, large family size, exposure to psychopathology, and paternal criminality. These data suggest that psychosocial factors cannot account for the link between behavioral inhibition and maternal psychopathology. Rather, the data bolster the contention that behavioral inhibition is quite heritable, with estimates ranging from 0.40 to 0.70 in twin studies [119–121].

Masi and colleagues [88] have found that the siblings of anxious adolescents, although free of psychopathology, also showed significantly higher levels of emotionality and shyness compared with the siblings of the children in two control groups. This suggests a shared genetic diathesis that can predispose a child to psychopathology. Indeed, high levels of emotionality were found in both the mothers and fathers of the anxious-depressed children. However, without a precipitating event or insult, this predisposition may not cross the line into a psychiatric diagnosis.

Overall, the data suggest that children who have inherited an inhibited temperament and are more sensitive to adversity factors may find it particularly daunting when challenged by a poor parenting environment colored by psychopathology. Yet, although the presence of a parent with panic disorder will predispose a child for panic disorder and other anxiety disorders [115–122], not all children will become ill. As such, additional features either internal or external to the child must be brought into the equation to more effectively assess risk and apply needed interventions [83].

Escalona [123] points out that simply noting the presence of an environmental stressor is not sufficient for understanding the impact on the child or child's response to the stressor. Rather, researchers and theorists must work to capture the child's "effective experience." As such, a second line of research has looked at child-centered variables to understand the relationships between early temperament and anxiety. The most heavily examined phenomenon involves individual differences in attentional or effortful control.

Attentional or effortful control

Flexible cognition and attention requires the ability to carry out two opposing processes: selecting goal-related stimuli for processing and detecting potentially significant and often unpredictable events [124]. Individuals must simultaneously and selectively deploy attention and filter out distracters outside of this realm, although at the same time they must allow for changes in the outer realm to intrude on the focus of attention when potentially significant. This delicate balance allows individuals to proceed through their daily activities without undue burden or disturbance. When the balance is lost, a cascading effect of successive cognitive and affective processes can lead to patterns of behavior that are maladaptive or disordered.

A number of researchers have suggested that among children with temperamental behavioral inhibition, children who are able to harness attentional control mechanisms can mitigate underlying reactive tendencies and avoid deleterious effects. In contrast, behaviorally inhibited children with poor control skills would be more beholden to initial affective reactions to external stimuli and would be more likely to show symptoms of anxiety. Thus, the coping resources available to the child may moderate the physiologic and behavioral correlates of temperament [125].

When these coping mechanisms are ineffective, negative characteristics often linked to anxiety are then observed. For example, when presented with ambiguous situations, young socially anxious children perceive threat more quickly and report more negative feelings [126]. Anxious children also have more negative cognitions and make lower estimates of their competency to cope with dangerous or stressful events [127]. In these cases, the child has proven unable to filter out the ambiguity and threat of the situation and focus on more positive and adaptive behaviors.

Temperamentally reactive children often react to threat or stress in two somewhat paradoxical ways. First, they show an avoidant coping style [94] and often retreat from direct engagement. Second, they will continue to monitor the potential threat, showing an attentional bias for such environmental stimuli. This could lead the anxious individual to find the environment more subjectively threatening.

Both trait anxious [128–130] and clinically anxious [131–133] adults appear to display an attentional bias toward threatening information. The data suggest that high- and low-trait anxious individuals show a similar quadratic function toward threat. That is, all individuals shift attention away from mild threat and toward intense threat. However, with stimuli of moderate intensity, the high-trait anxious individual will show a larger attentional bias toward the stimuli, relative to the low-trait anxious counterpart. This can be conceived of as a shift in phase for the function [134–136].

Although the data are preliminary, early findings indicate that anxiety-related attentional biases operate similarly in children and adults [137]. Parallel findings have been noted with clinically anxious [138,139], high-trait anxious [140]

(Vasey and Schippell, manuscript in preparation, 2002), and behaviorally in-hibited children [141]. For example, Vasey has found that in children with low effortful or attentional control, high levels of anxiety predicted a bias in favor of threat cues (M.W. Vasey, unpublished data, 2003). Interestingly, the relationship did not hold for children with good attentional control skills, suggesting that regulatory mechanisms can act as a buffer in the face of negative reactivity tempering the normal socioemotional consequences.

Rothbart and colleagues [142] have shown that individuals who are better equipped to regulate initial reactivity, particularly through the use of attentional mechanisms, are less likely to show prolonged periods of negative affect. For example, their data suggest that infants prone to distress are less adept at shifting attention away from a distressing stimulus and have difficulty engaging in self-soothing activity [142,143]. In addition, data from the present authors' tempera-ment cohort showed that mothers of 9-month old infants who show poor attentional control rate the infants as prone to distress and less likely to show spontaneous smiles (Pérez-Edgar, Martin, and Fox, manuscript in preparation, 2005). At age 4, these children also showed greater signs of social reticence.

As such, Mathews and MacLeod [144] suggest that the ability to effectively override initial reactive tendencies or biases is what distinguishes the healthy high-trait anxious individual from his or her counterpart who exhibits clinically relevant levels of anxiety. Lonigan and colleagues [5] have suggested that documenting the following six findings would help to empirically support the notion that effortful control moderates the relationship between affective reactivity and anxiety: (1) Negative affect, positive affect, and effortful control are shown to be distinct factors with significant stability over time; (2) there are unique relationships between negative affect and effortful control with anxiety; (3) the strength of the relationship between negative affect and anxiety is at least partially dependant on the individual's level of effortful control; (4) the strength of the effect of effortful control will vary with performance conditions, par-ticularly with respect to the timing of processing and response production; (5) effortful control does not moderate the relationship between negative affect and pre-attentional threat bias; and (6) a significant portion of the relationships between negative affect and effortful control with anxiety can be accounted for by attentional bias. Once systematic research programs are able to address each of these points, we should have a fuller picture of the role attention and attention regulation plays in the development and maintenance of anxiety.

Neural underpinnings

Paralleling the work examining reactivity and regulation in cognition and behavior, neuroscientists have begun to examine the balance between reactive neural structures (ie, the amygdala) and more regulatory structures (ie, the OFC). Although 20 years of work pointed to the role the amygdala may play in inhibited temperament [47,56], direct examination of this brain structure has only recently become available with the widespread adoption of MRI and functional MRI (fMRI) technology for research [145].

Previous work has linked the amygdala to the fear system. Fear induction through the injection of procaine [146] or cholecystokinin tetrapeptide (CCK4) [147] will produce amygdala activation in healthy adults. In addition, studies have demonstrated greater amygdalar activity to fearful versus happy [148] or neutral [149,150] facial expressions. Amygdalar activity also has been seen in response to threatening words [151], signals predicting shock [152], and aversive odors and tastes [153].

Individuals who have amygdalar damage but intact hippocampi do not acquire conditioned skin conductance responses (SCR) despite verbalizing the stimulus association [154]. In contrast, individuals who have an intact amygdala and damaged hippocampi cannot state the conditioned association while showing the expected SCR to the presentation of the conditioned stimulus [155]. The amygdala also activates when the contingencies between a stimulus and a negative outcome are unpredictable [156] or when the level of threat is ambiguous, requiring increased vigilance [157].

Recent work has suggested that the amygdala, beyond being integral to the fear system, also is involved in salience detection without regard to the hedonic value of the environmental stimulus. To that end, Baxter and colleagues [158] have noted that individuals with amygdalar damage are deficient in their ability to use information about positive and negative outcomes to guide their choice behavior. Indeed, the role of the amygdala in stimulus–reward learning might be just as important as its role in processing negative affect and fear conditioning [159], as can be seen in a series of studies examining reinforcement and learning in traditional Pavlovian paradigms [160,161].

Imaging studies of subjects who differ in temperament are still few in number. However, the first major study [162] has found that young adults (mean 22 years of age) categorized as inhibited in the second year of life showed significant bilateral amygdalar activation to the presentation of novel faces, versus fixation, relative to participants without a history of behavioral inhibition. Although imaging studies of anxious children are emerging only now, the recent work has been promising. For example, Monk and colleagues [163] have found that children fearful of an uncomfortable air puff to the larynx will show more right-sided amygdalar activation when faced with the threat of the upcoming air puff. In addition, children with anxiety disorders display hyper-responsive amygdalar activity compared with healthy children of the same age when viewing fearful versus neutral faces, particularly in the right hemisphere [164].

Potentially tempering reactivity within the amygdala is the orbital frontal cortex. The OFC is situated in the anterior and medial regions of the prefrontal cortex and is the only region in the prefrontal cortex that has strong reciprocal connections with the amygdala (Fig. 1) [165,166]. These connections may help explain the data suggesting that the amygdala also is closely involved in more complex social judgments, beyond the simple recognition of fear. For example, the amygdala appears to play a role in judging trustworthiness and approach-

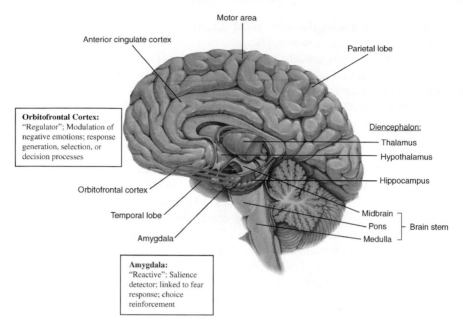

Fig. 1. Reciprocal connections between the amygdala and the orbitofrontal cortex (*black bars*). These connections may serve as the neural underpinnings for the relationships between reactivity and self-regulation noted in behavioral studies of temperament and anxiety.

ability, traits that require processing multiple complex cues [167]. In this regard, the OFC is linked to the modulation of negative emotions [168] and is critical for response generation, selection, or decision processes [161], as well as an adaptive change of behavior in the face of environmental consequences [169]. As such, according to Davidson and Irwin [170], damage to orbitofrontal areas "would not impair immediate reactivity to incentives, but...the capacity to sustain and anticipate such reactions when the immediate elicitors are not present." Similarly, the use of reinforcers to guide response selection also requires the interaction of the amygdala and OFC [158].

Animal and adult studies have correlated OFC damage with increased anxiety, affective lability, social disinhibition, and increased aggression [171–173]. Individuals with OFC lesions also appear to act more impulsively in both cognitive–behavioral tasks and in self-reported measures [174]. This impulsivity could be related to a tendency to respond rapidly to rewards and punishers without assessing the consequences sufficiently. It also points to a failure to self-regulate on the part of OFC patients. That is, although these individuals are fully aware of their impulsivity (or disinhibition and socially inappropriate behavior), they are unable to prevent themselves from acting out in such a manner.

Within the realm of anxiety disorders, multiple studies of adults with simple phobias document dysregulation of the orbitofrontal cortex during the presentation of symptom-arousing stimuli [175,176]. In social phobias, adults show increased amygdalar activity to neutral faces [177]. Increased amygdalar activation and decreased orbitofrontal cortex activity during a fear-provoking task [178] have also been documented.

Outstanding issues

Kagan and colleagues [90] have suggested that research is a "contest in which [nature] presents a sign and investigators try to determine its meaning, especially those features...that reveal the origin of the natural event." As noted here, the literature is beginning to suggest that a specific temperament accounts for a large amount of the variance in the development of anxiety disorders. Temperament may set the stage by shaping the child's early reactive and affective biases. It may then influence the child's ability to modify these inborn tendencies through individual differences in attentional and effortful regulation. These differences can be seen at the behavioral and psychophysiologic level, and preliminary work suggests that there are stable neural underpinnings for the observed differences.

If these observations prove correct, there are large implications for how researchers and clinicians should address the issue of childhood anxiety. However, there are a number of issues that first must be addressed before our understanding of the temperament-anxiety link may be usefully translated into effective, targeted interventions.

First, our constructs of temperament and anxiety must be carefully and fully defined. The lack of progress in this area may in part reflect the predominance of univariate and unidimensional approaches. In 2001, Kagan and colleagues [27] warned against assuming that anxiety and temperament are unitary natural phenomena that require only a simple consensus definition. In particular, the authors are concerned that the terms are traded back and forth within the literature without a solid grounding in the context in which they are experienced or observed. To study the phenomena most parsimoniously and parse out the root causes, the various forms of anxiety and temperament must be delineated. For example, the researcher must be careful to distinguish between the acute state of anxiety (eg, after a negative life event) and the chronic state of anxiety (eg, as part of a general personality trait), each of which may differ in their relationship to temperament and the added risk for the emergence of disorder.

From this point of view, the strongest data can be found in constructs that draw from multiple streams, including behavioral observation across contexts, parent- and child-reporting, and psychophysiology. This will allow researchers and clinicians to see fully the intersections between temperament and anxiety, better delineating which children are at greatest risk for future disorders and which shared traits, if any, are amenable to intervention.

Second, research must expand to encompass a broader time frame, examining the developmental trajectories of temperament and anxiety from infancy through middle childhood and adolescence and into adulthood. Because many of the studies to date that have examined the link between temperament and psychopathology has focused on fairly young children, it is possible that an additional or differing pattern of diagnoses will emerge over time with development and maturation. For example, it appears that the negative consequences of shyness or inhibition reach a peak in the adolescent years, in terms of difficult social encounters [179], poor self evaluations [180], and the emergence of compromising psychiatric problems [181]. To push the timeline even farther, the relationship between childhood or infant temperament and adult personality remains exceedingly unclear.

This suggests that the careful study of developmental trends in adolescence may prove an informative conduit, reinforcing the power of detailed longitudinal studies. Extended longitudinal studies will help confirm the long-term stability of psychopathology seen in adolescence. Presently, we do not know truly if the current findings are transient in nature, responding to the unique stressors of adolescence, or harbingers of life-long difficulty and disturbance.

Ollendick and Hirshfeld-Becker [182] suggest the following types of studies would be helpful in testing the viability of developmental psychopathology models of anxiety: (1) longitudinal prospective studies that identify temperamentally vulnerable children early in life and also monitor parental behavior and peer influences; (2) twin studies that assess both behavioral inhibition and childhood anxiety disorders; (3) adoption studies of at-risk children that assess both environmental and genetic risk factors; and (4) interventional studies of at-risk offspring who have behavioral inhibition.

This work also will help determine if the cognitive and neural measures noted above are markers for psychiatric vulnerability or are the actual symptoms of a disorder. Observed biologic differences across control and diagnostic groups should not be assumed to reflect a specific marker for the disorder; rather, the difference may point to a risk factor, or diathesis, that preceded the onset of the disorder and is shared with at-risk but healthy counterparts of the diagnostic group [145]. For example, several researchers have found decreased hippocampal volumes in individuals with PTSD [183], leading many investigators to propose that the decrease is a direct consequence of the individual's chronic state of stress [184,185]. However, recent studies examining twins discordant for PTSD have found that both twins show reduced hippocampal volumes, indicating that decreased size is a risk factor for PTSD, not a sign of the disorder [186].

If the link between temperament and anxiety does hold, targeted interventions must then tackle the question of how amenable core temperament traits may be to modification. There is some evidence that active attempts by parents to alter their child's worrisome temperament can nudge a child toward the mean in social behavior [70]. Preliminary data also indicate that early peer exposure through daily out-of-home care also can ameliorate early signs of inhibition [56]. In each case, systematic work is needed to test these relationships. Along these lines, Rapee [94] is currently testing an intervention protocol designed to decrease the likelihood of developing anxiety in inhibited children ages 3.5 to 4.5 years old. Preliminary data indicate that the intervention markedly decreases signs of inhibition and anxiety at a 1-year follow-up.

Summary

The broad range of issues touched on in this article highlights our view of temperament and psychopathology as complex, multidimensional phenomena that are embedded within multiple causative pathways and which, in turn, produce any number of developmental outcomes. As such, it seems clear that any future progress is almost wholly dependent on our ability to forge multi-disciplinary research programs that can address the link between temperament and anxiety from multiple levels of analysis across both time and contexts. This will allow the field to come closer to the larger goals shared across psychology: description, prediction, and intervention.

References

[1] Pine DS, Cohen P, Gurley D, et al. The risk for early-adulthood anxiety and depressive disorders in adolescents with anxiety and depressive disorders. Arch Gen Psychiatry 1998; 55:56–64.

[2] Rothbart MK. Differentiated measures of temperament and multiple pathways to childhood disorders. J Clin Child Adolesc Psychol 2004;33:82–7.

[3] Anthony JL, Lonigan CJ, Hooe ES, et al. An affect-based, hierarchical model of temperament and its relations with internalizing symptomatology. J Am Acad Child Adolesc Psychiatry 2002;31:480–90.

[4] Vasey MW, Dadds MR, editors. The developmental psychopathology of anxiety. New York: Oxford University Press; 2001.

[5] Lonigan CJ, Vasey MW, Phillips BM, et al. Temperament, anxiety, and the processing of threat-relevant stimuli. J Clin Child Adolesc Psychol 2004;33:8–20.

[6] Lerner RM, Hess LE, Nitz KA. Developmental perspective on psychopathology. In: Herson M, Last CG, editors. Handbook of child and adult psychopathology: a longitudinal perspective. Elmsford (NY): Pergamon Press; 1991. p. 9–32.

[7] Barlow DH, Chorpita BF, Turovsky J. Fear, panic, anxiety, and disorders of emotion. Nebr Symp Motiv 1996;43:251–328.

[8] Chua P, Dolan RJ. The neurobiology of anxiety and anxiety-related disorders: a functional neuroimaging perspective. In: Mazziotta JC, Toga AW, Frackowiak RSJ, editors. Brain mapping: the disorders. New York: Academic Press; 2000. p. 509–22.

[9] Greenberg PE, Sisitsky T, Kessler RC, et al. The economic burden of anxiety disorders in the 1990s. J Clin Psychiatry 1999;60:427–35.

[10] Gross C, Hen R. The developmental origins of anxiety. Nat Rev Neurosci 2004;5:545–52.

[11] Hettema JM, Neale MC, Kendler KS. A review and meta-analysis of the genetic epidemiology of anxiety disorders. Am J Psychiatry 2001;158:1568–78.

[12] Fyer AJ, Mannuzza S, Chapman TF, et al. Specificity in familial aggregation of phobic disorders. Arch Gen Psychiatry 1995;52:564–73.

[13] Mancini C, van Ameringen M, Szatmari P, et al. A high-risk study of the children of adults with social phobia. J Am Acad Child Adolesc Psychiatry 1996;35:1511–7.

[14] Cannon TD, Kaprio J, Lonnqvist J, et al. The genetic epidemiology of schizophrenia in a Finnish twin cohort: a population-based modeling study. Arch Gen Psychiatry 1998;55:67–74.

[15] Strauss CC, Last CG, Hersen M. Association between anxiety and depression in children and adolescents with anxiety disorders. J Abnorm Child Psychol 1998;16:57–68.

[16] Costello EJ, Angold A. Epidemiology. In: March J, editor. Anxiety disorders in children and adolescents. New York: Guilford; 1995. p. 109–24.

[17] Weissman MM, Myers JK, Harding PS. Psychiatric disorders in a US urban community. Am J Psychiatry 1978;135:459–62.

[18] Essau CA, Conradt J, Petermann F. Frequency and comorbidity of social phobia and social fears in adolescents. Behav Res Ther 1999;37:831–43.

[19] Fergusson DM, Horwood LJ, Lynskey MT. Prevalence and comorbidity of DSM-III-R diagnoses in a birth cohort of 15 year olds. J Am Acad Child Adolesc Psychiatry 1993;32: 1127–34.

[20] Heimberg R, Stin MB, Hiripi E, et al. Trends in the prevalence of social phobia in the United States: a synthetic cohort analysis of changes over four decades. Eur Psychiatry 2000; 15:29–37.

[21] McGee R, Feehan M, Williams S, et al. DSM-III disorders in a large sample of adolescents. J Am Acad Child Adolesc Psychiatry 1990;29:611–9.

[22] Last CG, Perrin S, Hersen M, et al. A prospective study of childhood anxiety disorders. J Am Acad Child Adolesc Psychiatry 1996;35:1502–10.

[23] Cole DA, Peeke LG, Martin JM, et al. A longitudinal look at the relation between depression and anxiety in children and adolescents. J Consult Clin Psychol 1998;66:451–60.

[24] Orvaschel H, Lewinsohn PM, Seeley JR. Continuity of psychopathology in a community sample of adolescents. J Am Acad Child Adolesc Psychiatry 1995;34:1525–35.

[25] Brady EU, Kendall PC. Comorbidity of anxiety and depression in children and adolescents. Psychol Bull 1992;111:244–55.

[26] Thomas A, Chess S. Temperament and development. New York: New York University Press; 1977.

[27] Kagan J, Snidman N, McManis M, et al. Temperamental contributions to the affect family of anxiety. Psychiatr Clin North Am 2001;24:677–88.

[28] Cairns RB. Social development: the origins and plasticity of social origins. San Francisco: Freeman; 1979.

[29] Lahey BB. Role of temperament in developmental models of psychopathology. J Clin Child Adolesc Psychol 2004;33:88–93.

[30] Prior M. Childhood temperament. J Child Psychol Psychiatry 1992;33:249–79.

[31] Rothbart MK, Ahadi SA. Temperament and the development of personality. J Abnorm Psychol 1994;103:55–66.

[32] Buss A. A theory of shyness. In: Jones WH, Cheek JM, Briggs SR, editors. Shyness: perspectives on research and treatment. New York: Plenum; 1986. p. 39–46.

[33] Watson D, Clark LA, Tellegen A. Development and validation of brief measures of positive and negative affect: the PANAS Scales. J Pers Soc Psychol 1988;54:1063–70.

[34] Ahadi SA, Rothbart MK, Ye R. Children's temperament in the US and China: similarities and differences. European Journal of Personality 1993;7:359–77.

[35] Angleitner A, Ostendorf F. Temperament and the big five factors of personality. In: Halverson Jr CF, Kohnstamm GA, editors. Developing structure of temperament and personality from infancy to adulthood. Hillsdale (NJ): Erlbaum; 1994. p. 69–90.

[36] Lonigan CJ, Carey MP, Finch Jr AJ. Anxiety and depression in children and adolescents: negative affectivity and the utility of self-reports. J Consult Clin Psychol 1994;62:1000–8.

[37] Roberts BW, DelVecchio WF. The rank-order consistency of personality traits from childhood to old age: a quantitative review of longitudinal studies. Psychol Bull 2000;126:3–25.

[38] Block J, Kremen A. IQ and ego-resiliency: clarifying their conceptual and empirical linkage and separateness. J Pers Soc Psychol 1996;70:349–61.

[39] Caspi A, Silva PA. Temperamental qualities at age 3 predict personality traits in young adulthood: longitudinal evidence from a birth cohort. Child Dev 1995;66:486–98.

[40] Derryberry D, Rothbart MK. Reactive and effortful processes in the organization of temperament. Dev Psychopathol 1997;9:633–52.

[41] Schmidt LA, Fox NA. The development and outcomes of childhood shyness: a multiple psychophysiological measure approach. In: Vasta R, editor. Annals of Child Development, Volume 13. Philadelphia: Kingsley; 1998. p. 1–20.

[42] Frick PJ, Morris AS. Temperament and developmental pathways to conduct problems. J Clin Child Adolesc Psychol 2004;33:54–68.
[43] Rothbart MK, Bates JE. Temperament. In: Damon W, Eisenberg N, editors. Handbook of child psychology: social, emotional, and personality development, Volume 3. New York: Wiley; 1998. p. 105–76.
[44] Garcia-Coll C, Kagan J, Reznick JS. Behavioral inhibition to the unfamiliar. Child Dev 1984;55:1005–19.
[45] Kagan J, Reznick S, Snidman N. The physiology and psychology of behavioral inhibition in children. Child Dev 1987;58:1459–73.
[46] Schmidt LA, Fox NA, Rubin KH, et al. Behavioral and neuroendocrine responses in shy children. Dev Psychobiol 1997;30:127–40.
[47] Kagan J, Reznick JS, Snidman N. Biological bases of childhood shyness. Science 1988; 240:167–71.
[48] Fox NA, Rubin KH, Calkins SD, et al. Frontal activation asymmetry and social competence at four years of age. Child Dev 1995;66:1770–84.
[49] Coplan RJ, Rubin KH, Fox NA, et al. Being alone, playing alone, and acting alone: distinguishing among reticence and passive and active solitude in young children. Child Dev 1994;65:129–37.
[50] Calkins SD, Fox NA, Marshall TR. Behavioral and physiological antecedents of inhibited and uninhibited behavior. Child Dev 1996;67:523–40.
[51] Marshall PJ, Stevenson-Hinde J. Behavioral inhibition, heart period, and respiratory sinus arrhythmia in young children. Dev Psychobiol 1998;3:283–92.
[52] Fox NA. Psychophysiological correlates of emotional reactivity during the first year of life. Dev Psychol 1989;25:364–72.
[53] Schmidt LA, Fox NA. Conceptual, biological, and behavioral distinctions among different categories of shy children. In: Schmidt LA, Schulkin J, editors. Extreme fear, shyness, and social phobia: origins, biological mechanisms, and clinical outcomes. Series in affective science. New York: Oxford University Press; 1999. p. 47–66.
[54] Bell MA, Fox NA. Brain development over the first year of life: relations between EEG frequency and coherence and cognitive and affective behaviors. In: Dawson G, Fischer KW, editors. Human behavior and the developing brain. New York: Guilford Press; 1994. p. 314–45.
[55] Davidson R. Asymmetric brain function, affective style, and psychopathology: the role of early experience and plasticity. Dev Psychopathol 1994;6:741–58.
[56] Fox NA, Henderson HA, Rubin KH, et al. Continuity and discontinuity of behavioral inhibition and exuberance: psychophysiological and behavioral influences across the first four years of life. Child Dev 2001;72:1–21.
[57] McManis MH, Kagan J, Snidman NC, et al. EEG asymmetry, power, and temperament in children. Dev Psychobiol 2002;40:169–77.
[58] Smoller JW, Rosenbaum JF, Biederman J, et al. Association of a genetic marker at the corticotropin-releasing hormone locus with behavioral inhibition. Biol Psychiatry 2003;54: 1376–81.
[59] Goldsmith HH, Lemery KS. Linking temperamental fearfulness and anxiety symptoms: a behavior-genetic perspective. Biol Psychiatry 2000;48:1199–209.
[60] Fordham K, Stevenson-Hinde J. Shyness, friendship quality, and adjustment during middle childhood. J Child Psychol Psychiatry 1999;40:757–68.
[61] Scarpa A, Raine A, Venables P, et al. The stability of inhibited/uninhibited temperament from ages 3 to 11 years in Mauritian children. J Abnorm Child Psychol 1995;23:607–18.
[62] Asendorpf JB. Beyond social withdrawal: shyness, unsociability, and peer avoidance. Hum Dev 1990;33:250–9.
[63] Asendorpf JB. The malleability of behavioral inhibition: a study of individual developmental functions. Dev Psychol 1994;30:912–9.
[64] Broberg A, Lamb M, Hwang P. Inhibition: its stability and correlates in sixteen- to forty-month-old children. Child Dev 1990;65:1153–63.

[65] Kerr M, Lambert WW, Stattin H, et al. Stability of inhibition in a Swedish longitudinal sample. Child Dev 1994;65:138–46.

[66] Kagan J. Galen's prophecy: temperament in human nature. New York: Basicbooks; 1994.

[67] Davis M, Walker DL, Lee Y. Roles of the amygdala and bed nucleus of the stria terminalis in fear and anxiety measured with the acoustic startle reflex. Ann N Y Acad Sci 1997;821: 305–31.

[68] Amaral DG, Price JL, Pitkanen A, et al. Anatomical organization of the primate amygdaloid complex. In: Aggleton JP, editor. The amygdala: neurobiological aspects of emotion, memory, and mental dysfunction. New York: Wiley; 1992. p. 1–66.

[69] Newman JD. The infant cry of primates. In: Lester BM, Boukydis CFZ, editors. Infant crying. New York: Plenum; 1985. p. 307–23.

[70] Kagan J, Reznick S, Clarke C, et al. Behavioral inhibition to the unfamiliar. Child Dev 1984; 55:2212–25.

[71] Neal JA, Edelmann RJ. The etiology of social phobia: toward a developmental profile. Clin Psychol Rev 2003;23:761–86.

[72] Eisenberg N, Fabes RA, Guthrie IK, et al. Dispositional emotionality and regulation: their role in predicting quality of social functioning. J Pers Soc Psychol 2000;78:136–57.

[73] Frick PJ. Integrating research on temperament and childhood psychopathology: its pitfalls and promise. J Clin Child Adolesc Psychol 2004;33:2–7.

[74] Zeanah CH, Boris NW, Scheeringa MS. Psychopathology in infancy. J Child Psychol Psychiatry 1997;38:81–99.

[75] Rutter M, Sroufe LA. Developmental psychopathology: concepts and challenges. Dev Psychopathol 2000;12:265–96.

[76] Kagan J, Snidman N. Early childhood predictors of adult anxiety disorders. Biol Psychiatry 1999;46:1536–41.

[77] Schwartz CE, Snidman NS, Kagan J. Adolescent social anxiety as an outcome of inhibited temperament in childhood. J Am Acad Child Adolesc Psychiatry 1999;53:1008–15.

[78] van Ameringen M, Mancini C, Oakman JM. The relationship of behavioral inhibition and shyness to anxiety disorder. J Nerv Ment Dis 1998;186:425–31.

[79] Fox NA, Pérez-Edgar K. Temperamental origins of irritability and social withdrawal. Presented at the 51st Annual Meeting of the American Academy of Child and Adolescent Psychiatry. Washington (DC), October 19–24, 2004.

[80] Rosenbaum JF, Biederman J, Gersten M, et al. Behavioral inhibition in children of parents with panic disorder and agoraphobia. Arch Gen Psychiatry 1988;45:463–70.

[81] Hirshfeld DR, Rosenbaum JF, Biederman J, et al. Stable behavioral inhibition and its association with anxiety disorder. J Am Acad Child Adolesc Psychiatry 1992;31:103–11.

[82] Schwartz CE, Snidman NS, Kagan J. Early childhood temperament as a determinant of externalizing behavior in adolescence. Dev Psychopathol 1996;8:527–37.

[83] Biederman J, Hirshfeld-Becker DR, Rosenbaum JF, et al. Further evidence of association between behavioral inhibition and social anxiety in children. Am J Psychiatry 2001;158: 1673–9.

[84] Biederman J, Rosenbaum JF, Bolduc-Murphy EA, et al. A three-year follow-up of children with and without behavioral inhibition. J Am Acad Child Adolesc Psychiatry 1993;32:814–21.

[85] Prior M, Smart D, Sanson A, et al. Does shy-inhibited temperament in childhood lead to anxiety problems in adolescence? J Am Acad Child Adolesc Psychiatry 2000;39:461–8.

[86] Schwartz CE, Wright CI, Shin LM, et al. Differential amygdalar response to novel versus newly familiar neutral faces: a functional MRI probe developed for studying inhibited temperament. Biol Psychiatry 2003;53:854–62.

[87] Lonigan CJ, Phillips BM, Hooe ES. Relations of positive and negative affectivity to anxiety and depression in children: evidence from a latent variable longitudinal study. J Consult Clin Psychol 2003;71:465–81.

[88] Masi G, Mucci M, Favilla L, et al. Temperament in adolescents with anxiety and depressive disorders and in their families. Child Psychiatry Hum Dev 2003;33:245–59.

[89] Buss AM, Plomin R. Temperament: early developing personality traits. Hillsdale (NJ): Erlbaum; 1984.

[90] Kagan J, Snidman N, McManis M, et al. One measure, one meaning: multiple measures, clearer meaning. Dev Psychopathol 2002;14:463–75.

[91] Hayward C, Killen JD, Kraemer HC, et al. Linking self-reported childhood behavioral inhibition to adolescent social phobia. J Am Acad Child Adolesc Psychiatry 1998;37:1308–16.

[92] Rosenbaum JF, Biederman J, Hirshfeld DR, et al. Further evidence of an association between behavioral inhibition and anxiety disorders: results from a family study of children from a non-clinical sample. J Psychiatr Res 1991;25:49–65.

[93] Hirshfeld-Becker DR, Biederman J, Calthrap S, et al. Behavioral inhibition and disinhibition as hypothesized precursors to psychopathology: implications for pediatric bipolar disorder. Biol Psychiatry 2003;53:985–99.

[94] Rapee RM. The development and modification of temperamental risk for anxiety disorders: prevention of a lifetime of anxiety? Biol Psychiatry 2002;52:947–57.

[95] Pine D. Pathophysiology of childhood anxiety disorders. Biol Psychiatry 1999;46:1555–66.

[96] Barrett PM, Rapee RM, Dadda MR, et al. Enhancement of cognitive style in anxious and aggressive children. J Abnorm Child Psychol 1996;24:187–203.

[97] Foa EB, Gilboa-Schechtman E, Amir N, et al. Memory bias in generalized social phobia: remembering negative emotional expressions. J Anxiety Disord 2000;14:501–19.

[98] Lundh LG, Ost LG. Recognition bias for critical faces in social phobics. Behav Res Ther 1996;34:787–94.

[99] Amir N, McNally RJ, Riemann BC, et al. Implicit memory bias for threat in panic disorder: application of the "white noise" paradigm. Behav Res Ther 1996;34:157–62.

[100] Hope DA, Rapee RM, Heimberg RG, et al. Representations of the self in social phobia: vulnerability to social threat. Cognit Ther Res 1990;14:177–89.

[101] Clark LA, Watson D, Mineka S. Temperament, personality, and the mood and anxiety disorders. J Abnorm Psychol 1994;103:103–16.

[102] Akiskal HS. The temperamental foundations of affective disorders. In: Mundt C, Goldstein MJ, editors. Interpersonal factors in the origin and course of affective disorders. London: Royal College of Psychiatrists; 1996. p. 3–30.

[103] Caldji C, Tannenbaum B, Sharma S, et al. Maternal care during infancy regulates the development of neural systems mediating the expression of fearfulness in rats. Proc Natl Acad Sci USA 1998;95:5335–40.

[104] Liu D, Dorio J, Day JC, et al. Maternal care, hippocampal synaptogenesis and cognitive development in rats. Nat Neurosci 2000;3:799–806.

[105] Francis D, Dorio J, Liu D, et al. Nongenomic transmission across generations of maternal behavior and stress responses in the rat. Science 1999;286:1155–8.

[106] Goldin PC. A review of children's reports of parent behaviors. Psychol Bull 1969;71:222–36.

[107] Parker G. A decade of research. Soc Psychiatry Psychiatr Epidemiol 1990;25:281–2.

[108] Shaw DS, Keenan K, Vondra JI. Developmental precursors of externalizing behavior: ages 1 to 3. Dev Psychol 1994;30:355–64.

[109] Calkins SD, Hungerford A, Dedmon SE. Mothers' interactions with temperamentally frustrated infants. Infant Ment Health J 2004;25:219–40.

[110] Rubin KH, Burgess KB, Hastings PD. Stability and social-behavioral consequences of toddlers' inhibited temperament and parenting behaviors. Child Dev 2002;73:483–95.

[111] Rubin KH, Hastings PD, Stewart SL, et al. The consistency and concomitants of inhibition: some of the children, all of the time. Child Dev 1997;68:467–83.

[112] Fox NA, Henderson HA, Marshall PJ, et al. Behavioral inhibition: linking biology and behavior within a developmental framework. Annu Rev Psychol 2005;56:235–62.

[113] Arcus DM. The experiential modification of temperamental bias in inhibited and uninhibited children. Cambridge (MA): Harvard University Press; 1991.

[114] Belsky J, Hsieh K-H, Crnic K. Mothering, fathering, and infant negativity as antecedents of

boys' externalizing problems and inhibition at age 3 years: differential susceptibility to rearing experience? Dev Psychopathol 1998;10:301–19.

[115] Biederman J, Rosenbaum JF, Bolduc EA, et al. A high-risk study of young children of parents with panic disorder and agoraphobia with and without comorbid major depression. Psychiatry Res 1991;37:333–48.

[116] Biederman J, Faraone SV, Hirshfeld-Becker DR, et al. Patterns of psychopathology and dysfunction in high-risk children of parents with panic disorder and major depression. Am J Psychiatry 2001;158:49–57.

[117] Rosenbaum JF, Biederman J, Hirshfeld DR, et al. A controlled study of behavioral inhibition in children of parents with panic disorder and depression. Am J Psychiatry 2000;157:2002–10.

[118] Hirshfeld-Becker DR, Biederman J, Faraone SV, et al. Lack of association between behavioral inhibition and psychosocial adversity factors in children at risk for anxiety disorders. Am J Psychiatry 2004;161:547–55.

[119] Robinson JL, Kagan J, Reznick JS, et al. The heritability of inhibited and uninhibited behavior: a twin study. Dev Psychol 1992;28:1030–7.

[120] Matheny Jr AP. Children's behavioral inhibition over age and across situations: genetic similarity for a trait during change. J Pers 1989;57:215–35.

[121] DiLalla L, Kagan J, Reznick J. Genetic etiology of behavioral inhibition among 2-year-old children. Infant Behavior and Development 1994;17:405–12.

[122] Beidel DC, Turner SM. At risk for anxiety. I: psychopathology in the offspring of anxious parents. J Am Acad Child Adolesc Psychiatry 1997;36:918–24.

[123] Escalona SK. The roots of individuality. Chicago: Aldine; 1964.

[124] Vuilleumier P, Armony JL, Driver J, et al. Effects of attention and emotion on face processing in the human brain: an event-related fMRI study. Neuron 2001;30:829–41.

[125] Nachmias M, Gunnar M, Mangelsdorf S, et al. Behavioral inhibition and stress reactivity: the moderating role of attachment security. Child Dev 1996;67:508–22.

[126] Muris P, Merckelbach H, Damsma E. Threat perception bias in nonreferred, socially anxious children. J Clin Child Adolesc Psychol 2000;29:348–59.

[127] Bogels SM, Zigterman D. Dysfunctional cognitions in children with social phobia, separation anxiety disorder, and generalized anxiety disorder. J Abnorm Child Psychol 2000;28:205–11.

[128] Fox E. Allocation of visual attention and anxiety. Cognition and Emotion 1993;7:207–15.

[129] MacLeod C, Mathews A. Anxiety and allocation of attention to threat. Q J Exp Psychol A 1988;40A:653–70.

[130] Mogg K, Bradley BP, Hallowell N. Attentional bias to threat: roles of trait anxiety, stressful events, and awareness. Q J Exp Psychol A 1994;47A:841–64.

[131] Bradley BP, Mogg K, White J, et al. Attentional bias for emotional faces in generalized anxiety disorder. Br J Clin Psychol 1999;58:267–78.

[132] MacLeod C, Mathews A. Biased cognitive operations in anxiety: accessibility of information or assignment of processing priorities? Behav Res Ther 1991;29:599–610.

[133] Mogg K, Mathews AM, Eysenck M. Attentional biases to threat in clinical anxiety states. Cognition and Emotion 1992;6:149–59.

[134] Mogg K, Bradley BP. A cognitive-motivational analysis of anxiety. Behav Res Ther 1998;36: 809–48.

[135] Mogg K, McNamara J, Powys M, et al. Selective attention to threat: a test of two cognitive models of anxiety. Cognition and Emotion 2000;14:375–99.

[136] Wilson E, MacLeod C. Contrasting two accounts of anxiety-linked attentional bias: selective attention to varying levels of stimulus threat intensity. J Abnorm Psychol 2003;112:212–8.

[137] Vasey MW. Anxiety-related attentional biases in childhood. Behav Change 1996;13:199–205.

[138] Vasey MW, Daleiden EL, Williams LL, et al. Biased attention in childhood anxiety disorders: a preliminary study. J Abnorm Child Psychol 1995;23:267–79.

[139] Taghavi MR, Neshat-Doost HT, Moradi AR, et al. Biases in visual attention in children and adolescents with clinical anxiety and mixed depression. J Abnorm Child Psychol 1999;27: 215–23.

[140] Schippell PL, Vasey MW, Cravens-Brown LM, et al. Suppressed attention to rejection, ridicule, and failure cues: a specific correlate of reactive but not proactive aggression in youth. J Clin Child Adolesc Psychol 2003;32:40–55.

[141] Pérez-Edgar K, Fox NA. A behavioral and electrophysiological study of children's selective attention under neutral and affective conditions. Journal of Cognition and Development 2005;6:89–116.

[142] Rothbart MK, Posner MI, Rosicky J. Orienting in normal and pathological development. Dev Psychopathol 1994;6:635–62.

[143] Ruddy MG. Attention shifting and temperament at 5 months. Infant Behavior and Development 1993;16:255–9.

[144] Mathews A, MacLeod C. Cognitive approaches to emotion and emotional disorders. Annu Rev Psychol 1994;45:25–50.

[145] Schwartz CE, Rauch SL. Temperament and its implication for neuroimaging of anxiety disorders. CNS Spectr 2004;9:284–91.

[146] Ketter TA, Andreason PJ, George MS, et al. Anterior paralimbic mediation of procaine-induced emotional and psychosensory experience. Arch Gen Psychiatry 1996;53:59–69.

[147] Benkelfat C, Bradwejn J, Ellenbogen M, et al. Functional neuroanatomy of CCK-4 induced anxiety in normal healthy volunteers. Am J Psychiatry 1995;152:1180–4.

[148] Morris J, Frith CD, Perrett D, et al. A differential neural response in the human amygdala to fearful and happy facial expressions. Nature 1996;383:812–5.

[149] Breiter HC, Etcoff NL, Whalen PJ, et al. Response and habituation of the human amygdala during visual processing of facial expressions. Neuron 1996;17:875–87.

[150] Whalen PJ, Rauch SL, Etcoff NL, et al. Masked presentations of emotional facial expressions modulate amygdala activity without explicit knowledge. J Neurosci 1998;18:411–8.

[151] Isenberg N, Silbersweig D, Engelien A, et al. Linguistic threat activates the human amygdala. Proc Natl Acad Sci USA 1999;96:10456–9.

[152] Funnark T, Fischer H, Wirk G, et al. The amygdala and individual differences in human fear conditioning. Neuroreport 1997;8:3957–60.

[153] Zald DH, Pardo JV. Emotion, olfaction, and the human amygdala: amygdala activation during aversive olfactory stimulation. Proc Natl Acad Sci USA 1997;94:4119–24.

[154] Bechara A, Tranel D, Damasio H, et al. Double dissociation of conditioning and declarative knowledge relative to the amygdala and hippocampus in humans. Science 1995;269:115–8.

[155] Fried I, Macdonald KA, Wilson CL. Single neuron activity in hippocampus and amygdala during recognition of faces and objects. Neuron 1997;18:875–87.

[156] LaBar KS, Gatenby JC, Gore JC, et al. Human amygdala activation during conditioned fear acquisition and extinction: a mixed-trial fMRI study. Neuron 1998;20:937–45.

[157] Whalen PJ. Fear, vigilance, and ambiguity: initial neuroimaging studies of the human amygdala. Current Directions in Psychological Science 1998;7:177–88.

[158] Baxter MG, Parker A, Lindner CCC, et al. Control of response selection by reinforcer value requires interaction of amygdala and orbital prefrontal cortex. J Neurosci 2000;20:4311–9.

[159] Baxter MG, Murray EA. The amygdala and reward. Nat Rev Neurosci 2002;3:563–73.

[160] Holland PC, Gallagher M. Amygdala-frontal interactions and reward expectancy. Curr Opin Neurobiol 2004;14:148–55.

[161] Pickens CL, Saddoris MP, Setlow B, et al. Different roles for orbitofrontal cortex and basolateral amygdala in a reinforcer devaluation task. J Neurosci 2003;23:11078–84.

[162] Schwartz CE, Wright CI, Shin LM, et al. Inhibited and uninhibited infants "grown up": adult amygdalar response to novelty. Science 2003;300:1952–3.

[163] Monk CS, Grillon C, Baas JMP, et al. A neuroimaging method for the study of threat in adolescents. Dev Psychobiol 2003;43:359–66.

[164] Thomas KM, Drevets WC, Dahl RE, et al. Amygdala response to fearful faces in anxious and depressed children. Arch Gen Psychiatry 2001;58:1057–63.

[165] Carmichael ST, Price JL. Limbic connections of the orbital and medial prefrontal cortex in macaque monkeys. J Comp Neurol 1995;363:615–41.

[166] Vasa RA, Grados M, Slomine B, et al. Neuroimaging correlates of anxiety after pediatric traumatic brain injury. Biol Psychiatry 2004;55:208–16.

[167] Adolphs R. Social cognition and the human brain. In: Cacioppo JT, Bernston GG, Adolphs R, et al, editors. Foundations in social neuroscience. Cambridge (MA): MIT Press; 2002. p. 313–31.

[168] Davidson RJ, Jackson DC, Kalin NH. Emotion, plasticity, context, and regulation: perspectives from affective neuroscience. Psychol Bull 2000;126:890–909.

[169] Bechara A, Damasio H, Damasio AR, et al. Different contributions of the human amygdala and ventromedial prefrontal cortex to decision-making. J Neurosci 1999;23:4311–9.

[170] Davidson RJ, Irwin W. The functional neuroanatomy of emotion and affective style. In: Cacioppo JT, Bernston GG, Adolphs R, et al, editors. Foundations in social neuroscience. Cambridge (MA): MIT Press; 2002. p. 473–90.

[171] Blumer D, Benson DF. Personality changes with frontal and temporal lobe lesions. In: Blumer D, Benson DF, editors. Psychiatric aspects of neurologic disease. New York: Grune & Stratton; 1975. p. 151–70.

[172] Butter CM, Snyder DR, McDonald JA. Effects of orbital frontal legions on aversive and aggressive behaviors in rhesus monkeys. J Comp Physiol Psychol 1970;72:132–44.

[173] Damasio H, Grabowski T, Frank R, et al. The return on Phineas Gage: clues about the brain from the skull of a famous patient. Science 1994;264:1102–5.

[174] Berlin HA, Rolls ET, Kischka U. Impulsivity, time perception, emotion, and reinforcement sensitivity in patients with orbitofrontal cortex lesions. Brain 2004;127:1108–26.

[175] Drevets W, Simpson J, Raichle M. Regional blood flow changes in response to phobic anxiety and habituation. J Cereb Blood Flow Metab 1995;15:S856.

[176] Fredrikson M, Fischer H, Wik G. Cerebral blood flow during anxiety provocation. J Clin Psychiatry 1997;58:16–21.

[177] Birbaumer N, Grodd W, Diedrich O, et al. fMRI reveals amygdala activation to human faces in social phobics. Neuroreport 1998;9:1223–6.

[178] Tillfors M, Furmark T, Marteinsdottir I, et al. Cerebral blood flow in subjects with social phobia during stressful speaking tasks: a PET study. Am J Psychiatry 2001;158:1220–6.

[179] Stewart SL, Rubin KH. The social problem-solving skills of anxious-withdrawn children. Dev Psychopathol 1995;7:323–36.

[180] Ollendick TH, King NJ, Frary RB. Fears in children and adolescents: reliability and generalizability across gender, age, and nationality. Behav Res Ther 1989;27:19–26.

[181] American Psychiatric Association. Diagnostic and statistical manual of mental disorders. 4th edition. Washington (DC): American Psychiatric Association; 1994.

[182] Ollendick TH, Hirshfeld-Becker DR. The developmental psychopathology of social anxiety disorder. Biol Psychiatry 2002;51:44–58.

[183] Bremner JD. Neuroimaging studies in post-traumatic stress disorder. Curr Psychiatry Rep 2002;4:254–63.

[184] Bremner JD. Alterations in brain structure and function associated with post-traumatic stress disorder. Semin Clin Neuropsychiatry 1999;4:249–55.

[185] Sapolsky RM. Why stress is bad for your brain. Science 1996;273:749–50.

[186] Gilbertson MW, Shenton ME, Ciszewski A, et al. Smaller hippocampal volume predicts pathologic vulnerability to psychological trauma. Nat Neurosci 2002;5:1242–7.

ELSEVIER
SAUNDERS

Child Adolesc Psychiatric Clin N Am
14 (2005) 707–726

CHILD AND
ADOLESCENT
PSYCHIATRIC CLINICS
OF NORTH AMERICA

A Genetic Epidemiologic Perspective on Comorbidity of Depression and Anxiety

Douglas E. Williamson, PhD*, Erika E. Forbes, PhD,
Ronald E. Dahl, MD, Neal D. Ryan, MD

*Department of Psychiatry, University of Pittsburgh, School of Medicine/Medical Center,
Western Psychiatric Institute and Clinic, Room E-723, 3811 O'Hara Street, Pittsburgh,
PA 15213, USA*

Comorbidity among the major psychiatric disorders has emerged specifically as a pervasive topic of theoretical and practical significance in child psychiatry as well as in psychiatry as a whole [1]. Depression and anxiety represent two of the most prevalent psychiatric disorders of childhood and are frequently comorbid [2]. Feinstein [3] first coined the term "comorbidity" and defined it as "any distinct additional clinical entity that has existed or that may occur during the clinical course of a patient who has the index disease under study" [3]. Although Feinstein used comorbidity to describe the coexistence of disease entities, comorbidity also has been used to describe the co-occurrence of symptoms of disease syndromes.

Comorbidity of depression and anxiety in population and clinical samples

To establish rates of comorbidity and to determine whether depression and anxiety are comorbid at a rate greater than chance, studies drawn from the population are necessary [2]. It is expected that higher rates of comorbidity will be found among clinical samples because of treatment bias, which increases the chance of being treated if more than one disorder is present [4]. Thus, for reasons

This work was supported by National Institute of Mental Health grants P01 MH41712 (to N.D. Ryan) and K01 MH001957 (to D.E. Williamson).
* Corresponding author.
E-mail address: WilliamsonDE@upmc.edu (D.E. Williamson).

that might be unrelated to the natural course of depressive disorders, rates of comorbidity would be expected to be higher in a clinical population.

Several community studies of children have assessed both depression and anxiety [5–9]. Results from these studies show that anxiety is highly prevalent among depressed children, with an estimated prevalence ranging from 38% [6,7] to 72% [5]. If anxiety were comorbid with depression only by chance, then the proportion of comorbid cases would be the product of the separate prevalence estimates. The expected prevalence of depression comorbid with anxiety in these studies, based on the conditional probabilities of the two, is less than 1%. Thus, population studies of depressed children suggest that anxiety disorders are highly comorbid in this age group and exceed the rate expected by chance alone.

Several studies based on clinical samples of depressed children and diagnostic criteria such as those found in the Diagnostic and Statistical Manual of Mental Disorders, Third Edition (DSM-III) have reported rates of comorbidity with anxiety disorders [10–15]. Estimates of the comorbidity of anxiety with depression ranged from as low as 11% [14] to as high as 86% [13].

Kovacs and colleagues [12] explored the rates of comorbid anxiety among depressed children. They found that approximately 43 (41%) of 104 children with an index episode of depression also met criteria for an anxiety disorder. The most frequent anxiety disorders found in children who have major depressive disorders (MDD) were separation anxiety disorder (41%) and overanxious disorder (13%) [12]. Depressed children with comorbid anxiety disorder were found to have an earlier age of onset of their depressive episode (9.6 ± 1.8 years of age) compared with purely depressed children (10.5 ± 1.9 years of age). Additionally, white children were found to be significantly more likely to have comorbid anxiety disorders compared with African-American children (odds ratio, 3.1; χ^2, 6.6; $P = .01$). Higher maternal symptom scores of psychopathology were associated with increased rates of comorbid anxiety among depressed children.

Age at onset of depression and anxiety

Although anxiety is highly comorbid among depressed children, the age at which the onset of depression and anxiety occur relative to one another has not been explored systematically. Interestingly, the study by Kovacs and colleagues [12] has shown that anxiety precedes the onset of depression in 67% of the comorbid cases [12]. This finding suggests a developmental sequence in the relationship between the two disorders, with comorbid depression and anxiety emerging first as anxiety. In support of the observation by Kovacs and colleagues [12], a 10-year longitudinal study of children of depressed parents showed that the risk for anxiety disorders peaked between 5 and 10 years of age, whereas the risk for depression peaked between 15 and 20 years of age [16]. Similarly, one study of depressed adults has shown that anxiety symptoms tended to precede the onset of depression in early adulthood by 5 to 7 years [17], and another study indicates that depression in early adulthood was predicted by characteristics of anxiety and depression 14 years earlier [18].

Evidence from studies of depressed adults suggests that depression is often preceded by anxiety and that this is more likely to be true among adults whose depression began before age 25 [19]. The onset of anxiety disorders preceded the onset of depression in 32% of the adults whose depression began before age 25, compared with 16% of the adults whose depression first occurred after age 25 [19]. Another study found that anxiety is more likely to precede the onset of a depressive episode than to follow the onset of depression [20]. Similarly, one study of depressed adults has shown that anxiety symptoms tends to precede the onset of depression in early adulthood by 5 to 7 years [17], and another study indicates that depression in early adulthood is predicted by characteristics of anxiety and depression 14 years earlier [18]. Considered together, these studies suggest an important role for development in the timing of the onset of depression and anxiety and point toward the importance of examining patterns of comorbidity in childhood. Intriguingly, results from a recent report [21] of twin girls suggest a shared genetic risk for anxiety expressed in childhood and for depression expressed during adolescence. If the typical pattern of comorbidity involves early anxiety and later depression, it may be that depression and anxiety are, at one level, a single disorder with the expression of different symptoms across development.

Theoretical considerations of comorbidity

The issue of whether depression and anxiety are comorbid because of artifacts of nosology or referral biases or whether they represent a meaningfully distinct syndrome has not been addressed adequately [22]. The failure to examine the presence of comorbid anxiety disorders in depressed children may lead to spurious associations between depression and anxiety disorders as well as other disorders among family members.

In psychiatry, comorbidity has been operationally defined as the simultaneous occurrence of two or more psychiatric disorders within the same person [23]. The concept of comorbidity was first described formally by Feinstein [3], and its importance was further elaborated by Kaplan and Feinstein [24]. These authors have described the pathogenic, diagnostic, and prognostic importance of comorbidity. Pathogenic comorbidity refers to the condition under which comorbidity results as a complication of the original disorder; for example, adults with panic disorder have been shown to be at increased risk for developing agoraphobia especially if their first panic attack occurred in a public setting or was viewed as humiliating [25]. Diagnostic comorbidity occurs when two disorders share the same pattern of symptoms; for example, the symptom of having difficulty concentrating is central to both depression and generalized anxiety disorder, thereby increasing the likelihood that the two disorders would co-occur in the same individual. Finally, prognostic comorbidity refers to a significant change in the future risk for disorders as determined by a comorbid disorder; for example, prospective studies have suggested that depressed children with comorbid conduct disorder may have a decreased risk for future episodes of depression [26].

Recently, the theoretical importance of comorbidity has been considered in greater detail [22,27]. Klein and Riso [27] have identified four broad categories that describe the causes for comorbidity: sampling procedures and base rates (chance, sampling bias, and population stratification); artifacts of diagnostic criteria (overlapping criteria and one disorder encompassing the other); diagnostic boundaries drawn in the wrong place (multiformity, heterogeneity, third independent disorder, and pure and comorbid disorders are different phases of the same disorder); and causal relationships between the comorbid disorders (one disorder is a risk factor for the other, and the two disorders are the result of overlapping causative processes).

To date, this approach has been applied to the comorbidity of depression and anxiety in two studies with adults. Examining these models among adult twins, the relationship between depression and generalized anxiety disorder was found to be best explained by three of Klein and Riso's models of comorbidity [27]. The possible models were that (1) the liabilities for depression and anxiety were correlated; (2) depression causes anxiety; and (3) there was reciprocal causation between depression and anxiety [28]. In a family study of adults, however, the relationship between depression and panic disorder best fit the model, suggesting that the two disorders were separate [29]. The relationship between depression and anxiety has never been tested with Klein and Riso's models among samples of children. It is important to examine the relationship between depression and anxiety early in development because it is likely that they may differ in meaningful ways with the adult-onset variants of these disorders.

Family genetic studies of depressed children

To examine the nature of the comorbidity between depression and anxiety, family genetic studies are useful to determine whether the two disorders share a common causative risk or whether one gives rise to the other [30]. To date, only two family studies of pediatric depression [31,32] have examined the familial aggregation of disorders based on the comorbidity of depression and anxiety in the child proband. Puig-Antich and colleagues [31] have reported that comorbid separation anxiety in depressed children is not associated with lifetime rates of depression or family history–research diagnostic criteria (FH-RDC) "Other" (in which anxiety disorders were classified) among their relatives. Similarly, in a family study of depressed adolescents, Williamson and colleagues [32] have reported that comorbid anxiety is not associated with an increased risk for depression among relatives. However, the risk for FH-RDC "Other" (in which the anxiety disorders were classified) psychiatric disorder was higher in the first-degree relatives of depressed adolescents who did not have a comorbid anxiety disorder (34% versus 18%). This finding suggests that depression and anxiety may co-segregate such that the two co-occur significantly more likely than because of chance.

Puig-Antich study of depressed and anxious children

Before his untimely death in December 1989, Joaquim Puig-Antich, MD, had collected detailed family data on depressed and anxious prepubertal children that remain unpublished. In this section, these family data are used in this section to explore the relationship between depression and anxiety. Lifetime episodes of DSM-III psychiatric disorders were assessed in the first-degree relatives (parents and siblings ≥6 years of age) of children ages 6 to 12 years old who had either depression (n = 67), anxiety (n = 17), or were normal controls (n = 72). The strengths of the Puig-Antich study include (1) the inclusion of both psychiatric and normal control children and their relatives; (2) the assessment of lifetime psychiatric disorders in relatives older than 6 years of age; (3) direct interviews with relatives; (4) the assessment of lifetime episodes of psychiatric disorders based on DSM-III criteria; (5) analyses examining the lifetime rates of psychiatric disorders in parents and siblings separately as well as all first-degree relatives; and (6) the systematic examination of depression and anxiety in children and their relatives.

Two previously identified analytic approaches were taken to explore the relationship between anxiety and depression. The primary aims of the current authors were to determine if depression and anxiety appear to be transmitted together or separately within families and whether depression with comorbid anxiety represents a third independent disorder [33,34]. Finally, we explored which theoretical model of comorbidity identified by Klein and Riso [27] best fit the data.

Sample

Depressed and anxious children aged 6 years 0 months to 12 years 11 months were recruited from the Child Depression Clinic at the New York State Psychiatric Institute, Columbia University, NY. Children presenting for treatment at the clinic who reported being sad, appeared to be sad, had suicidal ideation or behavior, refused to attend school, were nervous or afraid, or displayed ritualistic behavior were screened for inclusion into the study. If the initial screening indicated that the child had a diagnosis of major depression or any anxiety disorder then the child was invited to participate in a 2-week diagnostic screening protocol. The screening protocol included a diagnostic assessment with the Schedule for Affective Disorders and Schizophrenia for School-Age Children, Present Episode (K-SADS-P) [35]; a physical examination that included Tanner staging for pubertal development [36,37]; and, a second K-SADS-P assessment administered 10 to 14 days after the initial K-SADS-P assessment, covering the previous week, to ensure that the child continued to meet criteria for depression or anxiety.

Normal control children 6 years 0 months to 12 years 11 months of age were randomly selected and recruited from regular classrooms within the New York City metropolitan area. Children interested in participating discussed the project with and received their approval from their parents to participate. Prospective control children and their mothers were interviewed with the Schedule for Affective Disorders and Schizophrenia, Epidemiological Version (K-SADS-E) [38] about the presence of lifetime episodes of psychopathology in the child. Only children who had never met DSM-III criteria for any psychiatric disorder in their lifetimes were included in the study as normal controls.

Demographic characteristics of child probands

The demographic characteristics of the children are given in Table 1. Sixty-two children who had MDD were recruited, of whom 17 had an anxiety disorder (ANX), and 72 were normal control (NC) children. The three groups were comparable with regard to gender, age, religion, and socioeconomic status (SES). However, they differed significantly in ethnicity, with higher rates of Hispanic children in the control group than in the depressed and anxious groups. Although previous family studies have not found ethnicity to be differentially associated with lifetime rates of psychiatric disorders among relatives [31,32], ethnicity was modeled as a covariate in all analyses.

Table 1
Demographic characteristics of depressed, anxious, and normal control children

Demographic factors	MDD (n=62)	ANX (n=17)	NC (n=72)	Statistic	P value
Gender				$\chi^2 = 7.32$	NS
Females	20	8	37		
Males	42	9	35		
Ethnicity				FET	.0001
White	25	11	11		
African-American	16	1	36		
Other	21*	5*	25**		
Age (y)	9.7 ± 1.7	9.8 ± 1.3	9.8 ± 1.1	$F_{2,148} = 0.04$	NS
SES[a]	41.9 ± 16.2*	44.1 ± 17.7*·**	36.6 ± 12.8**	$F_{2,141} = 2.89$	.06
Religion[b]				FET	NS
Catholic	30	10	26		
Protestant	12	1	14		
Jewish	7	2	5		
Other	8	1	14		
None	3	3	9		

Abbreviations: FET, Fisher exact test; NS, not significant.
   [a] SES data not available for 3 MDD and 4 NC children.
   [b] Religion data not available for 2 MDD and 4 NC children.
   * Significantly different at the $P \leq .05$ level; ** Significantly different at the $P \leq .05$ level.
Data from Hollingshead AB. Four factor index of social status. New Haven (CT): Yale University Sociology Department; 1975.

Assessment of psychopathology in child probands

A child psychiatrist conducted the K-SADS-P, first interviewing the parent about the child's symptoms and then interviewing the child separately about her or his symptoms. The K-SADS-P [35] is a semi-structured diagnostic interview schedule designed to be used with children 6 to 17 years of age. It was adapted from the adult-based Schedule for Affective Disorders (SADS) [39] and designed for use in both clinical and research settings. Symptoms are rated on a six- or seven-point scale and reflect the degree of severity of the symptom anchored to specific criteria that are included for each symptom.

Based on separate reports from the parent and the child, the interviewer determined summary ratings for each symptom at its worst during the present psychopathologic episode and during the week before the interview. Final diagnoses were determined after a second child psychiatrist reviewed the K-SADS-P interview and reached consensus with the initial interviewer. The diagnoses of MDD and anxiety were made according to (DSM-III) criteria [40].

All normal controls were screened for the absence of lifetime episodes of psychopathology with the K-SADS-E [38], which was specifically designed to assess the presence of both current and past psychiatric disorders in children and adolescents ages 6 to 17 years old. Paralleling the administration of the K-SADS-P, the K-SADS-E was administered first to the parent and then to the child about the child's symptoms by an interviewer trained in child psychiatric interviewing. Unlike the K-SADS-P, symptoms are recorded as being either present or absent. Whenever there were discrepancies between the parent's and child's reports, the interviewer resolved the discrepancies by talking with the parent and child together. Summary symptom ratings were used for making all diagnoses. All occurrences of disorders were recorded, but only the symptoms for the current episode (if present) and the most severe past episode were documented in detail.

Assessment of psychopathology in first-degree relatives

The presence of lifetime psychopathology in all first-degree relatives (ie, siblings and parents) was assessed through a combination of the family study method, in which relatives are interviewed directly, and the family history method, in which informants provide information about other relatives. For a majority of the families, the proband's first-degree relatives were located within the New York City metropolitan area and were available to be interviewed directly. For relatives who were unable to be interviewed in person, telephone interviews were conducted. Telephone and face-to-face interviews have been shown to yield comparable reports of lifetime psychopathology for both Research and Diagnostic Criteria (RDC) and DSM-III diagnoses [41]. Relatives 18 years of age and older were assessed with the Schedule for Affective Disorders and Schizophrenia, Lifetime Version (SADS-L) [39], a structured clinical interview administered by interviewers with clinical training. The SADS-L assesses

symptoms and related criteria for making lifetime diagnoses according to
RDC [42]. Relatives aged 6 to 17 years (and their parents) were assessed with
the K-SADS-E.

Information about relatives who were not available to be interviewed directly
was collected using the family history method [43], a technique for obtaining
psychiatric diagnostic data through the use of "key" family informants that has
been widely used to examine the familial transmission of psychiatric disorders
(eg, Andreasen and colleagues, 1977 [43], and Mendlewicz and colleagues,
1975 [43a]). Adult relatives provided information about lifetime psychopathology in first-degree relatives who could not participate in psychiatric assessment.

Based on the collective diagnostic information provided by multiple informants from both direct and indirect interviews for each individual, information
was pooled to make the "best estimate" lifetime diagnoses based on DSM-III
criteria for each relative [44]. On a per-person basis, a panel of psychiatrists
reviewed the reported information from all informants and arrived at summary
or consensus lifetime diagnoses for each family member. All diagnoses were
made according to the degree of certainty (ie, possible, probable, or definite)
based on DSM-III criteria. Only diagnoses made at the probable or definite level
were counted. Additionally, all diagnoses among relatives were made blind to
the diagnostic status of the child proband.

Models and analytic strategy

Two somewhat parallel analytic strategies were taken to examine the
relationship between anxiety and depression in child probands and their first-
degree relatives. First, the analytic strategy of Pauls and colleagues [33,34],
which has been extended by Wickramaratne and Weissman [29], was used. In this
strategy, the relationship between depression and anxiety is examined using
logistic regression to determine if they are causally related or distinct, or whether
they form a third disorder with the two co-segregating together. As discussed by
Wickramaratne and Weissman [29], the co-segregation of depression and anxiety
can be examined among the first-degree relatives across the four proband groups.
If depression and anxiety form a third independent disorder, the two should co-
segregate among the relatives of probands with depression and anxiety but not
the other three proband groups. The Breslow-Day test for homogeneity of the
odds ratios across the four proband groups was used to test this hypothesis. If
the odds for depression and anxiety were different across groups as tested by the
Breslow-Day test and the two only co-segregated together within the comorbid
group, then this would indicate the presence of a third independent disorder.
Family ethnicity and gender of the child proband and the relative were included
as covariates.

The second analytic strategy consisted of examining the patterns of anxiety
and depression in first-degree relatives to determine which comorbidity model
likely fit the data. As indicated by Klein and Riso [27], if one is interested in the
type of comorbidity between two disorders, then the ideal family study would

consist of four diagnostic groups: probands with the pure form of disorder A; probands with the pure form of disorder B; probands with both A and B; and probands without either A or B. To date, two reports have used this approach to examine the relationship between depression and anxiety [28,29].

The predicted frequency of familial rates for depression and anxiety across the four groups for each comorbidity explanation are summarized in Table 2. To illustrate, comorbidity caused by population stratification occurs when each of the disorders being examined for comorbidity are associated with unique risk factors, while the risk factors tend to aggregate in similar subgroups of the population. Thus, even though the two disorders occur together only by chance, compared with the population as a whole, the rate of comorbidity appears to be higher than what is expected by chance.

If comorbidity were caused by population stratification, then the following relationships would be expected in family members for the four proband groups. The frequency of depression in relatives would be the same in depressed children with and without comorbid anxiety but would be greater than the frequency in

Table 2

Prediction of lifetime rates of depression and anxiety in child probands and their relatives according to Klein and Riso's (1993) models of comorbidity

Comorbidity models	Diagnoses in relatives	Expected relations in probands
Population stratification	MDD	MDD = MDD + ANX > ANX = NC
	MDD + ANX	MDD = MDD + ANX = ANX = NC
	ANX	ANX = MDD + ANX > MDD = NC
Overlapping diagnostic criteria	MDD	MDD > MDD + ANX > ANX = NC
	MDD + ANX	MDD = MDD + ANX = ANX > NC
	ANX	ANX > MDD + ANX > MDD = NC
One disorder encompassing another and multiformity	MDD	MDD = MDD + ANX > ANX = NC
	MDD + ANX	MDD = MDD + ANX > ANX = NC
	ANX	ANX > MDD = MDD + ANX = NC
Heterogeneity of the comorbid disorder	MDD	MDD > MDD + ANX > ANX = NC
	MDD + ANX	MDD = MDD + ANX = ANX = NC
	ANX	ANX > MDD + ANX > MDD = NC
Third independent disorder	MDD	MDD > MDD + ANX = ANX = NC
	MDD + ANX	MDD + ANX > MDD = ANX = NC
	ANX	ANX > MDD = MDD + ANX = NC
Different phases/alternative expression of the same disorder	MDD	MDD = MDD + ANX = ANX > NC
	MDD + ANX	MDD = MDD + ANX = ANX > NC
	ANX	MDD = MDD + ANX = ANX > NC
One disorder is a risk factor for the other	MDD	MDD = MDD + ANX = ANX > NC
	MDD + ANX	MDD = MDD + ANX = ANX > NC
	ANX	MDD = MDD + ANX = ANX = NC
Two disorders arise from overlapping causative processes	MDD	MDD = MDD + ANX > ANX > NC
	MDD + ANX	MDD = MDD + ANX = ANX > NC
	ANX	ANX = MDD + ANX > MDD > NC

Abbreviations: ANX, anxiety only; MDD, depression only; MDD + ANX, depression and comorbid anxiety.

Data from Klein DN, Riso LP. Psychiatric disorders: problems of boundaries and comorbidity. In: Costello CG, editor. Basic issues in psychopathology. New York: Guilford Press; 1993. p. 19–66.

relatives of anxious and normal control children. The frequency of depressed with comorbid anxiety disorder in relatives would be expected to be the same across the four proband groups. The frequency of ANX would be expected to be similar in the probands with anxiety and those with depressed with comorbid anxiety, which would, in turn, be greater than the frequency of in the depressed (MDD) and NC proband groups.

To explore these models for comorbidity posited by Klein and Riso [27], the analytic strategy employed by Wickramaratne and Weissman [29] was used. Accordingly, multinomial logit models allowing for nominal data with more than two categories and allowing for the inclusion of covariates (eg, age and gender of the relative) were used. The outcome variable was the diagnosis within the first-degree relatives (MDD, ANX, MDD plus ANX, or none) and was predicted by the same four-category diagnostic variable among the child probands. Covariates included ethnicity of the family as well as the gender of the child proband and the relative.

For all analyses examining the lifetime rates of psychiatric disorders in relatives, generalized estimating equations (GEE) with a logit link were used to account for the within family correlation of the observations [45,46]. Taking into account the within-family correlation will result in an increase in the efficiency of the estimators compared with analytic methods, assuming that each person within a family is independent from another [45]. The GEE methods have been shown to be robust and are correct even if the correlation matrix is misspecified [45]. The software package SUDAAN (Research Triangle Institute, Research Triangle Park, North Carolina) [47], developed specifically for the analysis of correlated data using GEE methods, will be used for this part of the analyses.

Examining the familial relationship between depression and anxiety among depressed children with and without comorbid anxiety

Depressed children were classified as having either depression only (n = 22) or having a comorbid anxiety disorder (n = 40). All children in the anxious group had anxiety only. The total number of assessed first-degree relatives for MDD only, MDD plus anxiety, anxiety only, and normal control probands were 66, 125, 51, and 198, respectively (Table 3).

First-degree relatives were classified into those having MDD only, MDD plus anxiety, anxiety only, and neither MDD nor anxiety. The distribution of MDD and anxiety among the first-degree relatives across the four proband groups

Table 3
Number of probands and relatives across the four proband groups

Proband groups	Probands (N)	Relatives (N)
MDD	22	66
MDD + ANX	40	125
ANX	17	51
NC	72	198

Table 4
Frequencies of major depressive and anxiety disorders among child probands and their first-degree relatives

Proband's diagnosis	Relative's diagnosis			
	MDD n (%)	MDD + ANX n (%)	ANX n (%)	None n (%)
MDD	18 (27.3)	7 (10.6)	6 (9.1)	35 (53.0)
MDD + ANX	32 (25.6)	26 (20.8)	14 (11.2)	53 (42.4)
ANX	5 (9.8)	10 (19.6)	6 (11.8)	30 (58.8)
NC	20 (10.1)	12 (6.1)	13 (6.6)	153 (77.3)

is detailed in Table 4. The information contained in Table 4 was used for examining the relationship between depression and anxiety among the child probands and their first-degree relatives.

To examine the relationship between depression and anxiety among the child probands and their first-degree relatives, we first computed the odds of a first-degree relative having MDD (with or without anxiety) and anxiety (with or without MDD) for each of the four proband groups (Table 5). Odds are calculated by dividing the total number of first-degree relatives having the disorder by the total number not having the disorder. For example, as indicated by Table 4, 25 of the first-degree relatives of MDD probands had MDD (7 with anxiety and 18 without), and 41 did not have MDD (6 had anxiety only, and 35 had neither anxiety nor MDD). Therefore, the odds that a first-degree relative of an MDD child proband has had a lifetime episode of MDD are 25/41 or 0.6098.

The ratio of the odds can then be compared across proband groups to determine whether a disorder is similarly likely among the first-degree relatives of two proband groups. The odds ratio is computed by dividing the odds of one group by the odds of the other. For example, the odds ratio for MDD among the first-degree relatives of MDD-only probands versus the first-degree relatives of normal control probands is 0.6098/0.1928 or 3.16, indicating a greater risk for MDD among the first-degree relatives of MDD children.

Table 5
Odds of major depressive disorder (with or without anxiety) and anxiety (with or without major depressive disorder) among first-degree relatives of the four proband groups

Proband's diagnosis	Relative's diagnosis	
	Odds for MDD[a]	Odds for ANX[b]
MDD	0.6098	0.2453
MDD + ANX	0.8657	0.4706
ANX	0.4167	0.4571
NC	0.1928	0.1445

[a] Proportion of relatives who have MDD divided by proportion of relatives who do not have MDD.

[b] Proportion of relatives who have ANX divided by proportion of relatives who do not have ANX.

Table 6

Adjusted odds ratios for major depressive disorder or anxiety among first-degree relatives by the four
proband groups

Proband's diagnosis	Relative's diagnosis	
	MDD OR (95% CI)	ANX OR (95% CI)
MDD vs		
MDD + ANX	0.70 (0.38–1.30)	0.70 (0.31–1.57)
ANX	1.69 (0.72–3.94)	0.56 (0.22–1.44)
NC	3.47 (1.77–6.80)**	1.72 (0.78–3.81)
MDD + ANX vs		
ANX	2.37 (1.11–5.06)**	0.84 (0.40–1.81)
NC	4.87 (2.79–8.51)**	2.70 (1.44–5.07)**
ANX vs		
NC	2.07 (0.97–4.41)*	3.08 (1.34–7.06)**

Odds ratios were adjusted for age, gender, ethnicity, and interview status of relative.
Abbreviations: CI, confidence interval; OR, odds ratio.
  * $P = .10$; ** $P = .05$.

A comparison of the adjusted odds ratios for all two-group comparisons
among the four proband groups is reported in Table 6. We computed odds ratios
for lifetime rates of MDD and lifetime rates of anxiety disorders in first-degree
relatives of the odds ratio for the difference in MDD among first-degree relatives
between the MDD only and the MDD plus ANX proband groups of 0.70, and the
corresponding 95% CI of 0.38 to 1.30 suggests that the risk for MDD in first-
degree relatives is the same for the two proband groups because the confidence
interval includes 1.

As for anxiety disorders, the first-degree relatives of depressed children with
comorbid anxiety had more comparable odds of having an anxiety disorder than
did the relatives of depressed children without a comorbid anxiety disorder (odds
ratio, 0.70; CI, 0.31–1.57) (see Table 6). Thus, from these data, it appears that the
risk for anxiety disorders tends to be the same for the first-degree relatives of
depressed children with and without comorbid anxiety disorders. Hence, anxiety
is similarly transmitted in the families of depressed children with and without
comorbid anxiety.

Pauls and colleagues [33,34] have suggested a third analytic step, which is
to examine whether MDD and anxiety co-segregate, thus representing a third
independent disorder. To test this, the odds of having depression and anxiety
within each relative were calculated for each of the four proband groups. As
shown in Table 7, the odds ratio for MDD to be associated with anxiety disorder
among the first-degree relatives was significant for all proband groups, with the
exception of the MDD group. Although they were not significant, the odds of
having anxiety in the presence of MDD was 2.27 among the relatives of
depressed only children, although this comparison failed to reach statistical
significance. Nonetheless, the analysis of the homogeneity of the odds ratios
across the four proband groups was not significant, indicating that co-segregation

Table 7
Co-segregation of major depressive disorder and anxiety in first-degree relatives across the four proband groups

Proband's diagnosis	Relative's diagnoses			Odds ratio (95% CI)	Statistic	P value
		ANX				
	MDD	Yes	No			
MDD	Yes	7	18	2.27 (0.66–7.76)	FET	NS
	No	6	35			
MDD + ANX	Yes	26	32	3.08 (1.40–6.74)	$\chi^2 = 7.12$	.0076
	No	14	53			
ANX	Yes	10	5	10.0 (2.50–39.98)	FET	.0009
	No	6	30			
NC	Yes	12	20	7.06 (2.84–17.59)	FET	.0001
	No	13	153			

Breslow-Day test for homogeneity of the odds ratio: $\chi^2 = 4.38$; degrees of freedom = 3; $P = .2232$. Estimate of the common odds ratio 4.20; 95% CI, 2.55–6.92; $P = .0001$.
Abbreviations: CI, confidence interval; FET, Fisher exact test; NS, not significant.

of depression and anxiety occurred similarly in the relatives of the four proband groups. Thus, the results of the above analyses suggest that depression and anxiety disorder are transmitted together among families. Furthermore, although depression and anxiety co-segregate among relatives, co-segregation is not limited only to the relatives of probands with depression and comorbid anxiety. Stated differently, the co-occurrence of depression and anxiety does not "breed true" within families, which would occur if the co-occurrence of the two disorders represented a third, independent disorder.

Examining Klein and Riso's models of comorbidity

Klein and Riso [27] have provided several models for explaining the relationship between two disorders and have posited the expected patterns of the two disorders using data from a family study (see Table 2). To explore the relationship between depression and anxiety among probands and their first-degree relatives, a multinomial logistic regression procedure was used that fits an exponential model for an outcome that has more than two categories. Thus, the classification of relatives having MDD only, MDD plus anxiety, anxiety only, and neither MDD nor anxiety could be examined by the proband's diagnosis similarly classified by the presence or absence of MDD and anxiety.

Paralleling the analytic approach described above, the odds for having MDD, MDD plus anxiety, or anxiety across the four proband groups are similarly calculated. For example, using the data provided in Table 4, 18 first-degree relatives of children with MDD only also had MDD only. Therefore, the corresponding odds are calculated as 18/35 or 0.5143. To calculate the odds ratio between proband groups of interest then involves simply dividing the two odds. For example, the odds ratio for MDD only among the first-degree relatives of

MDD only children compared with normal control children is 0.5143/0.1307 or 3.93. Odds ratios adjusted for demographic characteristics associated with the risk for MDD and anxiety are presented in Table 8.

Based on the odds ratios for MDD (without anxiety) shown in the first column of Table 8, the first-degree relatives of MDD children with and without a comorbid anxiety disorder had a similar risk. In turn, the risk for MDD only was significantly greater among the first-degree relatives of MDD children with and without a comorbid anxiety disorder than among the relatives of probands with anxiety only or the relatives of normal control probands, who did not differ from one another (see Table 8). Using the terminology shown in Table 2 to summarize this relationship, MDD (MDD only) in the first-degree relatives was distributed across the four proband groups as MDD, MDD plus ANX > ANX = NC. Thus, the conditions for two types of comorbidity, population stratification and one disorder encompassing another, were met for MDD only. Given the small number of children with anxiety only, it is also likely that the rates of MDD were underestimated in this group. Accordingly, it is likely that the following relationship exists: MDD = MDD plus ANX = ANX > NC. Thus, the condition of depression and anxiety representing different phases of alternative expression of the same disorder would be met.

For MDD plus anxiety among the first-degree relatives, the following relationships can be observed from the second column of Table 8. The MDD only probands did not differ from the MDD plus anxiety and anxiety only probands on the risk for MDD plus anxiety among first-degree relatives. The MDD only probands did have a trend toward an elevated risk for MDD plus anxiety among their relatives compared with normal control children (odds ratio,

Table 8

Adjusted odds ratios comparing odds for major depressive disorder only, major depressive disorder plus anxiety, and anxiety only among relatives of depressed only, depressed and anxious, anxious only, and normal control children

Proband's diagnosis	Relative's diagnosis		
	MDD OR (95% CI)	MDD + ANX OR (95% CI)	ANX OR (95% CI)
MDD vs			
MDD + ANX	0.8 (0.4–1.9)	0.5 (0.2–1.5)	0.9 (0.3–3.2)
ANX	4.0 (1.2–13.3)**	0.9 (0.2–2.9)	0.7 (0.2–3.1)
NC	3.8 (1.7–8.3)**	2.4 (0.8–7.0)*	2.5 (0.9–7.5)*
MDD + ANX vs			
ANX	4.7 (1.6–14.2)**	1.7 (0.6–4.6)	1.0 (0.3–3.0)
NC	4.9 (2.4–10.1)**	5.4 (2.3–12.6)**	2.9 (1.2–7.1)**
ANX vs			
NC	1.0 (0.3–3.2)	3.2 (1.1–9.4)**	2.8 (0.9–8.9)*

Odds ratios were adjusted for age, gender, ethnicity, and interview status of relative.
Abbreviations: CI, confidence interval; OR, odds ratio.
    * $P = .10$; ** $P = .05$.

2.4; $P \leq .07$). The MDD plus anxiety and anxiety only proband groups did not differ from one another in the risk for MDD plus anxiety in first-degree relatives, but both groups were significantly different from the risk for MDD plus anxiety in the relatives of normal controls. Thus, for MDD plus ANX among first-degree relatives, the proband groups were found to have MDD = MDD plus ANX = ANX > NC. This pattern fits three of the models for comorbidity: overlapping diagnostic criteria, different phases or alternative expressions of the same disorders, or two disorders arising from overlapping causative processes.

Finally, a comparison of the rates of anxiety among only the first-degree relatives across the four proband groups showed the following relationships. The depressed only, depressed plus anxiety, and anxiety only probands did not significantly differ from one another on the risk for anxiety disorder only among their first-degree relatives (see Table 8). The risk for anxiety disorders among the relatives of these three proband groups were either significantly different or tended to be different compared with the relatives of normal controls (see Table 8). Thus, for anxiety (ANX) among only the relatives, the relationships across the four proband groups can be algebraically represented as MDD = MDD plus ANX = ANX > NC. Comparing this pattern to the types of comorbidity illustrated in Table 4 shows that depression and anxiety may be different phases or alternative expressions of the same disorder.

Limitations of the Puig-Antich study

One of the limitations is that the three groups were not matched on demographic characteristics. As noted by Kendler [48], the ideal family study would consist of cases and controls that were similar with regard to demographic characteristics. Matching cases and controls on demographic characteristics enables the investigator to be certain that the between-group differences are not merely the result of a bias reflected in differences in the demographic composition of the groups. In the Puig-Antich study, normal control children were more likely to be nonwhite and lower SES, and they had younger relatives compared with the depressed and anxious children. The familial aggregation of disorders could have resulted from the between-group differences for each of these factors. However, the use of logistical regression analyses that controlled for various proband and demographic characteristics minimizes the chance that imbalances solely in demographic characteristics explain the between-group differences reported in this study. The imbalance found among depressed, anxious, and normal control children did not result in colinearity between the diagnostic groups and the various demographic characteristics. As a result, demographic characteristics could be controlled statistically. It is likely that controlling for these factors resulted in unbiased between-group estimates for all disorders.

A second limitation is the small number of participants in the anxious group. The smaller sample could have resulted in inflating both type I and type II errors.

Future family studies of depression and anxiety in children would benefit from the inclusion of larger samples of probands.

A third limitation is that probands were recruited from a clinical population and not chosen randomly from the population. It is possible that parents of depressed children with depression or an anxiety disorder more readily bring their child for treatment, resulting in a spurious finding of familial aggregation of depression and anxiety. However, evidence from population studies similarly supports the familial aggregation of depression [49,50], suggesting that the finding is not purely an artifact of sampling.

Depression and anxiety co-segregate in families

In the Puig-Antich study, analyses based on the methodologic approach of Pauls and colleagues [33,34] has shown that depression and anxiety in children are associated with an elevated risk for both depression and anxiety among their first-degree relatives. Further analyses has shown that depression and anxiety significantly co-occurred within first-degree relatives (ie, co-segregated) but did so regardless of whether the proband had either disorder alone, both disorders together, or neither disorder. Thus, depression and anxiety were found to significantly co-segregate, but each disorder did not "breed true" within the families of depressed and comorbid anxious children. Relatives of depressed children and relatives of anxious children were similarly likely to experience depression or anxiety. The one other family study of prepubertal children that examined the effect of comorbid anxiety among depressed probands has reported that the first-degree relatives of depressed children with and without comorbid anxiety did not differ with regard to the risk for depression nor anxiety [31]. These results are consistent with data from the Puig-Antich study, showing a general transmission of both depression and anxiety regardless of whether the child proband has a depression or an anxiety disorder. Unfortunately, the authors of the previous study did not explore whether depression and anxiety co-segregated together within relatives and whether the co-segregation was unique to the comorbid depressed and anxious group.

Studies of adult probands with affective disorders have consistently shown an increased risk for depression and anxiety in their children [16,51,52]. In agreement, behavior-genetic studies of adults have shown that depression and anxiety share primarily additive genetic components [53,54]. Behavior-genetic studies of children and adolescents have shown that the expression of depressive and anxious symptoms share an underlying genetic risk that accounts for nearly 80% of the variance between the two [55,56]. Interestingly, studies of both adults [53] and children [57] have suggested that the underlying genetic risk for each is differentially expressed as depression or anxiety, contingent on being exposed to different environmental stressors. Stressful events representing threat have been linked with anxiety [57,58], whereas loss events have been associated with depression [57,59].

Comorbidity model fit

In the Puig-Antich study, the theoretical models of comorbidity between depression and anxiety [27] were examined using multinomial logit models as described by Wickramaratne and Weissman [29]. Results of these analyses have shown that the model that was most consistent with the data is the model that identifies depression and anxiety as different phases or alternative expressions of the same disorder. To date, two studies of depressed adults have been reported that have examined the theoretical models of comorbidity for depression and anxiety [28,29]. In the study by Neale and Kendler [28], the results from a sample of female-female twin pairs has suggested that comorbidity of depression and generalized anxiety disorder fit three of the comorbidity models: (1) correlated liabilities between the two; (2) depression-induced generalized anxiety; and (3) reciprocal causation between the two [28]. In a family study of depression and panic disorder in adults, the comorbidity of the two was found to be explained best by the model that identifies them as heterogeneous disorders [29]. Differences in the best-fitting comorbidity models across reports, including the current one, likely reflect differences in the type of anxiety disorder being examined as well as developmental variations in the expression of the two disorders. Namely, the current study included a variety of anxiety disorders and was limited to children, whereas the previous studies included only adults.

The conclusion that depression and anxiety are different phases or alternative expressions of the same underlying disorder overlays directly onto the developmental literature, suggesting that anxiety disorders precede the onset of a depressive episode, especially for early-onset depression [18–20,60]. For example, one report showed that individuals who become depressed before the age of 25 are more likely to have their depressive episode preceded by an anxiety disorder, compared with those individuals who become depressed later in life [19]. These findings are consistent with those reported by Kovacs and colleagues [12], who found that in 67% of the depressed children with comorbid anxiety, the anxiety disorder preceded the onset of the depressive disorder. Notably, one recent report [21] has found that anxiety and depression expressed at different developmental periods share genetic risk. Anxiety, especially overanxious disorder, during childhood and depression during adolescence were shown to share the same genetic risk.

Clinical implications

Current research indicates that there is a strong relationship between depression and anxiety that first appears during childhood. Both depression and anxiety co-segregate in families, indicating that the familial risk for the two disorders is shared. There is evidence that depression and anxiety among prepubertal children and their first-degree relatives is a result of the two disorders being different phases or alternative expression of a single underlying disorder.

Epidemiologic and clinical studies have shown that anxiety often precedes the onset of depression. As such, it appears that the two disorders share a common underlying genetic pathway that may be expressed differentially across development, likely as a result of being exposed to unique stressors. The fact that selective serotonin reuptake inhibitors have been shown to effectively treat both depression and anxiety underscores the shared causes between the two. From a preventive health perspective, children with depressed or anxious relatives are at increased risk for developing anxiety or depression. In addition, anxious children are at increased risk for developing depression particularly during adolescence.

References

[1] Sabshin M. Comorbidity: a central concern of psychiatry in the 1990s. Hosp Community Psychiatry 1991;42(4):345.

[2] Angold A, Costello EJ. Depressive comorbidity in children and adolescents: empirical, theoretical, and methodological issues. Am J Psychiatry 1993;150(12):1779–91.

[3] Feinstein AR. The pre-therapeutic classification of comorbidity in chronic disease. J Chronic Dis 1970;23:455–68.

[4] Berkson J. Limitations of the application of fourfold table analysis to hospital data. Biometrics 1946;1:35–67.

[5] Anderson JC, Williams S, McGee R, et al. DSM-III disorders in preadolescent children: prevalence in a large sample from the general population. Arch Gen Psychiatry 1987;44(1):69–76.

[6] Bird HR, Canino G, Rubio-Stipec M, et al. Estimates of the prevalence of childhood maladjustment in a community survey in Puerto Rico: the use of combined measures. Arch Gen Psychiatry 1988;45(12):1120–6.

[7] Costello EJ, Costello AJ, Edelbrock C, et al. Psychiatric disorders in pediatric primary care: prevalence and risk factors. Arch Gen Psychiatry 1988;45(12):1107–16.

[8] Fleming JE, Offord DR, Boyle MH. Prevalence of childhood and adolescent depression in the community: Ontario Child Health Study. Br J Psychiatry 1989;155:647–54.

[9] Velez CN, Johnson J, Cohen P. A longitudinal analysis of selected risk factors for childhood psychopathology. J Am Acad Child Adolesc Psychiatry 1989;28(6):861–4.

[10] Alessi NE, Magen J. Comorbidity of other psychiatric disturbances in depressed, psychiatrically hospitalized children. Am J Psychiatry 1988;145(12):1582–4.

[11] Hershberg SG, Carlson GA, Cantwell DP, et al. Anxiety and depressive disorders in psychiatrically disturbed children. J Clin Psychiatry 1982;43(9):358–61.

[12] Kovacs M, Gatsonis C, Paulauskas SL, et al. Depressive disorders in childhood: IV. a longitudinal study of comorbidity with and risk for anxiety disorders. Arch Gen Psychiatry 1989;46(9):776–82.

[13] Geller B, Chestnut EC, Miller MD, et al. Preliminary data on DSM-III associated features of major depressive disorder in children and adolescents. Am J Psychiatry 1985;142(5):643–4.

[14] Mitchell J, McCauley E, Burke PM, et al. Phenomenology of depression in children and adolescents. J Am Acad Child Adolesc Psychiatry 1988;27(1):12–20.

[15] Puig-Antich J. The use of RDC criteria for major depressive disorder in children and adolescents. J Am Acad Child Adolesc Psychiatry 1982;21(3):291–3.

[16] Weissman MM, Warner V, Wickramaratne P, et al. Offspring of depressed parents: 10 years later. Arch Gen Psychiatry 1997;54(10):932–40.

[17] Ernst C, Schmid G, Angst J. The Zurich Study, XVI: early antecedents of depression: a longitudinal prospective study on incidence in young adults. Eur Arch Psychiatry Clin Neurosci 1992;242(2–3):142–51.

[18] Roza SJ, Hofstra MB, van der Ende J, et al. Stable prediction of mood and anxiety disorders based on behavioral and emotional problems in childhood: a 14-year follow-up during childhood, adolescence, and young adulthood. Am J Psychiatry 2003;160(12):2116–21.

[19] Parker G, Wilhelm K, Asghari A. Early onset depression: the relevance of anxiety. Soc Psychiatry Psychiatr Epidemiol 1997;32(1):30–7.

[20] Rohde P, Lewinsohn PM, Seeley JR. Comorbidity of unipolar depression: II. comorbidity with other mental disorders in adolescents and adults. J Abnorm Psychol 1991;100(2):214–22.

[21] Silberg J, Rutter M, Neale M, et al. Genetic moderation of environmental risk for depression and anxiety in adolescent girls. Br J Psychiatry 2001;179:116–21.

[22] Caron C, Rutter M. Comorbidity in child psychopathology: concepts, issues and research strategies. J Child Psychol Psychiatry 1991;32(7):1063–80.

[23] Maser JD, Cloninger CR, editors. Comorbidity of mood and anxiety disorders. Washington (DC): American Psychiatric Press, Inc.; 1990.

[24] Kaplan MH, Feinstein AR. The importance of classifying initial co-morbidity in evaluating the outcome of diabetes mellitus. J Chronic Dis 1974;27(7–8):387–404.

[25] Amering M, Katschnig H, Berger P, et al. Embarrassment about the first panic attack predicts agoraphobia in panic disorder patients. Behav Res Ther 1997;35(6):517–21.

[26] Harrington R, Fudge H, Rutter M, et al. Adult outcomes of childhood and adolescent depression: I. psychiatric status. Arch Gen Psychiatry 1990;47(5):465–73.

[27] Klein DN, Riso LP. Psychiatric disorders: problems of boundaries and comorbidity. In: Costello CG, editor. Basic issues in psychopathology. New York: Guilford Press; 1993. p. 19–66.

[28] Neale MC, Kendler KS. Models of comorbidity for multifactorial disorders. Am J Hum Genet 1995;57(4):935–53.

[29] Wickramaratne PJ, Weissman MM. Using family studies to understand comorbidity. Eur Arch Psychiatry Clin Neurosci 1993;243(3–4):150–7.

[30] Coryell W. Anxiety secondary to depression. Psychiatr Clin North Am 1990;13(4):685–98.

[31] Puig-Antich J, Goetz D, Davies M, et al. A controlled family history study of prepubertal major depressive disorder. Arch Gen Psychiatry 1989;46(5):406–18.

[32] Williamson DE, Ryan ND, Birmaher B, et al. A case-control family history study of depression in adolescents. J Am Acad Child Adolesc Psychiatry 1995;34(12):1596–607.

[33] Pauls DL, Hurst CR, Kruger SD, et al. Gilles de la Tourette's syndrome and attention deficit disorder with hyperactivity: evidence against a genetic relationship. Arch Gen Psychiatry 1986;43(12):1177–9.

[34] Pauls DL, Towbin KE, Leckman JF, et al. Gilles de la Tourette's syndrome and obsessive-compulsive disorder: evidence supporting a genetic relationship. Arch Gen Psychiatry 1986; 43(12):1180–2.

[35] Chambers WJ, Puig-Antich J, Hirsch M, et al. The assessment of affective disorders in children and adolescents by semistructured interview: test-retest reliability of the schedule for affective disorders and schizophrenia for school-age children, present episode version. Arch Gen Psychiatry 1985;42(7):696–702.

[36] Marshall WA, Tanner JM. Variations in pattern of pubertal changes in girls. Arch Dis Child 1969;44(235):291–303.

[37] Marshall WA, Tanner JM. Variations in the pattern of pubertal changes in boys. Arch Dis Child 1970;45(239):13–23.

[38] Orvaschel H, Puig-Antich J, Chambers W, et al. Retrospective assessment of prepubertal major depression with the Kiddie-SADS-e. J Am Acad Child Adolesc Psychiatry 1982;21(4):392–7.

[39] Endicott J, Spitzer RL. A diagnostic interview: the schedule for affective disorders and schizophrenia. Arch Gen Psychiatry 1978;35(7):837–44.

[40] American Psychiatric Association. Diagnostic and statistical manual of mental disorders. 3rd edition. Washington (DC): American Psychiatric Association; 1980.

[41] Sobin C, Weissman MM, Goldstein RB, et al. Diagnostic interviewing for family studies: comparing telephone and face-to-face methods for the diagnosis of lifetime psychiatric disorders. Psychiatr Genet 1993;3(4):227–33.

[42] Spitzer RL, Endicott J, Robins E. Research diagnostic criteria: rationale and reliability. Arch Gen Psychiatry 1978;35(6):773–82.

[43] Andreasen NC, Endicott J, Spitzer RL, et al. The family history method using diagnostic criteria: reliability and validity. Arch Gen Psychiatry 1977;34(10):1229–35.

[43a] Mendlewicz J, Fleiss JL, Cataldo M, et al. Accuracy of the family history method in affective illness: comparison with direct interviews in family studies. Arch Gen Psych 1975;32(3): 309–14.

[44] Leckman JF, Sholomskas D, Thompson WD, et al. Best estimate of lifetime psychiatric diagnosis: a methodological study. Arch Gen Psychiatry 1982;39(8):879–83.

[45] Liang KY, Zeger SL. Longitudinal data analysis using generalized linear models. Biometrika 1986;73:343–55.

[46] Zeger SL, Liang KY. An overview of methods for the analysis of longitudinal data. Stat Med 1986;11(14–15):1825–39.

[47] Shah BV, Barnwell BG, Bieler GS. SUDAAN user's manual, release 7.5. Research Triangle Park (NC): Research Triangle Institute; 1997.

[48] Kendler KS. The super-normal control group in psychiatric genetics: possible artifactual evidence for coaggregation. Psychiatr Genet 1990;1:45–53.

[49] Bridge JA, Brent D, Johnson BA, et al. Familial aggregation of psychiatric disorders in a community sample of adolescents. J Am Acad Child Adolesc Psychiatry 1997;36(5):628–36.

[50] Goodyer IM, Cooper PJ, Vize CM, et al. Depression in 11–16-year-old girls: the role of past parental psychopathology and exposure to recent life events. J Child Psychol Psychiatry 1993;34(7):1103–15.

[51] Warner V, Mufson L, Weissman MM. Offspring at high and low risk for depression and anxiety: mechanisms of psychiatric disorder. J Am Acad Child Adolesc Psychiatry 1995; 34(6):786–97.

[52] Warner V, Weissman MM, Mufson L, et al. Grandparents, parents, and grandchildren at high risk for depression: a three-generation study. J Am Acad Child Adolesc Psychiatry 1999; 38(3):289–96.

[53] Kendler KS, Heath AC, Martin NG, et al. Symptoms of anxiety and symptoms of depression: same genes, different environments? Arch Gen Psychiatry 1987;44(5):451–7.

[54] Kendler KS, Neale MC, Kessler RC, et al. Major depression and generalized anxiety disorder: same genes, (partly) different environments? Arch Gen Psychiatry 1992;49(9):716–22.

[55] Eley TC, Stevenson J. Using genetic analyses to clarify the distinction between depressive and anxious symptoms in children. J Abnorm Child Psychol 1999;27(2):105–14.

[56] Thapar A, McGuffin P. Anxiety and depressive symptoms in childhood–a genetic study of comorbidity. J Child Psychol Psychiatry 1997;38(6):651–6.

[57] Eley TC, Stevenson J. Specific life events and chronic experiences differentially associated with depression and anxiety in young twins. J Abnorm Child Psychol 2000;28(4):383–94.

[58] Finlay-Jones R, Brown GW. Types of stressful life event and the onset of anxiety and depressive disorders. Psychol Med 1981;11(4):803–15.

[59] Brown GW, Harris TO, Hepworth C. Loss, humiliation and entrapment among women developing depression: a patient and non-patient comparison. Psychol Med 1995;25(1):7–21.

[60] Giaconia RM, Reinherz HZ, Silverman AB, et al. Ages of onset of psychiatric disorders in a community population of older adolescents. J Am Acad Child Adolesc Psychiatry 1994;33(5): 706–17.

ELSEVIER
SAUNDERS

Child Adolesc Psychiatric Clin N Am
14 (2005) 727–743

CHILD AND
ADOLESCENT
PSYCHIATRIC CLINICS
OF NORTH AMERICA

Obsessive-Compulsive Disorder

Henrietta L. Leonard, MD*, Chelsea M. Ale, BA,
Jennifer B. Freeman, PhD, Abbe M. Garcia, PhD,
Janet S. Ng, BA

*The Pediatric Anxiety Research Clinic (PARC) at the Bradley Hasbro Research Center,
Rhode Island Hospital, Coro West 2, One Hoppin Street, Providence, RI 02906, USA*

Obsessive-compulsive disorder (OCD), as defined by the Diagnostic and Statistical Manual of Mental Disorders, Fourth Edition (DSM-IV) [1], is characterized by recurrent obsessions or compulsions that are distressful or interfere in one's life. Obsessions are defined as persistent thoughts, images, or impulses that are ego-dystonic, intrusive, and, for the most part, senseless. "Compulsions are repetitive, purposeful, and intentional behaviors that are performed in response to an obsession, according to certain rules, or in a stereotyped fashion." [1]

In general, compulsions are meant to relieve (or neutralize) anxiety or to prevent a dreaded event. An adolescent or adult may recognize that the ritual is unreasonable or excessive, but that is not necessarily true for the young child. Often, children and adolescents will attempt to hide their rituals, although with more severe symptoms, this usually is not possible. To meet diagnostic criteria for the disorder, the person must experience distress, spend more than 1 hour per day in either obsessions or compulsions, or there must be significant interference in one's life [1]. This article reviews the phenomenology, causes, treatment, and outcome of children and adolescents with OCD.

Clinical presentation

Typically, there is a specific list of obsessions and compulsions. Many of the symptoms can be understood as excessive worries about danger, separation, and contamination, which result in rituals of washing, checking, and hoarding. The

---

* Corresponding author.
E-mail address: Henrietta_Leonard@Brown.edu (H.L. Leonard).

1056-4993/05/$ – see front matter © 2005 Elsevier Inc. All rights reserved.
doi:10.1016/j.chc.2005.06.002
childpsych.theclinics.com

most common obsessions include excessive concerns about contamination (dirt, germs, and illness), harm coming to the self or others (eg, parents might be kidnapped), doing the right thing (ie, scrupulosity), reassurance, or intrusive sexual thoughts. Sometimes the need ("urge") for evenness, order, or exactness may be described, with an accompanying feeling of "incompleteness." The most common rituals are washing, repeating, checking, counting, touching, arranging, and hoarding [2]. Obsessions and compulsions seen in adults are similar to those seen in children, but the obsessions are more age appropriate (eg, children worry that they may be kidnapped or that their parents may be killed). It is not unusual for the OCD symptoms to change over time, and most children will have had most of the symptoms at some time in the course of their illness [3].

For individuals with a childhood onset of OCD, boys may be more likely to have a prepubertal onset and girls a pubertal onset. The male/female ratio tends to equalize in adolescence, and there are more women with OCD in adulthood than there are men [4]. Those individuals who have early onset OCD have a higher rate of tic disorders and may have a higher rate of comorbid attention deficit hyperactivity disorder (ADHD) [5]. In the children with the OCD-ADHD-tic disorder triad, the onset of the tic disorder may precede the onset of the OCD by several years [6–8]. It is hypothesized that the early onset OCD may represent a unique subtype. Family studies suggest that the children who have an early onset of OCD (before 9 years of age) have a higher rate of first-degree relatives with OCD or a tic disorder (eg, have a higher "genetic loading") than those with later onset [9].

Despite a specific core set of OC symptoms, systematic phenomenologic studies have found significant heterogeneity among children and adolescents with OCD; for example, the onset may be abrupt or insidious and may or may not be related to a clear precipitant. In a large phenomenologic study, one third of the children and adolescents reported that certain stimuli seemed to trigger their illness [7]. Pediatric OCD may follow a waxing and waning course, a chronic stable course, or may be characterized by dramatic exacerbations and remissions [6,7,10–12]. Current research is studyding whether the course of illness (chronic with some fluctuations versus abrupt severe exacerbations with remission) will prove meaningful as a means of categorizing subtypes.

Most early attempts to develop subtypes of OCD were based on the specific content of the obsessions and compulsions experienced by a patient. An important core of consistent symptom presentation appears to extend across both the life span and cultures [11,12]. However, as with adults, 90% of children in the National Institutes of Mental Health (NIMH) study reported that their obsessions and compulsions changed in both content and severity over time [3,7]. Thus, it appears unlikely that consideration of the content of obsessions of compulsions alone will lead to an identification of specific disorder subtypes.

Several studies have reported that compared with those subjects without tics, OCD patients with a comorbid tic disorder may have a greater incidence of symmetry, exactness, and aggressive obsessions as well as touching, rubbing, staring, and blinking rituals, whereas contamination worries and cleaning compulsions were reported to be more common in patients with non-tic related OCD [13,14]. These two putative subtypes also may differ in other important respects; compared with OCD without tics, tic-associated OCD may be more familial and more common in boys and early onset cases.

Increasing evidence suggests that early or prepubertal onset OCD is a unique subtype of the disorder. Proposed subtypes, which are neither necessarily mutually exclusive nor distinct, include early onset OCD, tic-related OCD, and streptococcal-precipitated OCD. Patients with an onset of OCD before age 9 are more likely to have a subtype that is familial and related to tic disorders [9]. Patients with OCD and a comorbid tic disorder may be more likely to have compulsions with more sensory phenomena and may need to perform the compulsions until they are "just right" [15]. Early onset OCD is associated with male preponderance, comorbidity with ADHD and other disorders, frequent absence of insight, and increased family loading for OCD [5]. The age at onset may help to identify developmental subtypes [16].

Pediatric autoimmune neuropsychiatric disorders associated with streptococcal infection

A subgroup of children with a pediatric onset of either OCD or a tic disorder has been described as having pediatric autoimmune neuropsychiatric disorders associated with streptococcal infection (PANDAS). These children have an abrupt onset of symptoms after a group A β-hemolytic streptococcal (GABHS) infection, and their course of illness is characterized by dramatic, acute worsening of symptoms with periods of remission. Only recently, with parallel studies of Sydenham's chorea [7,17,18], was this subgroup noted to have an onset of symptoms after GABHS infection [18].

The PANDAS subgroup is defined by five clinical characteristics: (1) the presence of OCD or a tic disorder; (2) a prepubertal symptom onset; (3) a dramatic onset and acute exacerbations with an episodic course of symptom severity; (4) temporal association between symptom exacerbations and GABHS infections; and (5) associated neurologic abnormalities (eg, choreiform movements) [2]. Fifty children meeting these criteria were systematically evaluated at the NIMH [2]. Identifying this subtype is important because they require a different assessment and treatment. In a child who has an acute onset of OCD or tics or has had a dramatic deterioration, medical illnesses (including seemingly benign upper respiratory infections) in the months prior should be considered carefully. Obtaining a throat culture, an antistreptolysin O titer, and anti-DNase B streptococcal titer may help to diagnose such an infection, even in the absence of clinical symptoms of pharyngitis [2,19]. The most obvious presentation to a pediatric or primary care office may be separation anxiety, worry, or increased urinary frequency [19]. For a recent review of the PANDAS subtype, the reader is referred to a study by Snider and Swedo [20].

Associated disorders

Patients with Tourette's disorder may have OCD or associated obsessive-compulsive symptoms [21–24]. In clinical practice, it is sometimes difficult to categorize a behavior as a ritual or a tic. Generally, if an action is preceded by a specific cognition, then it is considered to be a compulsive ritual; however, some complex motor tics may be preceded by a sensation or "urge." It may be impossible to distinguish a complex motor tic from a compulsive ritual, especially in patients with both OCD and Tourette's disorder. However, it is important to attempt to make the distinction, because they are treated differently.

The assessment of comorbidity is crucial for effective treatment planning, because other diagnoses are common in children and adolescents with OCD [5,7]. In the 70 consecutive children with OCD studied at the NIMH, comorbidity was common, with 18 children (26%) having no other psychiatric diagnosis [7,12]. Geller and colleagues [5] studied 30 consecutively referred pediatric OCD patients and found higher rates of comorbidity, with only one patient (3%) having no other diagnosis. Diagnoses shown to commonly co-occur with OCD include major depression and other mood disorders, multiple anxiety disorders, tic disorders, and disruptive behavior disorders, particularly attention-deficit hyperactivity disorder and oppositional defiant disorder; of these, only tic disorders are believed to have a shared genetic origin with OCD [9,24], and the relationship with ADHD merits further study [5,25]. Thus, comorbidity in OCD is common and frequently requires its own diagnostic and treatment interventions.

Differential diagnosis

When evaluating a child with recurrent thoughts or repetitive behaviors, it is important to consider whether the symptoms are developmentally appropriate. Developmental rituals of childhood are normal at certain ages, although they may be performed in a stereotypic or rule-bound fashion. The specific contents of developmental rituals do not typically resemble OCD rituals. Additionally, OCD rituals are associated with a later age at onset and usually are more dramatic, persistent, and distressing [26,27].

The differential diagnosis of OCD includes a number of disorders with obsessional features and "compulsive" behaviors, including depressive and anxiety disorders, eating disorders, somatoform disorders, and tic disorders. Obsessions differ in content, from the ruminations or brooding thoughts seen in major depression or dysthymia and from worries specific to everyday or real-life problems, as seen in other anxiety disorders (eg, separation anxiety disorder and specific phobia). In anorexia and bulimia, obsessive thoughts are limited to issues of food and weight. In body dysmorphic disorder, the obsessive concern is limited to an imagined flaw in one's physical appearance [28]. If the obsessions or compulsions are particularly bizarre and seen by the patient as reasonable, a diagnosis of psychosis should be considered.

Epidemiology

Estimates of the prevalence of OCD in children and adolescents have varied greatly, and most figures are probably low owing to the secrecy manifested by patients with the disorder. The Isle of Wight study [29], the first epidemiologic study, reported "mixed obsessional/anxiety disorders" in 7 of 2199 (0.3%) in a survey of 10- and 11-year-old children. In a whole-population adolescent epidemiologic study of OCD, Flament and colleagues (1988) reported a (weighted point) prevalence rate of 0.8% and a lifetime prevalence of 1.9% [30]. These figures suggest that OCD is a relatively common psychiatric disorder in adolescents. This rate is compatible with the estimated prevalence in the general population [31] and the finding that at least one third to one half of adults with OCD experienced the onset during childhood [4].

Causes

The serotonin hypothesis of OCD was initially based primarily on the effectiveness of the serotonin reuptake inhibitors in treating this disorder [32]. It is unlikely that just one neurotransmitter system can explain the complex findings in OCD. Neurobiological causes include neuroanatomical, neurophysiologic, and neuroimmunologic associations with metabolic abnormalities [33]. Several lines of research have implicated a neuroethologic model for the underlying explanation of OCD, resulting in fixed action patterns (obsessions and compulsions) that are inappropriately released [34].

Hormonal dysregulation also has been implicated as a cause of OCD. Notably, the male/female ratio for cases with an onset before the age of 10 years is 7:1, whereas subsequently it shifted to 1:1.5 after puberty. In a large epidemiologic study, the boys with OCD were shorter and had a flatter growth curve than normal and psychiatric controls, and the authors speculated that there may be a subtle neuroendocrine dysfunction in OCD [35].

There is a clear association between OCD and several basal ganglia illnesses, specifically Tourette's Syndrome (TS), postencephalitic Parkinson's disease, and Huntington's chorea [17,32]. Swedo and colleagues [17] have hypothesized that Sydenham's chorea, an autoimmune inflammation of the basal ganglia triggered by streptococcal infection, may represent a medical model for OCD. In the 11 children studied, nine (82%) had obsessive-compulsive symptoms, which started several days to weeks before the chorea was observed. The authors suggested that the obsessive-compulsive symptoms were accompanying manifestations of Sydenham's chorea, and those symptoms required medical care in some cases. Subsequently, several studies of patients who have Sydenham's chorea have confirmed this association [20]. Further support for basal ganglia involvement comes from anatomic observations, psychosurgery, and brain imaging studies [33,36].

Systematic studies support a genetic transmission for many OCD patients. Lenane and colleagues [37] have reported an increased rate (20%) of OCD in the first-degree relatives of 46 OCD probands. Thirty percent of the child probands had a first-degree family member with a lifetime history of OCD. When the histories of the parent and the child were examined, the specific OCD symptoms were dissimilar, suggesting that modeling or learning models did not account for this familial transmission.

Supporting a relationship between TS and OCD is the comorbidity of the disorder in affected individuals. There is an increased rate of tics in OCD probands [9,24,38,39]. Systematic family studies have led Pauls and colleagues [39] to hypothesize initially that some forms of OCD may represent alternative expressions of the genes responsible for TS. Pauls and colleagues [9,38,39] have reported an increased rate of OCD in the first-degree relatives of TS probands over that of the control sample of adoptee relatives, regardless of the OCD status of the TS probands. Despite large ongoing genetic studies, the gene for OCD or TS has not been identified.

One of the most interesting lines of work concerns the PANDAS subgroup [2]. The cause of OCD and tics in the PANDAS subgroup is unknown but is theorized to occur as a result of post-streptococcal autoimmunity in a manner similar to that of Sydenham's chorea. The working hypothesis for the patho-physiology begins with a Group A beta-hemolytic streptococcal (GAS) infection in a susceptible host that results in the production of antibodies (to GAS), which cross-react with the cellular components of the basal ganglia. The neuropsychiatric symptoms are hypothesized to arise from an interaction of these antibodies with neurons of the basal ganglia. Studies are underway to determine the specific parts of the basal ganglia that may be involved, as well as the cellular and humoral immune responses [20].

Treatment

Psychosocial treatments: behavioral therapy

Cognitive-behavioral treatments (CBT) are used clinically with much success in children with OCD, although its efficacy had been based predominantly on adult treatment studies and open trials [40], until the large Pediatric OCD Treatment Study (POTS) [41] combined treatment comparison was published. Authors of the expert consensus guidelines [42] and American Academy of Child and Adolescent Psychiatry (AACAP) practice parameters for OCD [43] consider CBT, specifically exposure with response prevention (ERP), an important intervention, and recommend starting with CBT or CBT plus selective serotonin reuptake inhibitors (SSRI), depending on the severity and comorbidity.

Exposure-based behavioral interventions came from the theoretical framework of instrumental condition, and the cognitive interventions are both used in OCD treatment [44]. ERP involves therapist-assisted in vivo exposure to feared situations, imaginal exposure to feared disasters, and instructions to refrain from rituals and avoidance behaviors. For the exposure exercises to be successful, the patient must have the information that corrects the distortion of the cognition (eg, that a situation is dangerous if its safety cannot be proven). Adjunctive interventions, including family involvement in treatment, anxiety management, training, cognitive restructuring, contingency management, and supportive therapy may enhance the efficacy of ERP through increasing treatment compliance and motivation [45].

A review of uncontrolled CBT treatment trials to that date report that the majority of patients were responders, with a mean Child Yale-Brown OC Scale (CY-BOCS) decrease from 50% to 67%. A consistent problem that complicates the interpretation of the findings of many of the uncontrolled studies is that some patients were receiving SSRI before and during the course of CBT, and therefore the separate effects of the CBT cannot be determined [46]. Additionally, there may have been ascertainment biases in enrolling patients and families, with those who were motivated for behavior therapy treatment.

March and colleagues [47] have reported on the manualized, structured CBT open protocol in 15 youth ages 8 to 18 years old. There were significant differences from pre- to post-treatment, with a mean reduction in symptom severity of approximately 50%. Sixty-seven of the patients showed more than 50% symptom improvement (which was maintained at follow-up). Only 20% were nonresponders. At the end of treatment, 40% of patients were rated as asymptomatic, and 60% of patients were rated as asymptomatic at follow-up. Forty percent of the sample was able to discontinue medication with booster sessions. This work led to a manual for children and adolescents with OCD (8–17 years old) [48], consisting of 14 visits over 12 weeks, spread out over five phases: psychoeducation, cognitive training, mapping OCD, exposure and response prevention, and relapse prevention and generalization training. Other investigators have applied similar models using gradual exposure, as reviewed by Piacentini [45]. The manual by March and Mulle [48] used in the POTS study [41] and those results are detailed below under combined treatments.

Pilot studies that have included a follow-up evaluation [47,49] support the durability of CBT, with therapeutic gains maintained for up to 9 months post-treatment. The consistent impression in the field is that CBT may provide larger and more long lasting symptom improvement than that seen with medication.

Psychosocial treatment: other psychotherapeutic modalities

Behavioral family intervention

Cognitive, developmental, and symptom differences, and most specifically the "embeddedness" in the family context play an important role in assessing and treating early onset OCD. Freeman and colleagues [50] have proposed that the family context is an important vehicle for treatment delivery, and behavioral family intervention (BFI) is an important paradigm in the treatment of childhood disorders [51]. Behavioral family intervention involves parents, teachers, and significant others as "behavior change agents" or "mediators." By dealing with the affective and cognitive aspects of the parent-child relationship as well as the targets of intervention, BFI is likened to a "cognitive-behavioral family intervention." Freeman and colleagues [50] have developed a BFI manualized treatment for children and their families with OCD, and initial pilot results seem promising. This suggests that a different conceptual approach is needed for younger children and that treatment designed for older children cannot be just extrapolated downward. A 12-week controlled study comparing BFI to relaxation therapy is ongoing.

Family therapy

An assessment of the family usually is a necessary component of an evaluation of an adolescent with OCD [52]. By dealing with the specific family dynamic issues and their resulting obstacles to engage in treatment, the family can participate in the OCD treatment plan of the identified patient in constructive and positive ways. Although there are no systematic studies of family therapy, family therapy may be useful to address issues of family discord, marital difficulties, and inappropriate roles or boundaries, which interfere with the adolescent's ability to participate in treatment for his or her OCD [52].

Dynamically oriented individual therapy

Jenike [53] has reviewed the psychotherapeutic interventions for OCD and concluded that the "traditional psychodynamic psychotherapy is not an effective treatment for obsessions or rituals in patients meeting criteria for OCD as defined in the DSM-III-R; there are no reports in the modern psychiatric literature of patients who stopped ritualizing when treated with this method alone." However, psychodynamic psychotherapy may play an adjunctive role in addressing both general and specific issues in the patient's life, such as how OCD affects the individual's self-esteem, personal relationships and outlook, and by encouraging compliance other therapies that focus more directly on the OCD symptoms.

Pharmacologic treatment of obsessive-compulsive disorder

The systematic efficacy studies of SSRI for the treatment of pediatric OCD form the largest body of work in the pharmacotherapy of childhood psychiatric disorders, other than that of ADHD. A review of the systematic studies supports the acute efficacy of clomipramine and SSRI in the treatment of children and adolescents with OCD.

The tricyclic antidepressant, clomipramine, a SRI (with an active metabolite with noradrenergic reuptake inhibition) was the first medication to be studied systematically in children and adolescents with OCD. Three studies have supported the efficacy of clomipramine for pediatric OCD [54–56]. Flament and colleagues [55] have reported that in 23 youths in a 10-week double blind, placebo-controlled crossover study, clomipramine (in doses of 3 mg/kg) was significantly more effective than placebo in decreasing OCD symptoms at week 5.

In an 8-week multicenter double blind parallel comparison, DeVeaugh-Geiss and colleagues [54] reported that clomipramine was superior to placebo for the treatment of OCD in youth. This study led to the first Food and Drug Administration (FDA) approval of a SRI in pediatric OCD (children aged 10 years and older). Clomipramine was found to be generally well tolerated and has an anticholinergic-adverse effects profile. Periodic EKGs are obtained during ongoing clinical care because of concerns about tachycardia and prolongation of the QTc interval.

To address whether the serotonergic specificity of clomipramine was critical, a double blind crossover comparison of clomipramine versus desipramine (a selective noradrenergic reuptake inhibitor without serotonergic activity) was completed in 48 children and adolescents with OCD [56]. In this 12-week double blind design, clomipramine (targeting 3 mg/kg/day and not exceeding 5 mg/kg/day) was significantly better than desipramine in decreasing the OCD symptoms at week 5. This study concluded that the serotonergic reuptake inhibition may be critical.

The SSRI (which include citalopram, escitalopram, fluoxetine, fluvoxamine, paroxetine, and sertraline) has emerged as the first-line pharmacotherapeutic agent for OCD. SSRIs have the advantage over clomipramine of having a generally more tolerable side effect profile (with few anticholinergic effects), a safer profile in overdoses, and do not require EKG monitoring. The expert consensus guidelines authors [42] suggest that clomipramine be used when a patient has failed two or three adequate trials of a SSRI in combination with CBT. A meta-analysis of systematic studies in pediatric OCD has reported that clomipramine was significantly superior to each of the SSRIs but that the SSRIs were comparably effective [57].

Systematic efficacy studies have shown that fluoxetine, fluvoxamine, and sertraline were each superior to placebo for children and adolescents with OCD [16,41,58–60]. Open studies support the use of citalopram and paroxetine. [61,62]. Sertraline has FDA-approved indication for the treatment of OCD in children ages 6 years and older; fluvoxamine is approved for children ages 8 years and older; and fluoxetine is approved for children 8 years and older.

March and colleagues [59] have reported on 187 children and adolescents (ages 6 to 17 years of age) with OCD studied in a randomized double blind placebo-controlled 8-week trial of sertraline (forced titration to 200 mg/day) versus placebo. Patients receiving sertraline compared with those receiving placebo showed significantly greater improvement on the CY-BOCS, the NIMH Obsessive Compulsive Scale, and the Clinical Global Improvement (CGI) scale. Significant differences (with intent-to-treat analyses) between the two groups were seen as early as week 3 and continued for the entire study. Similarly, in the POTS [41] four-arm 12-week combined treatment study, sertraline was superior to placebo.

Riddle and colleagues [60] have reported the safety and efficacy of fluvoxamine for 120 youth (ages 8 to 17 years old) with OCD in a randomized, controlled study in which they received either fluvoxamine (50–200 mg/day) or placebo for 10 weeks. Patients in the fluvoxamine group showed a significant improvement (on CY-BOCS) in comparison with the placebo group. In the fluvoxamine group, 42% of patients were responders (defined as a 25% decrease in CY-BOCS) in comparison with 26% in the placebo group, and this was significantly different.

Geller and colleagues [16] randomized 103 youth with OCD to either fluoxetine (starting at 10 mg/day) or placebo for 8 weeks. Intent-to-treat analyses reported that those in the fluoxetine group had significantly better improvement on CY-BOCs than did the placebo group. Fluoxetine (20–60 mg/day) was effective and well tolerated in the pediatric group. In the other systematic study of fluoxetine, Liebowitz and colleagues [58] randomized 43 patients to either fluoxetine or placebo for 8 weeks. Responders then went into an 8-week maintenance phase. The fluoxetine dosage was fixed at 60 mg/day for 6 weeks and then could be increased to 80 mg/day. At week 8, fluoxetine was not significantly better than placebo on the CY-BOCs or CGI-I scale; authors attributed this to either low power or short duration of treatment. The fluoxetine group continued to improve during the maintenance phase such that at week 16, 57% of the fluoxetine patients compared with 27% of the placebo patients (using data at week 8) were much or very much improved. The authors conclude that fluoxetine's effect took more than 8 weeks to develop.

A review of adverse effects of the SSRIs suggests that dropouts from blinded active medication assignment usually are less than 13%, and in many studies, there are no significant differences between the number of dropouts in the active and placebo arm [46]. Generally, the most common side effects seen with the SSRIs include sedation, nausea, diarrhea, insomnia, anorexia, tremor, sexual dysfunction, and hyperstimulation [46,60]. Rare adverse reactions include apathy syndrome, serotonin syndrome, extrapyramidal symptoms, and hypomania. Children and adolescents may be more vulnerable to agitation or activation while receiving SSRIs than adults are, but this reaction has only recently received study. The FDA concluded that children and adolescents on antidepressants may potentially develop suicidality, worsening of symptoms, anxiety, agitation, panic, insomnia, irritability, hostility, impulsivity, akathisia, and hypomania. In late 2004, the FDA added a "black box" warning to describe the potential increased risk of suicidality in children and adolescents who are given antidepressants. The FDA has recommended that children and adolescents be assessed frequently while receiving SSRI, to watch for an emerging worsening of symptoms or "activation."

How much do pediatric patients improve with pharmacotherapy alone? In general, a 30% to 40% reduction in OCD symptoms, which corresponds to an average six-point decrease on the CY-BOCS, is reported in the medication treatment group in the SSRI controlled studies [46]. A meta-analysis (of 12 studies with 1044 subjects) has reported the pooled standardized mean difference for results of all medication studies was 0.46 and showed a significant difference between drug and placebo treatment. Although significant, the overall effect sizes for medication were modest [57]. This, coupled with increasing scrutiny of the safety of the SSRIs, has led to further interest in CBT for the treatment of OCD.

The limited durability of pharmacotherapy, which often is seen clinically, has not been well studied. A double blind study of desipramine substitution in adolescents receiving long-term clomipramine maintenance reported that eight of nine patients relapsed when they were switched to desipramine, compared with two of 11 who continued taking clomipramine [63]. It is likely that medications have less durability than CBT, but until follow-up data are analyzed (for example from the POTS [41]), this is not well delineated. Interestingly, Cook and colleagues [64] have reported that in a long-term open treatment with sertraline (52-week extension study after a 12-week double blind trial) was effective and that improvement continued to be seen in the long term, although concomitant psychotherapy was allowed.

Although the number of studies on medication augmentation for partial responders to SSRIs are few, at this point, CBT would be the first choice for an "augmenting agent." There is a three-site systematic trial studying partial responders to SSRIs who are randomized to different doses of CBT [65], but in the absence of such data, the general clinical consensus is that CBT should be considered. Unfortunately, the availability of trained therapists is some-times limited, and some children are too sick or not motivated to participate. In considering medication augmentation, the adult studies support the trial of neuroleptic augmentation in SRI nonresponders or partial responders [66]. In a controlled risperidone versus placebo SRI augmentation study, risperidone addition was superior in reducing OCD symptoms. With increasing concerns about weight gain and increased risk of a metabolic syndrome, the atypical neuroleptics are being used more judiciously.

Combined treatments

The expert consensus guidelines [42] and the AACAP practice parameters for children who have OCD [43] recommend starting treatment with CBT or CBT plus an SSRI, depending on severity and comorbidity. Both guidelines recommend that patients started on SSRI monotherapy, who are partial responders, should have a trial of CBT.

The relative efficacy of medication, of CBT, and the combination have just been studied in a large randomized controlled trial [41]. One hundred and twelve patients, aged 7 through 17 years with a primary diagnosis of OCD were randomized to sertraline alone, pill placebo, CBT alone, or combined CBT and sertraline. Ninety-seven (87%) of the patients completed the full 12-week study. Predetermined primary outcome variables included change in CY-BOCS over 12 weeks (continuous) and remission status (dichotomous) (the responder being defined as a CY-BOCS of 10 or less). All three active treatments were each superior to placebo. Combined treatment ($P = .001$), CBT alone ($P = .003$), and sertraline alone ($P = .007$) proved statistically superior to placebo. Importantly, combined treatment proved superior to CBT alone ($P = .008$) and to sertraline alone ($P = .006$). Of note, CBT alone and sertraline alone did not differ significantly from one another. The remission rate (dichotomous variable) for combined treatment did not differ from that for CBT alone, but it did differ from sertraline alone and from placebo. The effect size for combined treatment, CBT alone, and sertraline alone were 1.4, 0.97, and 0.67, respectively. Sertraline was generally well tolerated, with adverse effects in at least 5% of patients treated and with an incidence at least two times that seen in patients treated with placebo. Two patients treated with sertraline experienced behavioral activation, but no patient became suicidal or attempted suicide. Patients treated with CBT, either alone or in combination with medication, showed a substantially higher probability of improvement, with the edge going to combination treatment over CBT alone at one site but not in the other. The authors conclude that children with OCD should begin treatment with the combination of CBT plus a SSRI or CBT alone.

Investigational treatments

Hypotheses concerning whether Sydenham's Chorea (SC) and PANDAS might share similarities in their pathophysiology led to the question whether penicillin prophylaxis would reduce neuropsychiatric symptom exacerbation in children with PANDAS by preventing streptococcal infection. An 8-month double blind placebo-controlled crossover trial comparing oral penicillin V (250-mg, twice daily) and placebo was conducted in 37 children [67]. There was no significant between-phase difference in either the OCD or tic symptom severity; however, penicillin administration failed to provide adequate prophylaxis against GABHS (as evidenced by the fact that 14 of 35 GABHS infections occurred during the penicillin phase). A number of children received antibiotic treatment multiple times during the placebo phase. The authors concluded that because of the failure to achieve an acceptable level of streptococcal prophylaxis, no conclusions could be drawn regarding the efficacy of penicillin prophylaxis in preventing tic or OCD symptom exacerbation.

In a subsequent study, the NIMH group compared antibiotic prophylaxis with azithromycin (250 mg, twice daily, once per week, with placebo administered twice daily on the other 6 days) or penicillin V-K (250 mg, twice daily) for 12 months [68]. Twenty three children with PANDAS were enrolled in this double blind randomized, controlled trial. Rates of streptococcal infections and neuropsychiatric symptom exacerbations were compared between the study year and the baseline year before entry (collected retrospectively). Significant decreases in streptococcal infections during the study year were found, with a mean of 0.1 infections per subject compared with the baseline year, with 1.9 infections in the penicillin group and 2.4 infections in the azithromycin group ($P \leq .01$). Significant decreases in neuropsychiatric exacerbations during the study year were also found, with a mean of 0.5 exacerbations per subject in the penicillin group and 0.8 exacerbations in the azithromycin group, compared with the baseline year, with 2.0 exacerbations in the penicillin group and 1.8 exacerbations in the azithromycin group ($P \leq .01$). The authors concluded that penicillin and azithromycin prophylaxis were found to be effective in decreasing streptococcal infections and neuropsychiatric symptom exacerbation in the PANDAS subgroup. The authors caution that there was a small sample size and lack of placebo control and that other evidence suggests that azithromycin prophylaxis should not be routinely recommended for PANDAS children (eg, macrolide-resistant *Streptococci*). Penicillin prophylaxis may be considered for children who meet all criteria for PANDAS criteria and who have an ongoing risk of streptococcal exposure.

If post-streptococcal autoimmunity is the cause of the exacerbations in this subgroup, then children with PANDAS may benefit from immunomodulatory therapies that have been shown in preliminary findings to treat symptoms of SC. Children with severe infection-triggered exacerbations of OCD or tic disorders were randomly assigned to plasma exchange (five single-volume exchanges over 2 weeks), intravenous immunoglobulin (IVIG) (1 g/kg, daily on 2 consecutive days), or placebo (saline solution given in the same manner as IVIG) [69]. Plasma exchange and IVIG were both effective in lessening of symptom severity for this group of children. Ratings were completed at 1 month, and symptom gains were maintained at 1 year. It should be noted that these children were much more significantly impaired than the average child with OCD or tics was, and therefore, these invasive interventions were considered. These interventions are investigational and should be considered in the context of research approved by a Human Investigations Committee and not in the context of routine clinical care.

Prognosis

Long-term outcome data have been limited by a few large systematic studies. A meta-analysis of sixteen samples followed for 1 to 15 years have reported that long-term persistence of pediatric OCD may be lower than reported previously [70]. Pooled mean persistence rates were 41% for full OCD and 60% for full or subthreshold OCD. Earlier age of onset, increased OCD duration, and inpatient (versus outpatient) status predicted greater persistence. Comorbid psychiatric illness and poor initial treatment response were poor prognostic factors.

The long-term medication studies, which are confounded by intercurrent treatment and by dropouts, suggest modest incremental improvement but not normalization over 52 weeks of SRI treatment [64]. The relapse rate after SSRI discontinuation has not been reported systematically but is suspected to be high. One assumes that with the development of new treatments (SSRIs and CBT) that more children will be able to access treatment earlier and are more likely to improve. As to whether this will improve long-term outcome remains to be studied.

Research questions

The PANDAS subtype remains one of the most interesting areas of research study. If children with this subtype could be identified early in their illness, would they have a different course or outcome? Genetic vulnerabilities as well as the identification of immune processes remain open and important areas of study.

One of the critical, unanswered questions is the long-term relative efficacy and durability of a SSRI, CBT, and their use in combination. The POTS [41] has provided important relative efficacy for the short-term treatment. What are the predictors for response for each of the different modalities? It has been reported that the availability of these two treatment modalities will improve the long-term prognosis, but a long-term comparison is required.

References

[1] American Psychiatric Association. Diagnostic and statistical manual of mental disorders. 4th edition. Washington (DC): American Psychiatric Association; 1994.

[2] Swedo SE, Leonard HL, Garvey MA, et al. Pediatric autoimmune neuropsychiatric disorders associated with streptococcal infections: clinical description of the first 50 cases. Am J Psychiatry 1998;155:264–71.

[3] Rettew DC, Swedo SE, Leonard HL, et al. Obsessions and compulsions across time in 79 children and adolescents with obsessive-compulsive disorder. J Am Acad Child Adolesc Psychiatry 1992;31:1050–6.

[4] Rasmussen SA, Eisen J. Epidemiology of obsessive compulsive disorder. J Clin Psychiatry 1990;51:10–3.

[5] Geller DA, Biederman J, Griffin S, et al. Comorbidity of juvenile obsessive-compulsive disorder with disruptive behavior disorders. J Am Acad Child Adolesc Psychiatry 1996;35:1637–46.

[6] Geller DA, Biederman J, Jones J, et al. Is juvenile obsessive-compulsive disorder a developmental subtype of the disorder? A review of the pediatric literature. J Am Acad Child Adolesc Psychiatry 1998;37:420–7.

[7] Swedo SE, Rapoport JL, Leonard HL, et al. Obsessive compulsive disorders in children and adolescents: clinical phenomenology of 70 consecutive cases. Arch Gen Psychiatry 1989;46:335–43.

[8] Leckman JF, Zhang H, Vitale A, et al. Course of tic severity in Tourette syndrome: the first two decades. Pediatrics 1998;102:14–9.

[9] Pauls D, Alsobrook JP, Goodman WK, et al. A family study of obsessive-compulsive disorder. Am J Psychiatry 1995;152:76–84.

[10] Flament MF, Koby E, Rapoport JL, et al. Childhood obsessive-compulsive disorder: a prospective follow-up study. J Child Psychol Psychiatry 1990;31:363–80.

[11] Hanna GL. Demographic and clinical features of obsessive-compulsive disorder in children and adolescents. J Am Acad Child Adolesc Psychiatry 1995;34:19–27.

[12] Thomsen PH. Obsessive-compulsive disorder in children and adolescents: predictors in childhood for long term phenomenological course. Acta Psychiatr Scand 1995;92:255–9.

[13] Holzer JC, Goodman WK, McDougle CJ, et al. Obsessive-compulsive disorder with and without a chronic tic disorder. Br J Psychiatry 1994;164:469–73.

[14] Leckman JF, Peterson BS, Anderson GM, et al. Pathogenesis of Tourette's syndrome. J Child Psychol Psychiatry 1997;38:119–42.

[15] Leckman JF, Walker DE, Goodman WK, et al. "Just right" perceptions associated with compulsive behavior in Tourette's syndrome. Am J Psychiatry 1994;151:675–80.

[16] Geller DA, Hoog SL, Heiligenstein JH, et al. Fluoxetine treatment for obsessive-compulsive disorder in children and adolescents: a placebo-controlled clinical trial. J Am Acad Child Adolesc Psychiatry 2001;40:773–9.

[17] Swedo SE, Leonard HL, Schapiro MB, et al. Sydenham's chorea: physical and psychological symptoms of St. Vitus dance. Pediatrics 1993;91:706–13.

[18] Swedo SE. Sydenham's chorea: a model for childhood autoimmune neuropsychiatric disorders. JAMA 1994;272:1788–91.

[19] Murphy ML, Pichichero ME. Prospective identification and treatment of children with pediatric autoimmune neuropsychiatric disorder associated with group A streptococcal infection (PANDAS). Arch Pediatr Adolesc Med 2002;156:356–61.

[20] Snider L, Swedo SE. PANDAS: current status and directions for research. Mol Psychiatry 2004;9:900–7.

[21] Cohen DJ, Leckman JF. Developmental psychopathology and neurobiology of Tourette's syndrome. J Am Acad Child Adolesc Psychiatry 1994;33:2–15.

[22] Frankel M, Cummings JL, Robertson MM, et al. Obsessions and compulsions in Gilles de la Tourette's syndrome. Neurology 1986;36:378–82.

[23] Leckman JF, Peterson BS. The Pathogenesis of Tourette's syndrome: epigenetic factors active in early CNS development. Biol Psychiatry 1993;34:425–7.

[24] Leonard HL, Lenane MC, Swedo SE, et al. Tics and Tourette's disorder: a 2- to 7-year follow-up of 54 obsessive-compulsive children. Am J Psychiatry 1992;149:1244–51.

[25] Pauls D, Leckman JF, Cohen DJ. Familial relationship between Gilles de la Tourette's syndrome, attention deficit disorder, learning disabilities, speech disorders, and stuttering. J Am Acad Child Adolesc Psychiatry 1993;32:1044–50.

[26] Leonard HL, Rapoport JL. Treatment of anxiety disorders in children and adolescents: handbook of anxiety, Volume 4. Elsevier Science Publishing; 1990.

[27] Evans DW, Leckman JF, Carter A, et al. Ritual, habit, and perfectionism: the prevalence and development of compulsive-like behavior in normal young children. Child Dev 1997;68:58–68.

[28] Phillips KA, Atala KD, Albertini RS. Case study: body dysmorphic disorder in adolescents. J Am Acad Child Adolesc Psychiatry 1995;34:1216–20.

[29] Rutter M, Tizard J, Whitmore K. Education, health, and behavior. London: Longmans; 1970.

[30] Flament MF, Whitaker A, Rapoport JL, et al. An epidemiological study of obsessive-compulsive disorder in adolescence. J Am Acad Child Adolesc Psychiatry 1988;27:764–71.

[31] Karno M, Golding MA, Sorenson SB, et al. The epidemiology of obsessive-compulsive disorder in five US communities. Arch Gen Psychiatry 1988;45:1094–9.

[32] Rauch SL, Jenike MA. Neurobiological models of obsessive-compulsive disorder. Psychosomatics 1993;34:20–32.

[33] Saxena S, Rauch SL. Functional neuroimaging and the neuroanatomy of obsessive-compulsive disorder. Psychiatr Clin North Am 2000;23:563–86.

[34] Leckman JF, Mayes LC. Understanding developmental psychopathology: how useful are evolutionary accounts? J Am Acad Child Adolesc Psychiatry 1998;37:1011–21.

[35] Hamburger S, Swedo SE, Whitaker A, et al. Growth rate in adolescents with obsessive-compulsive disorder. Am J Psychiatry 1989;146:652–5.

[36] Rauch SL, Whalen PJ, Curran T, et al. Probing striato-thalmic function in obsessive-compulsive disorder and Tourette syndrome using neuroimaging methods. Adv Neurol 2001;85:207–24.

[37] Lenane MC, Swedo SE, Leonard HL, et al. Psychiatric disorders in first degree relatives of children and adolescents with obsessive compulsive disorder. J Am Acad Child Adolesc Psychiatry 1990;29:407–12.

[38] Pauls DL, Raymond CL, Stevenson JM, et al. A family study of Gilles de la Tourette syndrome. Hum Genet 1991;48:154–63.

[39] Pauls DL, Leckman JF. The inheritance of Gilles de la Tourette's syndrome and associated behaviors. N Engl J Med 1986;315:993–7.

[40] March J. Cognitive-behavioral psychotherapy for children and adolescents with OCD: a review and recommendations for treatment. J Am Acad Child Adolesc Psychiatry 1995;34:7–18.

[41] Team POTS. Cognitive-behavior therapy, sertraline, and their combination for children and adolescents with obsessive-compulsive disorder. JAMA 2004;292:1969–76.

[42] March JS, Frances A, Carpenter D, et al. Expert consensus guidelines: treatment of obsessive-compulsive disorder. J Clin Psychiatry 1997;58:2–72.

[43] King RA, Leonard HL, March J. Practice parameters for the assessment and treatment of children

and adolescents with obsessive-compulsive disorder. J Am Acad Child Adolesc Psychiatry 1998;37:27S–45S.

[44] Foa EB, Kozak MJ. Emotional processing of fear: exposure to corrective information. Psychol Bull 1986;99:20–35.

[45] Piacentini J. Cognitive behavioral therapy of childhood OCD. Child Adolesc Psychiatr Clin N Am 1999;8:599–616.

[46] March J, Curry JF. Predicting the outcome of treatment. J Abnorm Child Psychol 1998;26: 39–51.

[47] March J, Mulle K, Herbel B. Behavioral psychotherapy for children and adolescents with obsessive-compulsive disorder: an open trial of a new protocol-driven treatment package. J Am Acad Child Adolesc Psychiatry 1994;33:333–41.

[48] March J, Mulle K. OCD in children and adolescents: a cognitive-behavioral treatment manual. New York: Guilford Press; 1998.

[49] Franklin ME, Kozak MJ, Cashman LA, et al. Cognitive-behavioral treatment of pediatric obsessive-compulsive disorder: an open clinical trial. J Am Acad Child Adolesc Psychiatry 1998;37:412–9.

[50] Freeman J, Garcia A, Fucci C, et al. Family-based treatment of early-onset obsessive-compulsive disorder. J Child Adolesc Psychopharmacol 2003;13:S71–80.

[51] Barrett PM, Dadds MR, Rapee RM. Family treatment of childhood anxiety: a controlled trial. J Consult Clin Psychol 1996;64:333–42.

[52] Lenane M. Families and obsessive compulsive disorder. In: Rapoport JL, editor. Obsessive compulsive disorder in children and adolescents. Washington (DC): American Psychiatric Press; 1989. p. 237–49.

[53] Jenike M. Psychotherapy of obsessive compulsive personality disorder. In: Jenike M, Baer L, Minichiello WE, editors. Obsessive-compulsive disorders: theory and management. Chicago: Year Book Medical; 1990. p. 295–305.

[54] DeVeaugh-Geiss J, Moroz G, Biederman J, et al. Clomipramine hydrochloride in childhood and adolescent obsessive-compulsive disorder: a multicenter trial. J Am Acad Child Adolesc Psychiatry 1992;31:45–9.

[55] Flament MF, Rapoport JL, Berg CJ, et al. Clomipramine treatment of childhood obsessive-compulsive disorder. Arch Gen Psychiatry 1985;42:977–83.

[56] Leonard HL, Swedo SE, Rapoport JL, et al. Treatment of obsessive-compulsive disorder with clomipramine and desipramine in children and adolescents. Arch Gen Psychiatry 1989;46: 1088–92.

[57] Geller DA, Biederman J, Stewart SE, et al. Which SSRI? A meta-analysis of pharmacotherapy trials in pediatric obsessive-compulsive disorder. Am J Psychiatry 2003;160:1919–28.

[58] Liebowitz MR, Turner SM, Piacentini J, et al. Fluoxetine in children and adolescents with OCD: a placebo-controlled trial. J Am Acad Child Adolesc Psychiatry 2002;41:1431–8.

[59] March JS, Biederman J, Wolkow R, et al. Sertraline in children and adolescents with obsessive-compulsive disorder: a multicenter randomized controlled trial. JAMA 1998;280:1752–6.

[60] Riddle MA, Reeve EA, Yaryura-Tobias JA, et al. Fluvoxamine for children and adolescents with obsessive-compulsive disorder: a randomized, controlled, multicenter trial. J Am Acad Child Adolesc Psychiatry 2001;40:222–9.

[61] Rosenberg DR, Stewart CM, Fitzgerald KD, et al. Paroxetine open-label treatment of pediatric outpatients with obsessive-compulsive disorder. J Am Acad Child Adolesc Psychiatry 1999;38: 1180–5.

[62] Thomsen PH, Ebbesen C, Persson C. Long-term experience with citalopram in the treatment of adolescent OCD. J Am Acad Child Adolesc Psychiatry 2001;40:895–902.

[63] Leonard HL, Swedo SE, Lenane MC, Rettew DC, et al. A double-blind desipramine substitution during long-term clomipramine treatment in children and adolescents with obsessive-compulsive disorder. Arch Gen Psychiatry 2001;48:922–7.

[64] Cook EH, Wagner KD, March JS, et al. Long-term sertraline treatment of children and adolescents with obsessive-compulsive disorder. J Am Acad Child Adolesc Psychiatry 2001;40: 1175–81.

[65] March J, Franklin ME, Leonard HL. Communications regarding treatment of pediatric OCD: augmentation of partial response (POTSII). Available at: https://email.brown.edu/exchweb/bin/redir.asp?URL=http://www.clinicaltrials.gov/ct/show/NCT00074815?order=1.

[66] McDougle CJ, Epperson CN, Pelton GH, et al. A double-blind, placebo-controlled study of risperidone addition in serotonin reuptake inhibitor-refractory obsessive-compulsive disorder. Arch Gen Psychiatry 2000;57:794–801.

[67] Garvey MA, Perlmutter SJ, Allen AJ, et al. A pilot study of penicillin prophylaxis for neuropsychiatric exacerbations triggered by streptococcal infections. Biol Psychiatry 1999;45: 1564–71.

[68] Snider LA, Lougee L, Slattery M, et al. Antibiotic prophylaxis with azithromycin or penicillin for childhood-onset neuropsychiatric disorders. Biol Psychiatry 2005;57:788–92.

[69] Perlmutter SJ, Leitman SF, Garvey MA, et al. Therapeutic plasma exchange and intravenous immunoglobulin for obsessive-compulsive disorder and tic disorders in childhood. Lancet 1999;354:1153–8.

[70] Stewart SE, Geller DA, Jenike M, et al. Long-term outcome of pediatric obsessive-compulsive disorder: a meta-analysis and qualitative review of the literature. Acta Psychiatr Scand 2004;110: 4–13.

ELSEVIER
SAUNDERS

Child Adolesc Psychiatric Clin N Am
14 (2005) 745–772

CHILD AND
ADOLESCENT
PSYCHIATRIC CLINICS
OF NORTH AMERICA

Childhood Post-Traumatic Stress Disorder: An Overview

Michael D. De Bellis, MD, MPH[a,b,*], Thomas Van Dillen, PhD[a]

[a]Department of Psychiatry and Behavioral Sciences, Duke University Medical Center, Box 3613, Durham, NC 27710, USA
[b]Healthy Childhood Brain Development and Developmental Traumatology Research Program, Department of Psychiatry and Behavioral Sciences, Duke University Medical Center, Box 3613, Durham, NC 27710, USA

Children can experience trauma in many different forms. Trauma can include the experience of a one-time traumatic event, such as a dog bite, or the challenge of growing up with an abusing parent. Trauma can be divided into subtypes: interpersonal trauma and noninterpersonal trauma, chronic or long-lasting trauma, and acute or one-time-only experiences. Interpersonal types of trauma are of human design and include warfare and terrorism, witnessing domestic or community violence, and violent personal assault (eg, child physical and sexual abuse and neglect). These are the most common causes of post-traumatic stress disorder (PTSD) in children and adolescents. Noninterpersonal types of trauma include natural disasters, disasters related to human causality, accidents, or diagnosis with life-threatening illness. When trauma is of interpersonal origins, it is usually chronic and causes more severe and long-lasting PTSD symptoms.

This article presents an overview of PTSD as it relates to children and adolescents and provides a critical review of the pediatric PTSD literature regarding the definition, epidemiology, clinical presentation, assessment, neurobiologic foundation, and treatment of PTSD. The importance of developmental and neurobiologic factors is emphasized as well as how the interactions of these

This work was supported by National Institute of Mental Health grants RO1-MH63407, MINH/NIMDS RO1-MH61744, and K24 MH071434 (to M.D. De Bellis).

* Corresponding author. Department of Psychiatry and Behavioral Sciences, Duke University Medical Center, Box 3613, Durham, NC 27710.

E-mail address: debel002@mc.duke.edu (M.D. De Bellis).

factors are unique to children. A literature search was conduced using PsycINFO and Medline databases, using key words "PTSD," "post-traumatic stress," "children," and "adolescents." For each subject heading, a search was included with words pertaining to the topic; for instance, under the heading "a brief history of PTSD," post-traumatic stress disorder and history were searched. This was performed with each subsequent topic area. In addition, references cited in the studies retrieved were searched for relevant information. Only English language articles were retained. Articles were included that were primarily limited to the last 10 years, with some exceptions.

A brief history of post-traumatic stress disorder

Accounts of an individual's response to trauma that describe PTSD symptoms were written in ancient times. The scientific study of trauma and particularly the link between the traumatic experience and psychiatric illness by Jean Martin Charcot, in the mid-nineteenth century, characterized hysteria as a neurosis of the brain, triggered by psychic trauma in hereditarily predisposed individuals [1,2]. Charcot described how trauma-induced "choc nerveux" could put patients into a mental state similar to that induced by hypnosis. Charcot's early conceptualization of trauma brought to the forefront a long-debated question about the mind-body relationship in treating medical and mental disorders. In a little over 100 years, a vast body of evidence and related neurologic and psychologic theory set forth indisputably that mental events could indeed alter the physical state of the body. In addition, the conceptualization of PTSD brought the etiologic agent of disease outside of the individual rather than being conceived of as an inherent individual weakness.

Definition of post-traumatic stress disorder

As described in the Diagnostic and Statistical Manual of Mental Disorders, Fourth Edition, Revised (DSM-IV-R), the essential feature (criterion A) of PTSD is exposure to an extreme traumatic stressor, in which the person experienced, witnessed, or was confronted with an event or events that involved actual or threatened death or serious injury or a threat to the physical integrity of self or others; and responded with intense fear, helplessness, horror or, in children, disorganized or agitated behaviors [3]. The DSM-IV-R diagnosis of PTSD is made when criterion A is experienced and when three clusters of categorical symptoms are present for more than 1 month after the traumatic events: (1) intrusive re-experiencing of the traumas (criterion B); (2) persistent avoidance of stimuli associated with the traumas (criterion C); and (3) persistent symptoms of increased physiologic arousal (criterion D). Cluster B re-experiencing and intrusive symptoms can be conceptualized best as a classically conditioned response. An external or internal conditioned stimulus (eg, the traumatic reminder) activates unwanted and distressful recurrent and intrusive memories of the traumatic experiences (eg, the unconditioned stimulus). Intrusive phenomena take the form of nightmares or night terrors, dissociative flashback episodes, and psychologic distress and physical reactivity on exposure to traumatic reminders. In young children, these intrusive thoughts may be part of repetitive play or trauma-specific re-enactments or compulsive rituals. Distressing dreams of the event may occur several weeks after the traumatic event and become generalized nightmares involving monsters, rescuing others, or threats to self or others. Criterion C symptoms represent both avoidant and dissociative behaviors, and they can be conceived of as ways to control the pain and distress of re-experiencing symptoms. These behaviors include efforts to avoid thoughts, feelings, conversations, activities, places, people, and memories associated with the trauma, amnesia for the trauma, diminished interest in others, feelings of detachment from others, a restricted range of affect, and a sense of a foreshortened future. The DSM-IV-R acknowledges that it may be hard for children to report criterion C symptoms. Children with PTSD may show diminished interest in normal activities (eg, playing with friends), feeling detached or removed from others, and lack expression of positive emotions such as love, contentment, or happiness [4]. Avoidant symptoms should be carefully evaluated with reports from parents, teachers, and other caregivers. Criterion D hyperarousal symptoms consist of persistent symptoms of increased physiologic arousal. The criterion D cluster of symptoms does not need to have been present before or worsened significantly since the traumatic event. Symptoms include difficulty falling or staying asleep, irritable mood or angry outbursts, difficulty concentrating, hypervigilance, and exaggerated startle response. Children also may exhibit physical symptoms such as stomachaches and headaches. Criterion E requires that the symptoms impair functioning in school, socially, or with the family, and criterion F states that symptoms persist for at least 1 month. Of the reported PTSD symptoms in children, re-experiencing is most common [5], and symptoms of avoidance and numbing are the least reported PTSD symptoms [6].

Although the diagnostic picture of PTSD in children of latency age and adolescents is similar to that of adults [7], this is not the case in younger children. In an epidemiologic survey [8], a prevalence rate of 0.1% for PTSD (by DSM-III-R criteria) was seen in preschool-aged children. This is far below the rates of 3% to 6% found in other surveys that have included adolescents [9,10]. It is difficult to detect the presence of PTSD symptoms, such as hyperarousal, re-experiencing, and avoidance in children below the age of 4 years; therefore, an alternative set of criteria has been proposed [11], which was more sensitive developmentally and was based on behavior. Using these criteria in young children, a PTSD diagnosis rate of 26% was found in children who witnessed violence [12]. This was more consistent with PTSD rates of traumatized adults and older children and in contrast to a rate of 0% using DSM-IV criteria [12]. It also should be noted that PTSD symptoms are seen commonly within the first month of a trauma, may be a normal response to severe stress, and usually fade within 3 months after the trauma [13]. However, children and adolescents with subthreshold and threshold PTSD suffer similar clinical impairment and may require intervention [14]. Therefore, more empirical evidence using developmentally sensitive assessments is needed to determine the nature and extent of stress reactions in children.

Acute stress disorder

Because reactions to trauma appear to be different for different people and manifest in different ways, the diagnosis of PTSD was not suitable for some clinical presentations, especially in those individuals who did not demonstrate all the symptoms or were otherwise reacting normally to a traumatic or stressful event. To account for the continuum of symptom presentation and in an attempt to identify people who subsequently develop PTSD, the term acute stress disorder (ASD) was coined [15]. ASD describes trauma reactions that occur in the initial month following a trauma. In particular, the emphasis is on dissociative symptoms that occur within the first month after the stressful event. In addition to symptoms of re-experiencing, avoidance, and arousal, a diagnosis of ASD requires three of five dissociative symptoms. Dissociative symptoms are defined as disruptions in the usually integrated functions of consciousness, memory, identity, or perception of the environment that interfere with the associative integration of information [16]. Examples include emotional numbing, reduced awareness of surroundings, derealization, depersonalization, and dissociative amnesia.

The value of ASD as a predictor for later PTSD remains controversial. Recent research indicates that a diagnosis of ASD in adults identifies some people at risk for PTSD [17,18]. In one study [19] of children, a diagnosis of ASD predicted PTSD. Studies of traumatized adults show that some people who display subclinical ASD (ie, they do not experience dissociative symptoms) develop PTSD, whereas some people may not display any symptoms of ASD but still develop PTSD [20,21]. In a study [22] of injured children, ages 8 to 17 years, ASD was not a strong predictor of PTSD; rather, subsyndromal ASD (ie, meeting all ASD criteria except for dissociation symptoms) was a more effective predictor of PTSD. Pediatric studies of traumatized children show that the severity of self-reported ASD symptoms is associated with later PTSD symptom severity [19,22,23]. Overall, acute symptoms, including heart rate, cortisol levels, appraisals about the traumatic experience, and memory functioning may provide more powerful predictive capacity than the actual ASD diagnosis in adults [24]. However, it is unclear whether ASD, as currently described by the DSM-IV-R, is a sensitive predictor of PTSD in children or adults. In addition, published studies of acute stress reactions in children and adolescents has not paid sufficient attention to specific stressors characteristics, developmental factors, or level of parental stress in predicting ASD [25]. More research is warranted.

Incidence and prevalence of childhood post-traumatic stress disorder

The National Comorbidity Study (NCS) is the most comprehensive general population study of the rates of mental illness, including PTSD, of US individuals between the ages of 15 and 54 years [26]. The NCS found an overall prevalence of PTSD of 7.8%, with the rate for women (10.4%) more than twice that for men (5.0%). Rape and combat were the events that were most likely to lead to PTSD. Having a diagnosis of PTSD was associated with an increased likelihood of having a lifetime history of at least one other axis I disorder (ie, mood, other anxiety, and substance use disorders) in 88.3% of men and in 79% of women with PTSD [26]. Similar to adults, pediatric PTSD also is associated with high rates of comorbid mood and other anxiety disorders [27,28]. Children and adolescents manifest both externalizing and internalizing disorder symptoms after trauma [28]. High rates of comorbid mood, other anxiety disorders, and substance use disorders are seen in adolescents with PTSD [29,30].

PTSD lifetime prevalence rates for children and adolescents are believed to be similar to or even higher than those of adults who suffer from the same or similar traumas [31]. However, there are only a few community studies and national survey data on pediatric PTSD to date. Traumatic events are seen in a high percentage of US children. The National Center for PTSD [32] estimates that 15% to 43% of girls and 14% to 43% of boys have experienced at least one traumatic event. A longitudinal general population study of youth in western North Carolina, involving 4965 interviews with 1420 children and adolescents and their parents or guardians, reported that 25% children had experienced at least one DSM extreme stressor by age 16 [33]. A community sample estimated a DSM-III-R PTSD prevalence rate by the use of the NIMH Diagnostic Interview Schedule, Version III, Revised (DIS-III-R) of 6.3% in adolescents [34]. A nationally representative survey of adolescents that included diagnostic interviews found a current prevalence rate of PTSD of 5% in US adolescents under the age of 18 [35]. The prevalence rate was higher among females than males and the events most likely to yield PTSD were abuse and violence, often at the hands of family members.

However, most studies of PTSD rates in children and adolescents have been carried out with those exposed to trauma, in whom rates of PTSD in these at-risk children are much higher. Following is a review PTSD prevalence rates in traumatized children and adolescents.

Pediatric post-traumatic stress disorder rates and types of trauma

Natural and human disasters

The rates of PTSD in children who have experienced natural disasters have been estimated to range from 9% to 50% [36]. Consequences of natural disasters such as earthquakes and hurricanes include destruction of structures, loss of life, death of loved ones, and relocation, and may explain the wide range of PTSD rates in children. In 1972, the collapse of the Buffalo Creek Dam resulted in the flooding of a WV town, widespread destruction, a large loss of lives, and a 37% rate of "probable" pediatric PTSD based on symptom count [37]. Symptoms of intrusion were most common, followed by restricted affect, irritability, and anger. Older children and girls were more likely to receive a diagnosis of PTSD. The most predictive of PTSD across age groups was the stability of the home, including the level of parents functioning and adaptability, suggesting the importance of family stability in modulating PTSD symptoms. After Hurricane Andrew, a category 4 storm that affected the community of Dade County, FL, in 1992, killed 40 people, children reported severe to very severe levels of PTSD symptoms on the Child PTSD Reaction Index (PTSD-RI), 10 months after the hurricane. Eighteen percent of the sample reported all three symptom clusters, in which the overall re-experiencing rate was most frequently endorsed at 78.3%, hyperarousal rates were 49.3%, and rate of avoidance was the least common symptom at 24.2% [38]. At the 2-year follow-up, 70% of the children in high-impact areas continued to score in the moderate to severe range for PTSD [39]. Three months after Hurricane Hugo, a category 4 storm that killed 60 people, the prevalence of PTSD in exposed children and adolescents was 5% [40]. In contrast, Hurricane Mitch, which was classified as a category 5 storm, caused massive destruction in Nicaragua and Honduras, in 1998, killing approximately 10,000 people. Using the Child PTSD Reaction Index, a dose-of-exposure pattern, with the highest scores found in the most affected region, was seen 6 months after this storm [41]. The degree of impact, objective and subjective features, and thoughts of revenge accounted for 68% of the variance in severity of post-traumatic stress reaction. Girls presented with more severe PTSD reaction than boys; however, when subjective features of exposure (ie, fear, horror, and helplessness) were controlled for, this difference was no longer significant, suggesting girls may be more willing to endorse these items or may experience more subjective symptoms than boys do. In a study of 231 Armenian children, ages 8 to 16 years, 6 months after an earthquake that occurred during school hours, the rates of PTSD were high for all three cities that were chosen because of the varying proximity to the epicenter of the earthquake [42]. However, a year and a half later, an exposure effect was observed in which those children closest to the epicenter experienced the highest frequency of PTSD, at rates of 95% re-experiencing, 71% hyperarousal, and 26% avoidance, respectively [43]. Most of the PTSD symptoms reported included intrusions (ie, intrusive thoughts and images) and arousal (ie, difficulty concentrating and increased startle response), followed by avoidance and guilt (not a criteria of PTSD in DSM-III). The most severe symptoms reported by children was guilt, which exceeded that reported by comparably exposed Armenian adults, suggesting traumatized children are developmentally vulnerable to excessive self-blame.

Chronic illness and medical illness

Children living with a life-threatening illness may experience PTSD from the initial diagnosis (acute life threat) and the subsequent treatment (repetitive threat to life and physical well being) [44]. In a cross-sectional design [45] that examined pediatric cancer survivors diagnosed with leukemia (N = 23), physically abused adolescents (N = 27), and healthy adolescents (N = 23) as a comparison group, the lifetime PTSD rates in cancer survivors was 35%. In another cross-sectional study [46], children who were diagnosed with leukemia (41%), lymphoma (21.8%), sarcoma (15.4%), or other cancer (21.8%) had a lifetime PTSD prevalence rate of 20.5% after treatment. The risk factors for PTSD symptoms are subjective factors related to cancer or its treatment, such as beliefs about past and present life threat and perceived treatment intensity rather than objective medical data [47]. The general level of anxiety for both the child and parent strongly predict PTSD symptoms [47]. Other associated factors are family functioning and poor social or family support [47]. The experience of a life-threatening illness such as childhood cancer clearly affects the child and family, not only initially but years later. This disruption in the family also includes siblings [48]. On the initial diagnosis, nonaffected siblings often feel isolated and abandoned by parents and may become resentful, angry, anxious, depressed, have jealous feelings of the ill sibling, guilt, and fear of dying themselves [49]. School problems, avoidance, and other problems are common to siblings of pediatric cancer patients [49]. Although siblings clearly show that the experience of cancer in the family is a significant stressor that may increase the likelihood of sibling psychopathology, research has yet to determine the prevalence of PTSD in this population [50]. In a study [51] examining the psychosocial consequence of bone marrow transplants (BMT) on siblings (donor and nondonor), moderate levels of PTSD reactions have been reported in one third of the 44 siblings studied. The sibling donors who underwent the BMT procedure experienced more anxiety and lower self-esteem than the nondonor siblings did. However, symptoms of PTSD were equal for both the sibling donors and nondonors, suggesting that not only is the experience of donating bone marrow predictive of developing PTSD symptoms but the general experience of a chronic illness in the family also poses an increased risk for PTSD. The cancer experience disrupts the familial network, and PTSD symptoms may be seen in all family members. Investigations aimed at reducing the risk for PTSD in medically ill children and their families are needed.

Exposure to war and terrorism

In the last 20 years, systematic research has established that children exposed to violence represent a highly vulnerable population whose PTSD responses may be greater than those of adults [52]. War has the potential to affect children in many ways, including victimization, witnessing violent acts and experiencing homelessness, starvation, or loss of family and friends. In a study of children's trauma reactions and adjustment to the war in Bosnia, 41% of the 791 children, aged 6 to 16 years, had significant PTSD symptoms and adjustment problems, and the effects of violence and deprivation were additive [53]. War has a significant long-term impact on children. A longitudinal study [54] examined 234 children, aged 7 to 12 years, who lived in the Gaza strip. Using the Child

Post-Traumatic Stress Reaction Index, investigators found rates of PTSD symptoms of 40.6% after 1 year and 10% 18 months after military activities. Overall, the continuation of PTSD symptoms was predicted by the amount of traumatic exposure. In a longitudinal follow up study [55] of Khmer youths who had survived the horrors of the Pol Pot regime (1975–1979), PTSD persisted at a rate of 35% at the 12-year follow-up. However, survivors did not report major functional impairments. In contrast to the previous studies, the current diagnosis of PTSD in this sample was related to a specific traumatic incident and not to other forms of multiple stressors or loss. Consistent with the above findings, another study [56] found that in a sample of 224 children between the ages of 10 and 16 years, who were exposed to war and chronic violence in Lebanon (1975–1991), the types of violence were more predictive of PTSD than the number of war traumas.

The premise of terrorism is to instill fear and a sense of vulnerability by creating uncertainty through acts of unpredictable violence [57]. Rates of PTSD in children exposed to terrorist events range from 28% to 50% [58–61]. Psychologic effects of terrorism-induced trauma on children are similar to the effects of nonterrorist traumatic events. The severity of symptoms is associated with the type and degree of exposure to the trauma, ongoing loss and instability, and the level of the child's development [62]. Unique features of terrorism-induced PTSD in children include the profound effects of terrorism on adults and the resultant difficulties these may cause in providing support and reassurance to children [57]. Additionally, children and adolescents are particularly vulnerable to terrorism because of the profound psychologic effects on their and their parent's sense of safety in the world, which may often generalize to unrelated risks [63].

Two incidents of terrorism in the US that exemplify the research are the Oklahoma City bombing and the September 11, 2001, terrorist attacks. The bombing in Oklahoma City occurred in the Murrah Federal Building, in April 1995. The destruction was so vast that it damaged hundreds of buildings near the explosion. One hundred and sixty people lost their lives, including 19 children who were in the day-care center located on the second floor. A study [64] of middle and high school students revealed that 7 weeks after the bombing, 62.8% of the sample worried about the well being of their families and themselves, with girls reporting higher levels of PTSD symptoms than boys. Those students who reported that their parents or siblings were killed or injured exhibited more symptoms of PTSD than those who did not experience a personal loss [64]. Highly predictive of the total PTSD symptoms at 7 weeks were self reports of arousal level at the time of the blast [64]. Also, in the middle school sample, television exposure was shown to be a greater predictor of PTSD symptoms than either physical or emotional exposure [65]. Two years after the terrorist attack, almost 20% of the sample reported current bomb-related symptoms that impaired their function at home or school, and 16% of children who lived approximately 100 miles away from Oklahoma City reported significant PTSD symptoms [66]. The PTSD-RI and the Brief Symptom Inventory were administered using an internet web-based survey to a cross-sectional sample of 2273 adults living in the New York City and the Washington, DC, metropolitan areas 1 to 2 months after the September 11, 2001, attacks [67]. Adults reported symptoms of distress among children living in their households, including 19.8% of children who were having trouble sleeping, 29.9% who were described as irritable, grouchy, or easily upset, and 26.5% who were described as fearful of separation from their parents. Although proportionately more children were rated to be upset in the New York City metropolitan area (60.7%) than in Washington, DC, (57.3%) and the rest of the United States (48.0%), the differences were not statistically significant. Formal diagnostic studies of pediatric PTSD after the September 11, 2001, terrorist attacks are warranted.

Family violence: domestic violence and sexual and physical abuse

A nationally representative survey examining the prevalence rate of PTSD in adolescents found that the events most likely to yield PTSD were abuse and violence, frequently within the family and perpetrated by family members [68,69]. Children who witnessed domestic violence show elevated PTSD symptoms [70]. Children of battered women, ages 7 to 12 years, met the criteria for PTSD in 13% of the cases [71]. In a sample of 337 school-aged children between the ages of 6 and 12 years who were recruited from shelters and the community, 19% who witnessed family violence had PTSD and also showed high levels of symptoms characteristic of phobias, separation anxiety, and oppositional disorder [72]. In another study [73], psychologic measures indicated the rate of PTSD was 40% among Hawaiian children who witnessed domestic violence even when measured on average 2 years after the mother's leaving the abusive relationship. In this study, the majority of the children (60%) indicated that they had themselves experienced physical abuse, but very few (4%) admitted to sexual abuse. An important finding of this study is that there is not a relationship between the likelihood of PTSD in the mothers and the likelihood of PTSD in their children, suggesting that psychologic dysfunction in the children is likely caused by directly witnessing or experiencing abuse. Additionally, the combination of maternal depression, anger, and dissociation appears to interfere with an abused mother's ability to provide a sufficient context of safety, resulting in higher rates of children's dissociation. Realizing that many studies fail to use comparison groups of homes without wife abuse, a national representative survey of 6002 households by the method of random-digit dialing was conducted [74]. Of the 2733 respondents who were married or living together and had at least one child younger than 18 (6.8% were infants and 23% were age 14 or older), 456 reported wife abuse (2295 without wife abuse). Households reporting wife abuse had higher rates of all forms of violence toward children than homes without wife abuse did (physical child abuse 8.2% versus 3.3%; physical punishment 82.4% versus 57.6%; verbal child abuse 71.3% versus 52.1%; and physical abuse, physical punishment, or verbal abuse 89.9% versus 72.1%). Children age 14 or older (23%) versus children ages 1 through 13 (6.8%) were at greater risk of abuse. It is evident from these results that domestic violence often overlaps with other forms of victimization, leading to a higher risk for childhood PTSD.

In clinically referred samples, the reported incidence rates of PTSD resulting from sexual abuse range from 42% to 90% [75–77], 50% to 100% from witnessing domestic homicide [78], and as high as 50% from physical abuse [75]. Only a few studies have focused on assessing PTSD in nonclinically referred maltreated children. One study [79] has reported a 39% incidence rate of PTSD in a nonclinically referred maltreated sample who were interviewed within 8 weeks of the abuse or neglect disclosure. Approximately one third of the PTSD subjects who were re-examined from the original sample continued to meet PTSD criteria at the 2-year follow-up [80]. Another study [81] has reported prevalence rates of PTSD of 36.3% in nonclinically referred sexually abused children 60 days immediately following sexual abuse disclosure. To date, there are no studies that directly examine PTSD in neglected children. Although child neglect is not abuse, neglect may be perceived as traumatic. The degree of the traumatic experience perceived by the child will depend on the age and developmental attainment of the child at the time of the neglect. An unsupervised child is more likely to witness interpersonal traumas such as domestic and community violence or experience traumatic accidents. It is estimated that one third to one half of neglected children witness domestic violence leading to PTSD symptoms [82]. Childhood victims of abuse (sexual or physical) as well as neglect have been found to be at an increased risk for developing a lifetime history of PTSD when assessed prospectively in young adulthood [83]. Furthermore, these investigators found that childhood abuse and neglect predicted the number of lifetime PTSD symptoms. Partial PTSD responses that are clinically impairing also are seen in victims of childhood maltreatment who do not meet DSM-IV-R criteria for PTSD [14,84–88]. Thus, PTSD is commonly seen in maltreated children, especially during the period immediately following maltreatment disclosure. The identification of psychosocial and treatment-related factors, which lead to the remission of PTSD in maltreated children, is an important area of future investigation.

In many of the studies described above, the selection of participants for inclusion in the sample may not have been completely representative of the general population in the areas studied. For this reason, conclusions must be drawn tentatively. Therefore, empirical evidence of pediatric PTSD needs to be determined in a comprehensive general population study using developmentally sensitive assessments. However, these studies provide an excellent base from which additional studies might be conducted.

Risk factors for pediatric post-traumatic stress disorder

Factors that increase the risks of having PTSD before the traumatic experience include a history of poor social support and adverse life events, parental poverty, a history of childhood maltreatment, poor family functioning, a familial or genetic family history of psychiatric disorders, introversion or extreme behavioral inhibition, female gender, and poor health and previous mental illness [89]. Of these, genetics and the trauma experience may play a critical role. In a twin study

[90], genetic factors accounted for 13% to 30% of the variance in the re-experiencing cluster, 30% to 34% in the avoidance cluster, and 28% to 32% in the arousal cluster of PTSD symptoms in Vietnam veterans with combat-related PTSD. Although symptoms in the re-experiencing cluster and one symptom in the avoidance and numbing cluster were strongly associated with trauma exposure, the shared environment did not contribute to the development of the disorder. However, some authors believe that childhood trauma is causally and independently related to this increased risk for adult psychiatric, alcohol use, and substance use disorders. For example, a study of twins discordant for childhood sexual abuse exposure has shown that even after controlling for family background and parental psychopathology, the exposed twin suffered from an increased risk for adult psychopathology [91]. Risk factors for PTSD associated with the trauma are the degree of trauma exposure, the parent's and child's subjective sense of danger, and other related traumatic events such as loss [92]. Risk factors associated with PTSD after the trauma include a lack of social supports and continued negative life events, parental reactions, and lack of post-trauma interventions [92]. Clinical studies that focus on early prevention and clinical intervention after the trauma are needed to diminish the disability and chronicity associated with pediatric PTSD.

Assessment of post-traumatic stress disorder in children

Since 1980, there has been a great deal of attention devoted to the development of instruments for assessing pediatric PTSD. We will review empirically supported interviews used to assess PTSD as defined by the DSM-IV-R in children and adolescents, along with reliability and validity information. Unique to PTSD and ASD among the psychiatric disorders is that they require the process of an identifiable event, yet because of the limited verbal ability of younger children, the reliability and validity of their reports are difficult to ascertain without interviewing the parent. However, parents are better at describing their child's behavior than at identifying their child's internal states [93]. Therefore, a combination of sources is best to identify and characterize children's symptoms. Children and adolescents often have a broader range of clinically significant symptoms of internalizing and externalizing responses to trauma exposure that are beyond the PTSD diagnostic criteria [28,94]. Therefore, the use of a multidimensional evaluation, including structured and semistructured interviews, reports of others in the child's life, and objective behavioral measures, may best capture the symptom profile. Comorbidity also needs to be assessed carefully.

Of all the pediatric PTSD instruments, one of the most used widely is the Child PTSD-RI [95]. This 20-item child and adolescent report measure has an algorithm to determine DSM-IV-R PTSD diagnosis. The total severity score and subscale scores map directly onto DSM-IV-R criterion B (intrusion), criterion C (avoidance), and criterion D (arousal). The measure may be administered in the following three ways: (1) as a self-administered paper and pencil measure; (2) by a one-to-one verbal administration, in which the instructions and questions are read to the child; and (3) by administration to a group in a classroom setting. It also has been translated to other languages and used worldwide. The PTSD-RI has a convergent validity of 0.70 (the Schedule for Affective Disorders and Schizophrenia for School Aged Children [K-SADS] Epidemiologic [-E] version with a cut-off of 38 has a sensitivity of 0.93) and specificity of 0.87 in detecting PTSD. Internal consistency across versions reports have found Chronbach α coefficients fall in the range of 0.90. A test-retest reliability coefficient of 0.84 for the DSM-IV-R version has been reported [95].

The Clinician-Administered PTSD Scale for Children and Adolescents (CAPS-CA) is an interview instrument that was modified from the adult version [96]. It is appropriate for DSM-III-R– or DSM-IV-R–defined PTSD. The CAPS-CA also is used widely and has a moderate to high Cronbach α coefficient of 0.81, 0.75, and 0.79, respectively, for re-experiencing, avoidance and numbing, and increased arousal symptom clusters.

The Children's PTSD Inventory is a structured interview that has been well validated [97,98]. Moderate to high Cronbach α coefficients (0.53–0.89) were evident on the PTSD symptom clusters, and an α coefficient of 0.95 for the diagnostic level of PTSD was reported. Inter-rater intraclass correlation co-efficients (ICC) for the clusters ranged from 0.88 to 0.96 and to 0.98 for diag-nosis. Moderate to high κ coefficients (0.65–1.00) were reported for inter-rater reliability for the clusters and 0.98 for diagnosis. In terms of test-retest reliability, a 96.5% agreement (reliability) was evident for diagnosis and moderate to high κ (0.67–1.00) and ICC (0.66–0.93) coefficients were observed for symptom clusters. A test-retest κ coefficient of 0.87 and an ICC of 0.88 was observed at the diagnostic level. The Children's PTSD Inventory was validated with the Diag-nostic Interview for Children and Adolescents-Revised (DICA-R) and SCID PTSD diagnoses, and the Revised Children's Manifest Anxiety Scale, and Child Behavior Checklist Internalizing scale [97].

The Childhood PTSD Interview is another structured interview instrument that has been validated [99]. Kuder-Richardson formula 20 coefficients of 0.52, 0.80, 0.76, and 0.78 for the PTSD stress-exposure, re-experiencing, numbing and avoidance, and increased arousal symptom clusters, respectively, have been reported. A coefficient of 0.91 has been reported for the overall PTSD scale.

The following structured interviews are used widely. They offer an advantage in that they assess the majority of comorbid mental health symptoms in children and adolescents as well as PTSD.

The PTSD module form, the CAPA, has been used widely in epidemiologic studies. It is a structured interview that can be administered by nonclini-cians to parents and to children as young as age 6 years and is appropriate for DSM-III-R– or DSM-IV-R–defined axis I disorders. Internal consistency esti-mates range from 0.75 to 0.81 for the PTSD symptom clusters [100].

The DICA-R also has been used widely in epidemiologic and clinical studies in the US and other countries [101]. It is a structured interview that can be administered by nonclinicians and is appropriate for DSM-III-R– or DSM-IV-R–

defined axis I disorders. α coefficients of 0.44, 0.87, and 0.83 for DSM-IV-R DICA-R criteria of reactivity, re-experiencing, avoidance and numbing, respectively, and increased arousal subscores with an omnibus item pool of an α coefficient of 0.94 have been reported.

The National Institute of Mental Health Diagnostic Interview Schedule for Children Version IV (NIMH DISC-IV) is a highly structured diagnostic interview that can be administered by nonclinicians [102]. The interview has moderate to good validity across a number of childhood diagnoses, is available in both English and Spanish versions, and can be given through a computer interface.

The K-SADS Present and Lifetime (-PL) version is a semistructured diagnostic instrument based on both the Present episode [103] and Epidemiologic (lifetime) (H. Orvaschel and J. Puig-Antich, unpublished manuscript, 1987) versions of the K-SADS used to determine the child's current and lifetime history of psychiatric illness. It is a semistructured interview administered by clinicians and is appropriate for DSM-III-R– or DSM-IV-R–defined axis I disorders. The K-SADS-PL has good reliability and concurrent validity and is designed for subjects 6 to 18 year olds and their parents, and it includes a comprehensive PTSD interview [104]. Published K-SADS-PL inter-rater agreement in scoring screens and diagnoses are high (range 93%–100%), test-retest reliability κ coefficients for present and lifetime disorders were in the excellent range, from .77 to 1.00 for mood, anxiety, and oppositional defiant disorders, and in the good range for PTSD and attention deficit hyperactivity disorder (0.63–0.67). This interview instrument has been used extensively in psychobiologic studies of childhood mood and anxiety disorders.

It should be noted that children may be developmentally unable to use language to describe their experiences or to talk about complex feelings. Alternative criteria to assess PTSD in young children have been developed [11]. Clinicians may administer projective or objective psychometric tests such as the Rorschach or the Minnesota Multiphasic Personality Inventory-Adolescent version to infer PTSD symptoms. Although these measures do provide some assessment of various components of PTSD, they are not in themselves diagnostic of PTSD. Because so many symptoms of PTSD overlap with other childhood disorders such as depression, ADHD, conduct or oppositional disorders, and substance abuse, it is beneficial to the child to complete a thorough evaluation to characterize their emotional, social, cognitive, and personality functioning. It is important for the clinician to determine whether the traumatic event is the precipitating cause of the problem behaviors. This may require constructing a time line of symptoms and life events [105]. The child may not meet all the criteria outlined in the DSM-IV-R; for instance, the child may avoid (deny) a particular person, place, or object but be unable to express this. This may limit the requirement of three numbering or avoidant symptoms and therefore not meet the PTSD criteria. Furthermore, other symptoms may present in accordance with or separate from one another so that the coexistence of all cluster PTSD symptoms may not actually occur. However, children with chronic adjustment disorders may require treatment. More work is needed to help the trauma field design instruments to identify clinical presentation after a trauma that are developmentally sensitive.

Neurobiology of childhood post-traumatic stress disorder

The maturation of developing biological stress response systems and the brain parallel the progressive physical, behavioral, cognitive, and emotional stages of development. Following is a review of the relevant studies.

Trauma and developing biologic stress response systems

The locus ceruleus-norepinephrine-sympathetic nervous system (SNS) or catecholamine system, the serotonin system, and the hypothalamic-pituitary-adrenal (HPA) axis are three major neurobiologic stress response systems that significantly influence arousal, stress reactions, physical and cognitive development, emotional regulation, and brain development [30]. Animal research has demonstrated that early life stress leads to alterations in the HPA axis that persist into adulthood [106,107]. This stress response is characterized by the elevation in levels of catecholamines and cortisol levels, which may adversely affect brain development [108]. Catecholamines contribute to "fight or flight," dilation of the pupils, diaphoresis, renal inhibition, and a decrease in peripheral blood flow [109]. The activation of catecholamines and corticotrophin-releasing hormone (CRH) and factor (CRF) result in animal behaviors consistent with anxiety, hyperarousal, and hypervigilance (ie, the core symptoms of PTSD) [110].

In adult PTSD, it is hypothesized that the locus ceruleus-SNS-catecholamine system and HPA axis responses to stress become maladaptive, causing long-term negative consequences [111]. Results from adult combat-related PTSD studies suggest that there is increased sensitivity of the locus ceruleus-SNS-catecholamine system, most clearly evident under experimental conditions of stress or challenge and that these biologic responses are more pronounced among PTSD-diagnosed combat veterans, compared with healthy combat or noncombat controls. However, the limited data relevant to traumatized children suggest that the locus ceruleus-SNS-catecholamine system is dysregulated in traumatized children, who may suffer from depressive and PTSD symptoms but who may or may not have a diagnosis of PTSD. These symptoms include findings of elevated 24-hour urinary catecholamine concentrations in neglected male children who have severe clinical depression [112], sexually abused girls [113], and male and female children with abuse-related PTSD [114]. Furthermore, decreased platelet α_2-adrenergic receptors and increased heart rate after an orthostatic challenge have been found in physically and sexually abused children with PTSD, suggesting an enhancement of SNS tone in childhood PTSD [115]. Depressed women with histories of child abuse evidenced autonomic hyperarousal at baseline and hypersensitivity of the HPA axis in response to a social stressor [116].

Serotonin, regarded as a master control neurotransmitter of complex neuronal communication, plays complex roles in the regulation of emotions (mood) and behavior (aggression and impulsive dysregulation) [117]. In traumatized children, the dysregulation of serotonin may play a role not only in PTSD symptom development, but it also may increase the risk for known comorbid major depression and aggression. However, little is known about serotonin regulation in traumatized children. This is an area that warrants further investigation.

The HPA axis, the major neuroendocrine stress response system, is implicated in the pathophysiology of PTSD. Elevated levels of CRH or CRF with low 24-hour urine-free cortisol concentrations have been reported consistently in adult PTSD cases [110]. However, increased cortisol levels are found typically in traumatized young and latency age children. These symptoms include elevated salivary cortisol in 6- to 12-year-old children raised in Romanian orphanages for more than 8 months of their lives, compared with early adopted and Canadian-born children 6.5 years after adoption [118], elevated 24-hour urine-free cortisol in prepubertal maltreated children with PTSD [114], and elevated salivary cortisol in traumatized children with threshold and subthreshold PTSD symptoms [119]. Further studies examining mechanisms for chronic compensatory adaptation of the HPA axis in traumatized children and its relationship to PTSD symptoms are needed.

Trauma and the developing brain

Brain development during childhood and adolescence is characterized by progressive myelination and regressive pruning processes. There is an over-production of neurons in utero and then selective elimination of many of these neurons in early childhood [120]. The total brain volume increases until approximately the age of 10 months, with approximately 75% of the adult brain weight occurring by age 2 [121]. Active periods of myelination occur during adolescence [122]. In the developing brain, elevated levels of catecholamines and cortisol may lead to adverse brain development through the mechanisms of accelerated loss (or metabolism) of neurons [123–126], delays in myelination [127], abnormalities in developmentally appropriate pruning [128,129], or the inhibition of neurogenesis [130–133]. Stress also decreases brain-derived neurotrophic factor expression [134]. Thus, the traumatic experiences may have adverse influences on a child's brain maturation. Understanding the complexities of dysregulated or hyperactive biologic stress response systems may be the key to understanding the brain development and cognitive functioning of traumatized children.

Exposure to mild to moderate uncontrollable stress has been found to impair prefrontal cortical function (eg, executive functions) in studies of humans and animals, through catecholamine and indirectly through CRF-mediated mechanisms [135,136]. The medial prefrontal cortex inhibits activation of the amygdala and limbic-related circuitry involved in fearful behaviors [137]. Thus, the medial prefrontal cortex is involved in the extinction of conditioned fear responses [137], and its dysfunction is implicated in the pathophysiology of PTSD [138]. Functional neuroimaging studies in adults with PTSD suggest that the medial prefrontal regions are hyporesponsive and that the amygdala is hyper-responsive [139–144]. However, many of the studies in adult PTSD involved radiation using positron emission tomography scanning, a technique that is not feasible in children. Magnetic resonance spectroscopy (MRS) is a safe approach to measuring neuronal integrity in children. N-acetylaspartate (NAA), considered to be a marker of neuronal health or integrity, is measured by MRS through the N-acetyl signal in the proton (1H) spectrum. Low levels of NAA are associated with neuronal damage or loss [145]. A study [146] of 11 children with maltreatment-related PTSD has suggested that maltreated children and adolescents with PTSD have lower NAA/creatine ratios compared with controls matched for age, race, socioeconomic status, and IQ level. These findings suggest specifically a loss of neuronal integrity in the anterior cingulate region of the medial prefrontal cortex and thus implicate dysfunction of the prefrontal cortex in pediatric PTSD. Other studies using cognitive instruments have demonstrated deficits on measures of frontal executive functioning in pediatric PTSD. Compared with controls, children with PTSD demonstrated deficits on card sorting and word list generation tasks, were more susceptible to distraction, showed higher rates of impulsivity, and exhibited greater problems with sustained attention [147]. Although they are based on a small number of subjects, these findings are consistent with neuroimaging studies indicating medial prefrontal dysfunction in PTSD. Similarly, general memory deficits have been reported in children with PTSD [148]. In a large-scale twin study [149], which used 1116 monozygotic and dizygotic 5-year old twin pairs, exposure to domestic violence was associated with delayed intellectual development, showing a dose-response relationship. On average, children exposed to high levels of domestic violence had IQ scores eight points lower than children who were not exposed. Child exposure to domestic violence is associated with high rates of PTSD; however, this study did not assess for PTSD. Further research is necessary to ascertain how psychiatric symptoms interact with neuropsychologic deficits. However, more pediatric studies using cognitive instruments, functional (f)MRI, and MRS are needed to understand brain function in pediatric PTSD.

Unlike findings in adult PTSD, in which several studies have reported hippocampal atrophy [125], MRI studies of maltreated children suggest that child abuse-related PTSD is associated with global adverse brain development. In one research study [108], 43 maltreated children and adolescents with PTSD and 61 matched controls underwent comprehensive clinical assessments and an anatomic MRI brain scan. Maltreated subjects with PTSD had 7.0% smaller intracranial and 8.0% smaller cerebral volumes than controls did. The total midsagittal area of corpus callosum, a major area of myelination, and the middle and posterior regions of the corpus callosum were smaller in abused subjects. In contrast, right, left, and total lateral ventricles, and prefrontal cortical cerebrospinal fluid (CSF) volumes were proportionally larger than controls were, after adjustment for intracranial volume. In another study [150], which controlled for socioeconomic status, 28 psychotropic-naïve children and adolescents with abuse-related PTSD and 66 sociodemographically similar healthy controls underwent comprehensive clinical assessments and anatomic MRI brain scans. Compared with controls, subjects with PTSD had smaller intracranial, cerebral, prefrontal cortex, prefrontal cortical white matter, and right temporal lobe volumes, and areas of the corpus callosum and its subregions, and larger frontal lobe CSF volumes than controls did. The total midsagittal area of corpus callosum and middle and posterior regions remained smaller, whereas right, left, and total lateral ventricles and frontal lobe CSF volumes were proportionately larger than in controls, after adjustment for cerebral volume. Hence, myelinated areas of the brain appear particularly susceptible to the effects of early stress. In these two studies, the finding of positive correlations of intracranial and cerebral volumes with age of onset of PTSD trauma suggest that traumatic stress is associated with disproportionately negative consequences if it occurs during early childhood. The finding of negative correlations of intracranial and cerebral volumes with trauma duration suggest that childhood maltreatment has global and adverse influences on brain development that may be cumulative. In another study [151] from a separate research group, smaller brain and cerebral volumes also were observed in traumatized children with subthreshold PTSD and threshold PTSD, compared with archival controls. Interestingly, traumatized children and adolescents with PTSD or subthreshold PTSD showed no anatomical differences in limbic (hippocampal or amygdalar) structures, either cross-sectionally [108,150,151] or longitudinally [152]. Maltreated males with PTSD may show more evidence of adverse brain development than maltreated females with PTSD [153]. These findings may suggest that males are more vulnerable to the effects of severe stress in global brain structures than females are. Interestingly, in a study of a large sample of adult survivors of child abuse who were followed from childhood in a long-term prospective study [154] of early ($\leq$11 years old) child abuse or neglect, compared with sociodemographically matched controls, maltreated males demonstrated lower levels of a comprehensive measure of resilience as adults than maltreated females, indicating that males are more vulnerable to the long-term consequences of childhood trauma.

Understanding the complexities of dysregulated or hyperactive biologic stress response systems is the key to rational psychopharmacologic therapies for traumatized children. Because dysregulated biologic stress response systems can have profound adverse effects on brain development and cortical functioning, it is extremely important to down-regulate catecholamines and cortisol by damping down the activity of the fight-or-flight reaction and its indirect limbic (amygdalar) activation. This can be done in many ways. After the safety of the traumatized child is assured, effective psychotherapy and the use of antianxiety and antidepressant medications that target specific somatic symptoms can down-regulate hyperaroused biologic stress systems. Because treatment may alleviate the adverse physiologic effects of stress on a child's brain maturation, further neuroimaging studies before and after evidence-based interventions are warranted.

Treatment approaches for childhood post-traumatic stress disorder

The best available evidence for treating child adolescent PTSD supports trauma-focused psychotherapy with cognitive-behavioral therapy (CBT) approaches (B.E. Saunders, L. Berliner, and R.F. Hanson, unpublished manuscript, 2001) [155–159]. These approaches include exposure strategies that allow: (1) trauma processing and exposure to traumatic arousal in tolerable doses so that traumatic feelings can be mastered and integrated adaptively into the child's experience; (2) establishing a coherent narrative to promote habituation of conditioned anxiety; (3) learning to cope with unpleasant affect and physiologic sensation; (4) revising maladaptive cognitive schemas; (5) correcting cognitive distortions; (6) learning stress management and relaxation skills; and (7) facilitating cognitive or narrative restructuring. These components are identified as the preferred treatment for PTSD symptoms. CBT is provided typically in a brief (10–18 sessions) treatment model. Caregiver involvement is critical for successful treatment [160]. Play therapy, traditionally developed as a nondirective psychodynamic intervention, is used currently as a tool to help foster communication of trauma-related issues [161]. Play with drawings, dolls, toys, and games also can be effective when they are used as a vehicle for communicating cognitive behavioral strategies.

Results from a recent randomized controlled trial [162] of 229 children with sexual abuse-related PTSD symptoms, age 8 to 14 years, who were assigned randomly to either trauma-focused (TF-)CBT or child-centered therapy indicated that children assigned to TF-CBT, compared with those assigned to child-centered therapy, demonstrated more improvements with regard to PTSD depression, behavioral problems, shame, and abuse-related attributions. Parents also showed similar improvements of depression, distress related to abuse, and parenting practices. Of this sample, 89% met full DSM-IV-R PTSD diagnostic criteria, and more than 90% of the children had experienced traumatic events other than sexual abuse, including loss, exposure to violence, physical abuse, and accidents. Thus TF-CBT is efficacious in children who have been exposed to multiple traumas. Variants of CBT have been successfully used in traumatized children. Eye movement desensitization and reprocessing and massage therapy, a form of relaxation therapy, has shown to decrease PTSD symptoms in children who were victims of a natural disaster [163,164]. Little is known about the brain mechanisms that mediate clinical response to CBT. Theoretical models implicate top-down prefrontal mechanisms in depression and anxiety disorders because interventions focus on modifying of cognitive distortions, affective bias, and maladaptive information processing [165]. Further work in this area is warranted.

Psychotropic treatment

Some of the most common biologic abnormalities related to PTSD are adrenergic hyperactivity, HPA axis enhanced negative feedback, neurotransmitter alterations, including dopamine, epinephrine, and opioid dysregulation, elevated CRF levels, glutaminergic dysregulation, and increased thyroid activity [166]. Psychopharmacologic treatment and psychotherapy aimed at target symptoms of PTSD criterion B, C, and D symptoms provide a rational treatment of PTSD symptoms. Pharmacotherapy attempts to address these abnormalities by treating their corresponding symptoms were shown to be efficacious with adults and children. Recent studies show strong support for the efficacy of the serotonin reuptake inhibitor antidepressant and antiobsessive compulsive disorder medications, sertraline [167] and fluoxetine [168] in adult PTSD. Selective serotonin reuptake inhibitors (SSRI) have been found to be effective in treating overall PTSD symptoms and particularly effective with treatment trials of at least 8 weeks [169,170]. Antidepressants and antianxiety medications are used to decrease both avoidant and dissociative behavior. α agonists have been found to be effective for hyperarousal symptoms (ie, criterion D symptoms) [170].

However, it must be noted that there are few psychopharmacologic studies of PTSD in traumatized children. To date, there has been just one randomized double blind study [171] of the treatment with acutely traumatized children and adolescents. In this study, 25 children age 2 to 19 years old who were thermally injured and suffered ASD symptoms were studied prospectively for 1 week. Symptoms most commonly observed were re-experiencing the trauma, hyperarousal, and associated mood symptoms. No one symptom was more prevalent than another, and participants experienced between three and 11 total symptoms. Ten of the 12 (83%) children on a low dose of imipramine (1 mg/kg) versus five of 13 (38%) of the children administered chloral hydrate demonstrated remitting symptoms of ASD. Pharmacologic therapy was continued for 6 months with no rebound of ASD symptoms when they began to be weaned from the medication. Although it appears that imipramine is effective in treating ASD and PTSD, it also is associated with safety and cost issues. The authors pointed out that future studies may use less cardiotoxic medications such as fluoxetine or clonidine. Furthermore, methodologic limitations that restrict the applicability of the results include a small sample size and a large range of ages. In another study [172] conducted in 24 child burn patients, ages 6 to 16 years old, the relationship of morphine dose correlated with a decrease of PTSD symptoms based on a PTSD change score over a 6-month period. This reduction in symptoms remained after controlling for body surface area burned, children's report of pain, and length of hospital stay and suggest that the mechanism of action of morphine is on fear conditioning and memory consolidation. That is, morphine may have reduced the hyperadrenergic state by inhibiting the locus ceruleus and thus diminished fear conditioning by attenuating norepinephrine turnover in the amygdala. In an open trial [173], propranolol, a peripheral adrenergic blocker, was effective (up to 2.5 mg/kg) in decreasing PTSD symptoms in 11 sexually or physically abused children with PTSD. An open trial [174] of clonidine, a central α_2-adrenergic partial agonist, which dampens catecholamine transmission centrally by decreasing the activity of the locus ceruleus, reduced PTSD symptoms in seven maltreated children, ages 3 to 6 years old. Guanfacine, a longer acting and more selective central α_2-adrenergic partial agonist was found to be effective in decreasing nightmares in a single case study of a 7-year-old child [175]. In a case report [176], a maltreated boy with PTSD was followed prospectively using single voxel proton MRS measures of anterior cingulate N-acetylaspartate (NAA)/creatine ratios, a marker of neural integrity. Clonidine treatment was associated with NAA/creatine ratio increase and improvement in sleep measures on symptom remission, indicating that clonidine may improve anterior cingulate functioning and alleviate PTSD symptoms by removing the stress-mediated inhibition on the rate of anterior cingulate neurogenesis. Another study [177] compared outcomes in an 8-week open trial of citalopram, an SSRI, in children and adolescents as well as adults who had a diagnosis of PTSD. Twenty four children and adolescents, ages 10 to 18 years old, and 14 adults assessed for PTSD severity at baseline and every 2 weeks thereafter for 8 weeks. Children and adolescents demonstrated a greater reduction (54%) than adults (39%) did in CAPS-CA total scores between baseline and follow-up. Also, children and adolescents showed significant improvement in hyperarousal symptoms but not re-experiencing and avoidance symptoms, compared with adults. Unique to this study is that it examined 18 children who had delayed onset PTSD and six with acute PTSD. Overall, citalopram was found to decrease PTSD symptoms in children and adolescents equally as well as in adults.

A result of a survey found that 95% of the respondents prescribed medication for those diagnosed with PTSD despite not having any completed randomized controlled trials of psychotropic medications [178]. Overall, psychopharmacologic treatments should not be considered the primary or sole intervention for pediatric PTSD. More research on this issue is needed, making it an attractive area for future work.

Summary

There has been increasing research on PTSD in children over the past 20 years. What used to be thought of as a disorder associated primarily with combat soldiers has now made its way into mainstream society with the increased realization that no one is immune to its possible effects, especially children. Because of the interaction between trauma and development, children are particularly vulnerable to traumatic events. Although in the last 10 years there has been a proliferation of research on the biologic underpinnings of trauma exposure in children, little is understood about the risk or protective factors in children's response to trauma. Although trauma exposure may affect neurodevelopment, there has been little development in the way of diagnostic criteria, assessment, and treatment interventions that reflect this knowledge. More work is needed in the development of empirically based treatment interventions. Studies of pharmacologic treatments using well-developed, randomized, controlled clinical trials are needed to guide practitioners. Finally, the current research has implications for policy development. Policies that focus on a proactive rather than reactive approach would better serve child trauma victims. Because brain development is integrally related to environmental factors, active early intervention offers the greatest hope. Such an approach, coupled with the fact that children tend to strive toward growth, would be effective in addressing the devastating consequences of early trauma that may last well beyond the period of exposure.

References

[1] Birmes P, Hatton L, Brunet A, et al. Early historical literature for post-traumatic symptomatology. Stress & Health 2003;19:17–26.
[2] Van der Kolk BA, Weisaeth L, Van der Hart O. History of trauma in psychiatry. In: Van der Kolk BA, McFarlane AC, Weisaeth L, editors. Traumatic stress. New York: Guildford Press; 1996. p. 47–74.
[3] American Psychiatric Association. Diagnostic and statistical manual of mental disorders. 4th edition, revised. Washington (DC): American Psychiatric Association; 2000. p. 424–32.
[4] Keane TM, Barlow DH. Posttraumatic disorder. In: Barlow DH, editor. Anxiety and its disorders: the nature and treatment of anxiety and panic, Volume 2. New York: Guilford Press; 2002. p. 418–53.
[5] Weems CF, Silverman WK, La Greca AM. What do youth referred for anxiety problems worry about? worry and its relation to anxiety and anxiety disorders in children and adolescents. J Abnorm Child Psychol 2000;28(1):63–72.
[6] Lonigan CJ, Anthony JL, Shannon MP. Diagnostic efficacy of posttraumatic symptoms in children exposed to disaster. J Clin Child Psychol 1998;27(3):255–67.
[7] Pynoos RS, Eth S, editors. Witnessing acts of personal violence. Washington (DC): American Psychiatric Press; 1985.
[8] Lavigne JV, Gibbons RD, Christoffel KK, et al. Prevalence rates and correlates of psychiatric disorders among preschool children. J Am Acad Child Adolesc Psychiatry 1996;35:204–14.
[9] Cuffe SP, Addy CL, Garrison CZ, et al. Prevalence of PTSD in a community sample of older adolescents. J Am Acad Child Adolesc Psychiatry 1998;37:147–54.
[10] Reinherz HZ, Giaconia RM, Lefkowitz ES, et al. Prevalence of psychiatric disorders in a community population of older adolescents. J Am Acad Child Adolesc Psychiatry 1993;32: 369–77.
[11] Scheeringa MS, Zeanah CH, Drell MJ, et al. Two approaches to the diagnosis of posttraumatic stress disorder in infancy and early childhood. J Am Acad Child Adolesc Psychiatry 1995;34: 191–200.
[12] Scheeringa MS, Zeanah CH, Myers L, et al. New findings on alternative criteria for PTSD in preschool children. J Am Acad Child Adolesc Psychiatry 2003;42:561–70.
[13] Blank AS. The longitudinal course of posttraumatic stress disorder. In: Davidson JRT, Foa EB, editors. Posttraumatic stress disorder DSM-IV and beyond. Washington (DC): American Psychiatric Press; 1993. p. 3–22.
[14] Carrion VG, Weems CF, Ray RD, et al. Toward an empirical definition of pediatric PTSD: the phenomenology of PTSD symptoms in youth. J Am Acad Child Adolesc Psychiatry 2001;41:166–73.
[15] Koopman C, Classen C, Cardena E, et al. When disaster strikes, acute stress disorder may follow. J Trauma Stress 1995;8(1):29–46.
[16] Putnam FW. Dissociation in children and adolescents: a developmental perspective. New York: Guilford Press; 1997.
[17] Bryant RA, Harvey AG. A prospective study of psychophysiological arousal, acute stress disorder, and posttraumatic stress disorder. J Abnorm Psychol 2000;109(2):341–4.
[18] Brewin CR, Andrews B, Rose S, et al. Acute stress disorder and posttraumatic stress disorder in victims of violent crime. Am J Psychiatry 1999;156:360–6.

[19] Daviss WB, Mooney D, Racusin R, et al. Predicting posttraumatic stress after hospitalization for pediatric injury. J Am Acad Child Adolesc Psychiatry 2000;39:576–83.

[20] Harvey AG, Bryant RA. Memory for acute stress disorder symptoms: a two-year prospective study. J Nerv Ment Dis 2000;188(9):602–7.

[21] Harvey AG, Bryant RA. The relationship between acute stress disorder and posttraumatic stress disorder: a 2 year prospective evaluation. J Consult Clin Psychol 1999;67:985–8.

[22] Kassam-Adams N, Winston FK. Predicting child PTSD: the relationship between acute stress disorder and PTSD in injured children. J Am Acad Child Adolesc Psychiatry 2004;43(4):403–11.

[23] Fein J, Kassam-Adams N, Gavin M, et al. Persistence of posttraumatic stress in violently injured youth seen in the emergency department. Arch Pediatr Adolesc Med 2002;156:836–40.

[24] Harvey AG, Bryant RA. Acute stress disorder: a synthesis and critique. Psychol Bull 2002; 128(6):886–902.

[25] March JS. Acute stress disorder in youth: a multivariate prediction model. Biol Psychiatry 2003;53:809–16.

[26] Kessler RC, Sonnega A, Bromet E, et al. Posttraumatic stress disorder in the national comorbidity survey. Arch Gen Psychiatry 1995;52:1048–60.

[27] Pynoos RS, Steinberg AM, Wraith R. A developmental model of childhood traumatic stress. In: Cicchetti D, Cohen DJ, editors. Developmental psychopathology, Volume 2. New York: John Wiley & Sons, Inc.; 1995. p. 72–95.

[28] March JS, Amaya-Jackson L, Terry R, et al. Posttraumatic symptomatology in children and adolescents after an industrial fire. J Am Acad Child Adolesc Psychiatry 1997;36(8):1080–8.

[29] De Bellis MD. Developmental traumatology: a contributory mechanism for alcohol and substance use disorders. Psychoneuroendocrinology 2002;27:155–70.

[30] De Bellis MD. Developmental traumatology: the psychobiological development of maltreated children and its implications for research, treatment, and policy. Dev Psychopathol 2001; 13:537–61.

[31] Fletcher KE. Childhood posttraumatic stress disorder. In: Mash EJ, Barkley RA, editors. Child psychopathology. New York: Guilford Press; 1996. p. 242–76.

[32] Hamblen J. PTSD in children and adolescents. Department of Veterans Affairs National Center for Post Traumatic Stress Disorder. Available at: http://www.ncptsd.org/facts/specific/fs_children.html. Accessed November 2004.

[33] Costello EJ, Erkanli A, Fairbank JA, et al. The prevalence of potentially traumatic events in childhood and adolescence. J Trauma Stress 2002;15:99–112.

[34] Giaconia RM, Reinherz HZ, Silverman AB, et al. Trauma and posttraumatic stress disorder in a community population of older adolescents. J Am Acad Child Adolesc Psychiatry 1995;34: 1369–80.

[35] Kilpatrick DG, Saunders BE. Prevalence and consequences of child victimization: results from the National Survey of Adolescents. Washington (DC): National Institute of Justice; 1999.

[36] Vogel JM, Vernberg EM. Children's psychological responses to disasters. J Clin Child Psychol 1993;22:464–84.

[37] Green B, Grace M, Lindy J, et al. Buffalo Creek survivors in the second decade: comparison with unexposed and nonlitigant groups. J Appl Soc Psychol 1990;20:1033–50.

[38] La Greca AM, Silverman WK, Vernberg EM, et al. Symptoms of posttraumatic stress in children after Hurricane Andrew: a prospective study. J Consult Clin Psychol 1996;66:883–92.

[39] Shaw JA, Applegate B, Schorr C. Twenty-one month follow up study of school-age children exposed to Hurricane Andrew. J Am Acad Child Adolesc Psychiatry 1996;35:359–64.

[40] Garrison CZ, Weinrich MW, Hardin SB, et al. Posttraumatic stress disorder in adolescents after a hurricane. Am J Epidemiol 1993;138:522–30.

[41] Goenjian AK, Molina L, Steinberg AM, et al. Posttraumatic stress and depressive reactions among Nicaraguan adolescents after hurricane Mitch. Am J Psychiatry 2001;158:788–94.

[42] Pynoos RS, Goenjian A, Tashjian M, et al. Post-traumatic stress reactions in children after the 1988 Armenian earthquake. Br J Psychiatry 1993;163:239–47.

[43] Goenjian AK, Pynoos RS, Steinberg AM, et al. Psychiatric comorbidity in children after the 1988 earthquake in Armenia. J Am Acad Child Adolesc Psychiatry 1995;34(9):1174–84.

[44] Tribe O, Moro MR, Barbet T, et al. Posttraumatic stress symptoms after childhood cancer. Eur Child Adolesc Psychiatry 2003;12:255–64.

[45] Pelcovitz D, Libov BG, Mandel F, et al. Post-traumatic stress disorder and family functioning in adolescent cancer. J Trauma Stress 1998;11:205–11.

[46] Hobbie WL, Stuber M, Meeske K, et al. Symptoms of posttraumatic stress in young adult survivors of childhood cancer. J Clin Oncol 2000;18:4060–6.

[47] Meeske KA, Ruccione K, Globe DR, et al. Posttraumatic stress, quality of life and psychological distress in young adult survivors of childhood cancer. Oncol Nurs Forum 2001; 28:481–9.

[48] Houtzager BA, Grootenhuis MA, Last BF. Supportive groups for siblings of pediatric oncology patients: impact on anxiety. Psychooncology 2001;10:315–24.

[49] Spinetta JJ, Jankovic M, Eden T, et al. Guidelines for assistance to siblings of children with cancer: report of the SIOP working committee on psychosocial issues. Med Pediatr Oncol 1999; 33:395–8.

[50] Murray JS. Siblings of children with cancer: a review of the literature. J Pediatr Oncol Nurs 2000;16:25–34.

[51] Packman WL, Crittenden MR, Schaeffer E, et al. Psychological consequences of bone marrow transplantation in donor and nondonor siblings. J Dev Behav Pediatr 1997;18:244–53.

[52] Barenbaum J, Ruchkin V, Schwab-Stone M. The psychosocial aspects of children exposed to war: practice and policy initiatives. J Child Psychol Psychiatry 2004;45:41–62.

[53] Allwood MA, Bell-Dolan D, Husain SA. Children's trauma and adjustment reactions to violent and nonviolent war experiences. J Am Acad Child Adolesc Psychiatry 2002;41:450–7.

[54] Thabet AA, Vostanis P. Post traumatic stress disorder reactions in children of war: a longitudinal study. Child Abuse Negl 2000;24:291–8.

[55] Sack WH, Him C, Dickason D. Twelve year follow up of Khmer youths who suffered massive war trauma as children. J Am Acad Child Adolesc Psychiatry 1999;39:1173–9.

[56] Macksoud MS, Aber JL. The war experiences and psychosocial development of children in Lebanon, Child Dev 1996;67:70–88.

[57] Fremont WP. Childhood reactions to terrorism-induced trauma: a review of the past 10 years. J Am Acad Child Adolesc Psychiatry 2004;43:381–92.

[58] Laor N, Wolmer L, Mayes LC, et al. Israeli preschool children under SCUDs: a 30-month follow-up. J Am Acad Child Adolesc Psychiatry 1997;36:349–56.

[59] Laor N, Wolmer L, Cohen DJ. Mothers' functioning and children's symptoms 5 years after a SCUD missile attack. Am J Psychiatry 2001;158:1020–6.

[60] Pfefferbaum B, Nixon S, Tucker P. Posttraumatic stress response in bereaved children after Oklahoma City bombing. J Am Acad Child Adolesc Psychiatry 1999;38:1372–9.

[61] Sack WH, McSharry S, Clarke GN, et al. The Khmer adolescent project: I. epidemiologic findings in two generations of Cambodian refugees. J Nerv Ment Dis 1994;182:387–95.

[62] Wooding S, Raphael B. Psychological impact of disasters and terrorism on children and adolescents: experiences from Australia. Prehospital Disaster Med 2004;19:10–20.

[63] Halpern-Felcher BL, Millstein SL. The effects of terrorism on teens' perceptions of dying: the new world is riskier than ever. J Adolesc Health 2002;30:308–11.

[64] Gurwitch RH, Kees M, Becker SM. In the face of tragedy: placing children's reactions to trauma in a new context. Cognitive & Behavioral Practice 2002;9:286–95.

[65] Pfefferbaum B, Nixon S, Tivis R, et al. Television exposure in children after a terrorist incident. Psychiatry 2001;64:202–11.

[66] Pfefferbaum B, Seale T, McDonald N, et al. Posttraumatic stress two years after the Oklahoma City bombing in youths geographically distant from the explosion. Psychiatry 2000;63: 358–70.

[67] Schlenger WE, Caddell JM, et al. Psychological reactions to terrorist attacks: findings from the National Study of Americans' Reactions to September 11. JAMA 2002;288:581–8.

[68] Saunders BE, Kilpatrick DG, Hanson RF, et al. Prevalence, case characteristics, and long-term psychological correlates of child rape among women: a national survey. Child Maltreat 1999; 4:187–200.

[69] Boney-McCoy S, Finkelhor D. Psychological sequelae of violent victimization in a youth sample. J Consult Clin Psychol 1995;63:726–36.

[70] McCloskey LA, Figueredo AJ, et al. The effects of systemic family violence on children's mental health. Child Dev 1995;66:1239–61.

[71] Graham-Bermann SA, Levendosky AA. Traumatic stress symptoms in children of battered women. J Interpers Violence 1998;13:111–28.

[72] McCloskey LA, Walker M. Posttraumatic stress in children exposed to family violence and single-event trauma. J Am Acad Child Adolesc Psychiatry 2000;39:108–15.

[73] Chemtob CM, Carlson JG. Psychological effects of domestic violence on children and their mothers. International Journal of Stress Management 2004;11:209–26.

[74] Tijima EA. Risk factors for violence against children: comparing homes with and without wife abuse. J Interpers Violence 2002;12:122–49.

[75] Dubner AE, Motta RW. Sexually and physically abused foster care children and posttraumatic stress disorder. J Consult Clin Psychol 1999;67:367–73.

[76] Lipschitz DS, Winegar RK, Hartnick E, et al. Posttraumatic stress disorder in hospitalized adolescents: psychiatric comorbidity and clinical correlates. J Am Acad Child Adolesc Psychiatry 1999;38:385–92.

[77] McLeer SV, Callaghan M, Henry D, et al. Psychiatric disorders in sexually abused children. J Am Acad Child Adolesc Psychiatry 1994;33:313–9.

[78] Pynoos RS, Nader K. Children's memory and proximity to violence. J Am Acad Child Adolesc Psychiatry 1989;28:236–41.

[79] Famularo R, Fenton T, Kinscherff R. Child maltreatment and the development of post traumatic stress disorder. Am J Dis Child 1993;147:755–60.

[80] Famularo R, Fenton T, Augustyn M, et al. Persistence of pediatric post traumatic stress disorder after 2 years. Child Abuse Negl 1996;20:1245–8.

[81] McLeer SV, Dixon JF, Henry D, et al. Psychopathology in non-clinically referred sexually abused children. J Am Acad Child Adolesc Psychiatry 1998;37:1326–33.

[82] Lyon TD. Are battered women bad mothers? Rethinking the termination of abused women's parental rights for failure to protect. In: Dubowitz H, editor. Neglected children: research, practice, and policy. Thousand Oaks (CA): Sage Publications, Ltd.; 1999. p. 237–60.

[83] Widom CS. Posttraumatic stress disorder in abused and neglected children growing up. Am J Psychiatry 1999;156:1223–9.

[84] Armsworth MW, Holaday M. The effects of psychological trauma on children and adolescents. J Couns Dev 1993;72:49–56.

[85] Mannarino AP, Cohen JA, Berman SR. The relationship between preabuse factors and psychological symptomatology in sexually abused girls. Child Abuse Negl 1994;18:63–71.

[86] Wolfe DA, Sas L, Wekerle C. Factors associated with the development of posttraumatic stress disorder among victims of sexual abuse. Child Abuse Negl 1994;18:37–50.

[87] Wolfe J, Charney DS. Use of neuropsychological assessment in posttraumatic stress disorder: psychological assessment. J Consult Clin Psychol 1991;3:573–80.

[88] Hillary BE, Schare ML. Sexually and physically abused adolescents: an empirical search for PTSD. J Clin Psychol 1993;49:161–5.

[89] Davidson JRT, Fairbank JA. The epidemiology of posttraumatic stress disorder. In: Davidson JRT, Foa EB, editors. Posttraumatic stress disorder DSM-IV and beyond. Washington (DC): American Psychiatric Press; 1993. p. 147–69.

[90] True WR, Rice J, Eisen SA, et al. A twin study of genetic and environmental contributions to liability for posttraumatic stress symptoms. Arch Gen Psychiatry 1993;50:257–64.

[91] Kendler KS, Bulik CM, Silberg J, et al. Childhood sexual abuse and adult psychiatric and substance use disorders in women: an epidemiological and cotwin control study. Arch Gen Psychiatry 2000;57:953–9.

[92] Pynoos RS, Nader K. Mental health disturbances in children exposed to disaster: prevention intervention strategies. In: Goldston S, Yager J, Heinicke C, et al, editors. Preventing mental health disturbances in childhood. Washington (DC): American Psychiatric Press; 1990. p. 211–33.

[93] Loeber R, Green SM, Lahey BB. Mental health professionals' perception of the utility of children, mothers, and teachers as informants on childhood psychopathology. J Clin Child Psychol 1990;19(2):136–43.

[94] Kendall-Tackett KA, Williams LM, Finkelhor D. Impact of sexual abuse on children: a review and synthesis of recent empirical studies. Psychol Bull 1993;113(1):164–80.

[95] Steinberg AM, Brymer MJ, Decker KB, et al. The University of California at Los Angeles post-traumatic stress disorder reaction index. Curr Psychiatry Rep 2004;6:1–5.

[96] Newman E, Ribbe D. Psychometric review of the clinician administered PTSD scale for children. In: Stamm BH, editor. Measurement of stress, trauma, and adaptation. Lutherville (MD): Sidran Press; 1996. p. 106–14.

[97] Yasik AE, Saigh PA, Oberfield RA, et al. The validity of the children's PTSD inventory. J Trauma Stress 2001;14(1):81–94.

[98] Saigh PA, Yasik AE, Oberfield RA, et al. The childrens' PTSD inventory development and reliability. J Trauma Stress 2000;13(3):369–80.

[99] Fletcher K. Childhood PTSD interview-child form. In: Carlson E, editor. Trauma assessments: a clinician's guide. New York: Guilford Press; 1997. p. 248–50.

[100] Costello EJ, Angold A, March J, et al. Life events and post-traumatic stress: the development of a new measure for children and adolescents. Psychol Med 1998;28:1275–88.

[101] Reich W, Leacock N, Shanfeld C. Diagnostic interview for children and adolescents-revised (DICA-R). St. Louis (MO): Washington University; 1994.

[102] Shaffer D, Fisher P, Lucas CP, et al. NIMH diagnostic interview schedule for children version IV (NIMH DISC-IV): description, differences from previous versions, and reliability of some common diagnoses. J Am Acad Child Adolesc Psychiatry 2000;39:28–38.

[103] Chambers WJ, Puig-Antich J, Hirsch M, et al. The assessment of affective disorders in children and adolescents by semi-structured interview: test-retest reliability of the schedule for affective disorders and schizophrenia for school-age children, present episode version. Arch Gen Psychiatry 1985;42:696–702.

[104] Kaufman J, Birmaher B, Brent D, et al. Schedule for affective disorders and schizophrenia for school-age children-present and lifetime version (K-SADS-PL): initial reliability and validity data. J Am Acad Child Adolesc Psychiatry 1997;36:980–8.

[105] De Bellis MD. Posttraumatic stress disorder and acute stress disorder. In: Ammerman RT, Hersen M, editors. Handbook of prevention and treatment with children and adolescents. New York: John Wiley & Sons, Inc.; 1997. p. 455–94.

[106] McEwen B. The neurobiology of stress: from serendipity to clinical relevance. Brain Res 2000; 886(1–2):172–89.

[107] Meaney M. Maternal care, gene expression, and the transmission of individual differences in stress reactivity across generations. Annu Rev Neurosci 2001;24:1161–92.

[108] De Bellis MD, Keshavan M, Clark DB, et al. A.E. Bennett research award. developmental traumatology: II: brain development. Biol Psychiatry 1999;45:1271–84.

[109] Murburg MM, Ashleigh EA, Hommer DW, et al. Biology of catecholaminergic systems and their relevance to PTSD. In: Murburg MM, editor. Catecholamine function in posttraumatic stress disorder: emerging concepts. Washington (DC): American Psychiatric Press; 1994. p. 3–15.

[110] Southwick SS, Yehuda R, Wang S. Neuroendocrine alterations in posttraumatic stress disorder. Psychiatr Ann 1998;28:436–42.

[111] Southwick SM, Yehuda R, Morgan CA. Clinical studies of neurotransmitter alterations in post-traumatic stress disorder. In: Friedman MJ, Charney DS, Deutch AY, editors. Neurobiological and clinical consequences of stress: from normal adaptation to post-traumatic stress disorder. Philadelphia: Lippincott-Raven; 1995. p. 335–49.

[112] Queiroz EA, Lombardi AB, Santos Furtado CRH, et al. Biochemical correlate of depression in children. Arq Neuropsiquiatr 1991;49(4):418–25.

[113] De Bellis MD, Lefter L, Trickett PK, et al. Urinary catecholamine excretion in sexually abused girls. J Am Acad of Child and Adol Psych 1994;33:320–7.

[114] De Bellis MD, Baum A, Birmaher B, et al. A.E. Bennett Research Award developmental traumatology: I: biological stress systems. Biol Psychiatry 1999;45:1259–70.

[115] Perry BD, editor. Neurobiological sequelae of childhood trauma: PTSD in children. Washington (DC): American Psychiatric Press, Inc.; 1994.

[116] Heim C, Newport DJ, Heit S, et al. Pituitary-adrenal and autonomic responses to stress in women after sexual and physical abuse in childhood. JAMA 2000;284:592–7.

[117] Lesch KP, Moessner R. Genetically driven variation in serotonin update: is there a link to affective spectrum, neurodevelopmental and neurodegenerative disorders? Biol Psychiatry 1998;44:179–92.

[118] Gunnar MR, Morison SJ, Chisholm K, et al. Salivary cortisol levels in children adopted from Romanian orphanages. Dev Psychopathol 2001;13:611–28.

[119] Carrion VG, Weems CF, Ray RD, et al. Diurnal salivary cortisol in pediatric posttraumatic stress disorder. Biol Psychiatry 2002;51:575–82.

[120] Sowell ER, Trauner DA, Gamst A, et al. Development of cortical and subcortical brain structures in childhood and adolescence: a structural MRI study. Dev Med Child Neurol 2002; 44:4–16.

[121] Spreen O, Risser AH, Edgell D. Developmental neuropsychology. New York: Oxford University Press, Inc.; 1995.

[122] Paus T, Collins DL, Evans AC, et al. Maturation of white matter in the human brain: a review of magnetic resonance studies. Brain Res Bull 2001;54:255–66.

[123] Smythies JR. Oxidative reactions and schizophrenia: a review-discussion. Schizophr Res 1997;24:357–64.

[124] Simantov R, Blinder E, Ratovitski T, et al. Dopamine induced apoptosis in human neuronal cells: inhibition by nucleic acids antisense to the dopamine transporter. Neuroscience 1996;74: 39–50.

[125] Sapolsky RM. Glucocorticoids and hippocampal atrophy in neuropsychiatric disorders. Arch Gen Psychiatry 2000;57:925–35.

[126] Edwards E, Harkins K, Wright G, et al. Effects of bilateral adrenalectomy on the induction of learned helplessness. Neuropsychopharmacology 1990;3:109–14.

[127] Dunlop SA, Archer MA, Quinlivan JA, et al. Repeated prenatal corticosteroids delay myelination in the ovine central nervous system. J Matern Fetal Neonatal Med 1997;6:309–13.

[128] Todd RD. Neural development is regulated by classical neuro-transmitters: dopamine D2 receptor stimulation enhances neurite outgrowth. Biol Psychiatry 1992;31:794–807.

[129] Lauder JM. Neurotransmitters as morphogens. Prog Brain Res 1988;73:365–88.

[130] Tanapat P, Galea LA, Gould E. Stress inhibits the proliferation of granule cell precursors in the developing dentate gyrus. Int J Dev Neurosci 1998;16:235–9.

[131] Gould E, McEwen BS, Tanapat P, et al. Neurogenesis in the dentate gyrus of the adult tree shrew is regulated by psychosocial stress and NMDA receptor activation. J Neurosci 1997;17: 2492–8.

[132] Gould E, Tanapat P, Cameron HA. Adrenal steroids suppress granule cell death in the developing dentate gyrus through an NMDA receptor-dependent mechanism. Brain Res Dev Brain Res 1997;103:91–3.

[133] Gould E, Tanapat P, McEwen BS, et al. Proliferation of granule cell precursors in the dentate gyrus of adult monkeys is diminished by stress. Proc Natl Acad Sci U S A 1998;95:3168–71.

[134] Smith MA, Makino S, Kvetnansky R, et al. Effects of stress on neurotrophic factor expression in the rat brain. Ann N Y Acad Sci 1995;771:234–9.

[135] Arnsten AFT. The biology of being frazzled. Science 1998;280(5370):1711–2.

[136] Arnsten AFT, Goldman-Rakic PS. Noise stress impairs cortical function: evidence for a hyperdopaminergic mechanism. Arch Gen Psychiatry 1998;55:362–8.

[137] LeDoux J. Fear and the brain: where have we been, and where are we going? Biol Psychiatry 1998;44:1229–38.

[138] Hamner MB, Lorberbaum JP, George MS. Potential role of the anterior cingulate cortex in PTSD: review and hypothesis. Depress Anxiety 1999;9:1–14.

[139] Bremner JD, Narayan M, Staib L, et al. Neural correlates of memories of childhood sexual abuse in women with and without posttraumatic stress disorder. Am J Psychiatry 1999; 156:1787–95.

[140] Bremner JD, Staib L, Kaloupek D, et al. Neural correlates of exposure to traumatic pictures and sound in Vietnam combat veterans with and without posttraumatic stress disorder: a positron emission tomography study. Biol Psychiatry 1999;45:806–16.

[141] Lanius RA, Williamson PC, Boksman K, et al. Brain activation during script-driven imagery induced dissociative responses in PTSD: a functional magnetic resonance imaging investigation. Biol Psychiatry 2002;52:305–11.

[142] Shin LM, McNally RJ, Kosslyn SM, et al. Regional cerebral blood flow during script-imagery in childhood sexual abuse-related PTSD: a PET investigation. Am J Psychiatry 1999;156: 575–84.

[143] Shin LM, Orr SP, Carson MA, et al. Regional cerebral blood flow in the amygdala and medial prefrontal cortex during traumatic imagery in male and female Vietnam veterans with PTSD. Arch Gen Psychiatry 2004;61:168–76.

[144] Shin LM, Whalen PJ, Pitman RK, et al. An fMRI study of anterior cingulate function in posttraumatic stress disorder. Biol Psychiatry 2001;50:932–42.

[145] Prichard JW. MRS of the brain-prospects for clinical application. In: Young IR, Charles HC, editors. MR spectroscopy: clinical applications and techniques. London: The Livery House; 1996. p. 1–25.

[146] De Bellis MD, Keshavan MS, Spencer S, et al. N-acetylaspartate concentration in the anterior cingulate in maltreated children and adolescents with PTSD. Am J Psychiatry 2000;157: 1175–7.

[147] Beers SR, De Bellis MD. Neuropsychological function in children with maltreatment-related posttraumatic stress disorder. Am J Psychiatry 2002;159:483–6.

[148] Moradi AR, Doost HTN, Taghavi MR, et al. Everyday memory deficits in children and adolescents with PTSD: performance on the Rivermead behavioral memory test. J Child Psychol Psychiatry 1999;40:357–61.

[149] Koenen KC, Moffitt TE, Caspi A, et al. Domestic violence is associated with environmental suppression of IQ in young children. Dev Psychopathol 2003;15:297–311.

[150] De Bellis MD, Keshavan M, Shifflett H, et al. Brain structures in pediatric maltreatment-related ptsd: a sociodemographically matched study. Biol Psychiatry 2002;51:544–52.

[151] Carrion VG, Weems CF, Eliez S, et al. Attenuation of frontal asymmetry in pediatric posttraumatic stress disorder. Biol Psychiatry 2001;50:943–51.

[152] De Bellis MD, Hall J, Boring AM, et al. A pilot longitudinal study of hippocampal volumes in pediatric maltreatment-related posttraumatic stress disorder. Biol Psychiatry 2001;50:305–9.

[153] De Bellis MD, Keshavan MS. Sex differences in brain maturation in maltreatment-related pediatric posttraumatic stress disorder [special issue: brain development, sex differences, and stress: implications for psychopathology]. Neurosci Biobehav Rev 2003;27:103–17.

[154] McGloin JM, Widom CS. Resilience among abused and neglected children grown up. Dev Psychopathol 2001;13:1021–38.

[155] Deblinger E, Helfin AH. Cognitive behavioral interventions for treating sexually abused children. Thousand Oaks (CA): Sage Publications; 1996.

[156] Cohen JA for the work group on quality issues. Practice parameters for the assessment and treatment of children and adolescents with posttraumatic stress disorder. J Am Acad Child Adolesc Psychiatry 1998;37(Suppl 10):S4–26.

[157] Saigh PA. The behavioral treatment of child and adolescent posttraumatic stress disorder. Advances in Behavioral Research and Therapy 1992;14:247–75.

[158] March JS, Amaya-Jackson J, Murray MC, et al. Cognitive-behavioral psychotherapy for children and adolescents with posttraumatic stress disorder after a single-incident stressor. J Am Acad Child Adolesc Psychiatry 1998;37:585–93.

[159] Kolko DJ. Individual cognitive behavioral therapy and family therapy for physically abused children and their offending parents: a comparison of clinical outcomes. Child Maltreat 1996; 1:322–42.

[160] Cohen JA, Mannarino AP. Factors that mediate treatment outcome of sexually abused preschool children: six- and 12-month follow-up. J Am Acad Child Adolesc Psychiatry 1998;37:44–51.

[161] Gil E. The healing power of play. New York: Guilford Press; 1991.

[162] Cohen JA, Deblinger E, Mannarino AP, et al. A multisite, randomized controlled trial for children with sexual abuse-related PTSD symptoms. J Am Acad Child Adolesc Psychiatry 2004;43:393–402.

[163] Field T, Seligman S, Scafedi F, et al. Alleviating posttraumatic stress in children following Hurricane Andrew. J Appl Dev Psychol 1996;17:37–50.

[164] Chemtob CM, Narkashima JP, Hamada RS. Psychosocial intervention for postdisaster trauma symptoms in elementary school children. Arch Pediatr Adolesc Med 2002;156:211–6.

[165] Clark D, Beck AT, Afford B. Scientific foundations of cognitive theory and therapy of depression. New York: John Wiley & Sons; 1999.

[166] Cohen JA, Perel JM, DeBellis MD, et al. Treating traumatized children: clinical implications of the psychobiology of PTSD. Trauma Violence Abuse 2001;3(2):91–108.

[167] Brady K, Pearlstein T, Asnis GM, et al. Efficacy and safety of sertraline treatment of posttraumatic stress disorder: a randomized controlled trial. JAMA 2000;283:1837–44.

[168] van der Kolk BA, Dreyfuss D, Michaels M, et al. Fluoxetine in posttraumatic stress disorder. J Clin Psychiatry 1994;55:517–22.

[169] Sutherland SM, Davidson JRT. Pharmacotherapy for post-traumatic stress disorder. Psychiatr Clin North Am 1994;17(2):409–23.

[170] Taylor TL, Chemtob CM. Efficacy of treatment for child and adolescent traumatic stress. Arch Pediatr Adolesc Med 2004;158:786–91.

[171] Robert R, Blakeney PE, Villarreal C, et al. Imipramine treatment in pediatric burn patients with symptoms of acute stress disorder: a pilot study. J Am Acad Child Adolesc Psychiatry 1999;38:873–82.

[172] Saxe G, Stoddard F, Courtney D, et al. Relationship between acute morphine and the course of PTSD in children with burns. J Am Acad Child Adolesc Psychiatry 2001;40:915–21.

[173] Famularo R, Kinsherff R, Fenton T. Propranolol treatment for childhood posttraumatic stress disorder, acute type. Am J Dis Child 1988;142:1244–7.

[174] Harmon RJ, Riggs PD. Clonidine for posttraumatic stress disorder in preschool children. J Am Acad Child Adolesc Psychiatry 1996;35:1247–9.

[175] Horrigan JP. Guanfacine for posttraumatic stress disorder nightmares. J Am Acad Child Adolesc Psychiatry 1996;35:975–6.

[176] De Bellis MD, Keshavan MS, Harenski KA. Case study: anterior cingulate N-acetylaspartate concentrations during treatment in a maltreated child with PTSD. J Child Adolesc Psychopharmacol 2001;11:311–6.

[177] Seedat S, Stein DJ, Ziervogel C, et al. Comparison of response to a selective serotonin reuptake inhibitor in children, adolescents, and adults with PTSD. J Child Adolesc Psychopharmacol 2002;12:37–46.

[178] Cohen JA, Mannarino AP, Rogal SS. Treatment practices for childhood posttraumatic stress disorder. Child Abuse Negl 2001;25:123–36.

ELSEVIER
SAUNDERS

Child Adolesc Psychiatric Clin N Am
14 (2005) 773–795

CHILD AND
ADOLESCENT
PSYCHIATRIC CLINICS
OF NORTH AMERICA

Separation Anxiety Disorder, Panic Disorder, and School Refusal

Cynthia Suveg, PhD*, Sasha G. Aschenbrand, MA, Philip C. Kendall, PhD, ABPP

Department of Psychology, Temple University, Weiss Hall 1701 North 13th Street, Philadelphia, PA 19122, USA

Several studies attest to the relatively frequent, impairing, and chronic nature of anxiety in youth [1–6]. Consequently, there is a growing literature examining etiologic pathways to these disorders and efficacious treatments for them. This review examines separation anxiety disorder, a commonly occurring childhood anxiety disorder, and panic disorder (PD), a more rare anxiety disorder in youth. Finally, we examine school refusal, a problem once believed to be associated solely with anxiety but which may be tied to an internalizing or externalizing disorder or no disorder at all.

Separation anxiety disorder

Symptom picture

The essential feature of separation anxiety disorder (SAD) is excessive anxiety concerning separation from home or major attachment figures. This anxiety may be expressed through recurrent distress in anticipation of or on separation from attachment figures, a constant need to know the whereabouts of attachment figures, or extreme homesickness when away from home. When separated from attachment figures, children with SAD are often preoccupied with fears that harm will befall these people or themselves. They might also express fears of

This work was supported by National Institute of Mental Health grants MH 63747 and MH 64484.
* Corresponding author.
E-mail address: csuveg@temple.edu (C. Suveg).

being lost or kidnapped, have trouble leaving attachment figures to attend school or to go to friends' houses, or have difficulty being alone. Children with SAD often exhibit behavior characterized as "clingy," perhaps even following their parents around. These children also often have difficulty sleeping alone and might have nightmares concerning separation themes. Physical complaints, such as stomachaches, nausea, and headaches are common when separation occurs or is anticipated. To meet the criteria for a diagnosis of SAD, the anxiety must be beyond that which is to be expected for the child's developmental level, last longer than 4 weeks, begin before age 18 years, and cause significant distress or impairment in social, academic, or other important areas of functioning.

Epidemiology

Epidemiologic studies indicate a prevalence rate of 3% to 5% for SAD in children and adolescents [7–10]. Research suggests that the prevalence of SAD is higher in childhood than in adolescence [11–13]. In adolescents, studies suggest prevalence rates of 2% to 4%, with some suggestion that the prevalence rates are higher in younger than in older adolescents [14–17]. One study [18] found that SAD was the most prevalent disorder in a sample of children referred to an anxiety disorders specialty clinic, with a rate of 33%. Symptoms of separation anxiety failing to cause significant impairment also appear to be relatively common; one study [13] estimated a prevalence rate of 50% for subthreshold symptoms of separation anxiety in 8-year-old children.

The peak age of onset for SAD appears to be between the ages of 7 and 9 years [19]. Francis and colleagues [20] found that SAD appears to have different symptom expression in young children, older children, and adolescents. In this study, young children reported more SAD symptoms and more often endorsed nightmares involving separation themes than older children and adolescents did. Young children and older children also often presented with extreme distress on separation, whereas this symptom was infrequent in adolescents. However, all of the adolescents with SAD presented with physical complaints on school days.

Several studies have indicated that SAD is more common in girls than in boys [7,9,18], whereas other studies have found equal prevalence rates by gender [19,20]. Compton and colleagues [21], in an examination of sociodemographic variations in SAD and social phobia (SoP) in community and clinic samples, found that in both samples, children reporting a high number of SAD symptoms were likely to be between the ages of 8 and 12 years old and female. Considering race, rates of SAD have not been found to differ between white children and African-American or Hispanic children in samples of youth referred to anxiety disorders clinics [22,23]. However, in a community sample of children, African-American children reported more SAD symptoms than white children did [21]. A number of studies also have demonstrated an association between socioeconomic disadvantage and SAD [18,24].

Given that childhood anxiety disorders frequently are comorbid, it is important to discuss the similarities and differences among SAD, generalized anxiety disorder (GAD), and SoP. It may sometimes be difficult to parse out symptoms of SAD and GAD because both may involve worries about personal safety or the health or safety of important attachment figures. Similarly, SAD and social phobia may present with superficially similar features: both conditions are associated with a fear of situations often associated with people (ie, school or sleepovers). The distinguishing feature of SAD is that the fear is specifically related to separation experiences (the fear is greatly reduced when the child is with parents), whereas in the other anxiety disorders, the presence of an attachment figure usually has little impact on the fear.

Etiology

Biologic factors, genetics, and temperament have been investigated as potential contributors to the etiology of SAD. The genetic contribution to SAD has been studied primarily through research on familial aggregation of anxiety disorders, including top-down and bottom-up studies and twin studies of adult and childhood anxiety disorders. With regard to genetic studies, the conclusions drawn regarding the relative roles of genetic and environmental influences in SAD are mixed. Eaves and colleagues [25] investigated the etiology of SAD symptoms in female twins and found that the best model consisted of additive influences of genetic and nonshared environment. Topolski and colleagues [26], using the same sample, reported that genetic variation did not appear to make a major contribution to individual differences in SAD symptoms; in this study, the estimate of heredity for SAD was 4%, whereas the influence of shared environment, including family factors, was 40%. Contrary to these results, a recent study by Cronk and colleagues [27] found moderate heritability for risk for separation anxiety. Paternal absence was found to have an important influence in vulnerability for SAD, whereas the effect of socioeconomic disadvantage was less robust. The results of these studies may suggest that a diathesis to anxiety in general is inherited, rather than a vulnerability to a specific anxiety disorder. Moreover, the variability of results may reflect different genetic and environmental contributions according to age, gender, and type of anxiety.

Considering top-down studies, a large segment of the literature indicates an increased risk for anxiety disorders in youth whose parents have anxiety or mood disorders. Considering anxiety disorders in general, Beidel and Turner [28] found that the odds of meeting criteria for an anxiety disorder were five times greater for children of anxiety-disordered parents than for children of parents without a psychiatric disorder. Research also has investigated the degree of specificity of transmission of anxiety disorders in families. A review by Merikangas and colleagues [29] revealed that there is specificity of familial aggregation of anxiety disorders among parents and children. Considering SAD specifically, a number of studies have shown a relationship with both PD and major depressive disorder (MDD). For example, Weissman and colleagues [30] reported significantly higher rates of anxiety disorders, particularly SAD, in children of parents with major depression and PD than in children of normal controls. In a follow-up study of this sample, however, Mufson and colleagues [31] found that the children did not differ overall by parental diagnosis in the mean number of diagnoses or for the specific types of anxiety disorders. Another study examined the children of parents with MDD, PD (with and without MDD), and no diagnosis, finding that children of parents who had PD plus MDD had higher rates of SAD and panic spectrum disorders [32]. Capps and colleagues [33] found that the majority of children of agoraphobic parents, compared with children of parents with no history of psychopathology, met Diagnostic and Statistical Manual of Mental Disorders, Third Edition, Revised (DSM-III-R) diagnostic criteria for anxiety and depression. A more recent study by Biederman and colleagues [34] reported that both parental PD and parental MDD, individually or comorbidly, were associated with an increased risk for SAD, indicating that SAD may be related to both MDD and PD-agoraphobia (AG). As these studies show, the limited number of parents and children with pure cases of specific anxiety disorders precludes definitive conclusions regarding the diagnostic specificity of anxiety disorders within families.

With regard to bottom-up studies, Last and colleagues [35] compared maternal lifetime psychiatric illness for children with SAD or overanxious disorder (OAD) and for children who were psychiatrically disturbed but did not manifest an anxiety or affective disorder. Results indicated that the majority of mothers in each of the anxiety groups had a lifetime history of at least one anxiety disorder, and when compared with the control group, mothers of anxious children exhibited significantly higher rates of anxiety disorders.

Kagan and colleagues [36] have described the temperamental construct known as "behavioral inhibition to the unfamiliar," which is characterized by the consistent tendency to display fear and withdrawal in situations that are novel and unfamiliar. The literature suggests that social withdrawal in infancy is associated with later anxiety [37]. Biederman and colleagues [38] investigated the psychopathologic correlates of behavioral inhibition at a follow-up 3 years after their initial assessment in two samples of inhibited and uninhibited children. Results indicated that children with behavioral inhibition showed significantly higher rates of multiple anxiety disorders, avoidant disorder, SAD, and AG, compared with children without this trait. Whereas the initial assessments showed that the increased risk for anxiety disorders was accounted for by higher rates of avoidant disorder, OAD, and phobic disorder [39], the follow-up findings indicate that the increased risk was accounted for by higher rates of avoidant disorder and SAD. A further follow-up of the children as adolescents showed that there was a significant association between earlier classification of a child as inhibited and generalized social anxiety at adolescence but no association with specific fears, separation anxiety, or performance anxiety [40]. These data indicate that important aspects of an inhibited temperament are preserved from the second year of life to early adolescence, which predispose an adolescent to social anxiety.

Several studies have investigated the ventilatory physiology of children with anxiety disorders in an attempt to understand the biologic similarities between these disorders and adult anxiety disorders, including panic disorder. Research in this area has led to the hypothesis that CO_2hypersensitivity is a marker of biologic vulnerability for PD [41]. Pine and colleagues [42] compared the ventilatory physiology of children and adolescents with anxiety disorders, including PD, SoP, SAD, and OAD, with ventilatory physiology of psychiatrically healthy control subjects. The results provide some evidence of associations among SAD, PD, and CO_2-induced panic. Pine and colleagues [41] performed another ventilatory physiology study with 57 probands who have an anxiety disorder (social phobia, GAD, SAD, and PD) and 47 normal comparisons. The results indicated that childhood anxiety disorders, particularly SAD, were associated with CO_2 hypersensitivity, and SAD emerged as the only significant predictor of CO_2-induced panic. Another study in this area replicated the link between childhood anxiety disorders and CO_2 sensitivity but failed to obtain support for CO_2hypersensitivity as a familial risk marker for PD in youth [43].

Accumulated evidence supports the integral role of family and parenting behavior in youth anxiety. Although typically limited to maternal influences, findings in family functioning research cluster within several themes: (1) parents of anxious youth tend to be overly controlling and intrusive, overprotective, and less granting of psychologic autonomy and less accepting than parents of nonanxious youth [44–48a]; (2) higher levels of parental rejection and criticism are associated with higher levels of youth anxiety [49–52], but studies focusing on parental negative affect and degree of emotional warmth have been mixed [47,49,52–54]; (3) parents of anxious youth model and reinforce anxious or avoidant behavior [55,56]; and (4) families of anxious youth are more conflicting and less cohesive and have poor problem-solving and communication skills [57,58]. Unfortunately, because the majority of the aforementioned studies focus on childhood anxiety disorders as a group, we are uninformed about these issues with regard to families of children with SAD, specifically.

Developmental course

Klein [59] proposed that SAD in childhood is associated with panic disorder in adulthood. The affirmative evidence for the separation anxiety hypothesis has been shown in several retrospective studies, finding that patients with PDAG report childhood histories of SAD more often than patients with other disorders do and in biologic studies finding similar ventilatory physiology among patients with SAD and patients with PDAG [41,42,60,61]. In contrast, a number of retrospective studies and familial aggregation studies have found that patterns of anxiety disorders do not support a specific association between SAD and PDAG [31,62]. Although not specifically testing the separation anxiety hypothesis, some longitudinal data are available that support the link between SAD and PDAG [63,64]. The specificity of the posited SAD–PDAG relationship is complicated by the frequent comorbidity of PDAG with depression, suggesting that SAD may be a predisposition to affective disorders in general. Preliminary familial study evidence suggests that although both PDAG and MDD in the parent are associated with an increased risk of SAD in the child, the relationship seems to be slightly stronger between SAD and PDAG [31,32].

Recently, a 7.4-year follow-up was conducted of youth who had received treatment for an anxiety disorder in childhood. Those who were identified initially as SAD were compared with those identified initially with other anxiety disorders (GAD and SoP), and the frequency of panic disorder was examined [65]. SAD was predictive of more anxiety disorders 7.4 years later but not predictive specifically of panic disorder. This pattern held for cases whose treatment was deemed effective and for those whom treatment was less effective. Although studies of untreated SAD cases are needed, as well as studies that follow cases for even longer than 7 years, it appears that the developmental trajectory for SAD youth may be linked to adult anxiety disorder, although not automatically tied to PD.

Treatment

The efficacy of both psychotherapy and pharmacotherapy has been empirically evaluated for the treatment of childhood anxiety disorders. In general, both psychotherapy and medication trials have targeted broad collections of childhood anxiety disorders (SAD, GAD, and SoP), because of the hypothesized similarity in etiology and a demonstrated similarity in treatment response. Given that no published trials have evaluated the efficacy of psychotherapy versus pharmacotherapy, there is a critical need for head-to-head trials. Such trials will allow researchers to evaluate the relative efficacy of each treatment for childhood anxiety disorders. A trial evaluating the efficacy of sertraline, cognitive-behavioral therapy (CBT), CBT plus sertraline, and placebo for the treatment of SAD, GAD, and SoP is currently underway (Child and Adolescent Anxiety Multimodal Study).

Randomized clinical trials, however, have evaluated the efficacy of these treatments separately. There is a consensus that cognitive-behavioral therapy is a first-line treatment for childhood anxiety disorders, including SAD. According to the American Psychological Association guidelines for determining whether a treatment meets the criteria for being designated as "empirically-supported," CBT for youth diagnosed with anxiety disorders has been established as a "probably efficacious" treatment [66,67]. In CBT programs, children generally learn to recognize signs of anxiety, acquire relaxation skills, identify and modify anxious self-talk, and learn problem solving in anxiety-provoking situations. The educational portion of therapy is followed by a practice phase with exposure tasks in which children are exposed to a hierarchy of increasingly anxiety-provoking situations.

CBT has been found to be efficacious in treating anxiety disorders in children, using both an individualized, child-focused format [68,69] and a treatment program more integrally involving parents [70–76]. A group treatment of CBT for anxious youth also has been found to be efficacious in treating childhood anxiety disorders [77]. None of these studies has found specificity or differential treatment response for SAD relative to the other childhood anxiety disorders (eg, GAD and SoP). Kendall and colleagues [78–78b] reported that the presence of comorbid disorders, including SAD, does not appear to lead to differential treatment response.

As stated earlier, no published trials have evaluated the relative efficacy of CBT versus pharmacotherapy for SAD. However, several studies have been conducted to evaluate the efficacy of pharmacologic agents for SAD. Despite the effort, the field has yet to endorse a specific medication for SAD. Nevertheless, medications with Food and Drug Administration indications for adults with anxiety disorders are often used and said to be of some benefit for anxious children and adolescents [79]. Mixed results have been found for tricyclic antidepressants (TCA), including imipramine and clomipramine, in treating SAD [80–82]. Positive results from open clinical trials of selective serotonin reuptake inhibitors (SSRIs) with anxious children [83,84] led to a large controlled study of fluvoxamine, an SSRI, with children who have SAD, GAD, and social phobia. The overall improvement rate was 78% for fluvoxamine versus 29% for placebo [85]. A randomized clinical trial comparing sertraline, CBT, CBT plus sertraline, and pill placebo in the treatment of childhood anxiety disorders is currently underway. Based on current knowledge, CBT can be recommended as a treatment for anxious youth, with the potential use of medication, preferably with SSRIs, when it is appropriate [79].

Panic disorder

Symptom picture

Until recently, there was significant controversy about whether panic disorder existed in children and adolescents [86]. Some researchers questioned whether children had the cognitive ability to catastrophize the bodily sensations that characterize spontaneous panic attacks. However, with the recent surge of research on panic in youth, the issue has shifted from whether PD exists in youth to considerations of the phenomenology of panic in children and adolescents [87,88].

The defining feature of PD for both children and adults is the presence of recurrent, unexpected panic attacks, at least one of which is followed by 1 month or more of persistent worry about having another attack, the implications of the attack, or a significant change in behavior caused by the attack. Importantly, the panic attacks that define panic disorder are spontaneous; they are not cued solely by social situations, as would potentially be the case in social anxiety, or associated with a specific cue, as would be seen in specific phobia. Panic attacks, as defined by the DSM-IV-R [89] criteria, include both physiologic (eg, palpitations, sweating, and trembling) and cognitive symptoms (eg, fear of dying and fear of losing control), which usually reach a peak of intensity within 10 minutes. Some researchers have found that children and adolescents are more likely to experience physiologic rather than cognitive symptoms during a panic attack [87,90,91]. For example, in a study of 17 youth diagnosed with PD, 94% of the sample reported that they experienced palpitations, trembling, and flushes or chills during a panic attack [91]. In contrast, fear of dying and going crazy were reported by just 59% and 65% of the sample, respectively. Similarly, in a study of 20 youth who had PD, ages 8 to 17 years old, Kearney and colleagues [87] found that the most commonly reported panic symptoms were rapid heartbeat, nausea, hot or cold flashes, and shaking or jitteriness. The feelings or fear of going crazy and of dying were reported by 50% of the sample. The studies reviewed previously show that youth suffering from panic experience both cognitive and bodily symptoms. The cognitive symptoms experienced by youth should not be overlooked because the combination of symptoms likely adds to the overall terrifying nature of the panic experience.

Epidemiology

Given that research has only begun to explicate the nature of panic in youth, few epidemiologic studies are available, and of those that are available, there are methodologic limitations, diagnostic issues, and small sample sizes. With that stated, several studies using community samples estimate prevalence rates for PD in youth at less than 1% [2,92–96]. Prevalence rates using clinical samples are higher [97,98], suggesting that up to 10% of youth qualify for PD [91]. Although PD occurs relatively infrequently compared with other anxiety disorders among youth, many youth report that they experience panic symptoms [90]. In community sample studies, 20% or more of youth report experiencing a panic attack at some time in their lives [92,94].

In studies using samples of youth and retrospective reports by adults, the mean age of onset for PD ranges from mid-adolescence to mid-20s [91,94,99–101]. For example, in a study of 17 youth with PD, ages 9 to 18 years, Last and Strauss [91] found a mean age of onset of 15.6 years. Furthermore, mothers of the panic-disordered children who themselves qualified for panic disorder reported the onset of their own panic in late adolescence or early adulthood. However, larger epidemiologic studies found, based on retrospective reports, a mean age of onset for PD in the mid-20s [100,101].

Regarding gender, panic attacks occur equally in females and males [92,94], although PD occurs more frequently in females [90,91,94]. Compared with other anxiety disorders in youth, little is known about PD generally, and even less is known about the epidemiology or phenomenology of the disorder across racial and ethnic groups. Of those studies that were reviewed, many either did not report on the race or ethnicity of the sample [98], or included only white youth in the sample [87], or included a diverse sample but did not indicate that analyses examined racial or ethnic differences [94]. However, one study by Ginsburg and Drake [102] included low-income African-American youth and found a positive relationship between anxiety sensitivity and panic symptoms, a relationship that also has been found with white samples.

Comorbidity is high among youth with PD, with estimates indicating that anywhere from 50% to 90% of youth with PD suffer from a comorbid condition [91,92,98]. Comorbid conditions include not only anxiety and depressive disorders but externalizing disorders as well (eg, attention-deficit hyperactivity disorder (ADHD) and oppositional defiant disorder [91,98]). In a study specifically examining the relationship between PD and AG in 472 consecutively referred children and adolescents ages 4 to 18 years old, Biederman and colleagues [98] found that 65% of children with PD also meet criteria for AG and that the percentage was significantly greater than that for youth with other forms of psychopathology. The findings are consistent with other studies that also found that a significant percentage of adolescents with PD also met the criteria for AG [87]. A later report by Hayward and colleagues [93] using a nonclinical sample of children did not find a significant relationship between the presence of panic attacks and agoraphobic symptoms. As Hayward and colleagues and other investigators have discussed, the differences in findings may be explained by a referral bias in that those youth with both PD and AG are more likely to seek treatment than are those with just PD.

Etiology

Many etiologic studies now exist regarding anxiety disorders in youth, although fewer specifically examine the development of PD. For example, as reviewed in the etiology section of SAD, behavioral inhibition, the tendency to withdraw from unfamiliar situations or people, has been identified as a general risk factor for the development of anxiety disorders [103]. Parenting factors such as overprotective and controlling behaviors also have been associated with anxiety in youth, although these factors have not been related to discrete disorders. Given that these etiologic factors have already been discussed in the SAD etiology section and apply to PD, they will not be reviewed here. Rather, the discussion will focus only on the research related specifically to PD.

Extrapolating from the etiologic model of panic by Barlow [104], Mattis and Ollendick [105] proposed a developmental model of panic in children. In this model, both biologic (ie, aspects of temperament such as low self-regulatory ability and high distress reactivity) and psychologic (ie, insecure-ambivalent attachment to caregiver and failure to regulate distress through caregiver) vulnerabilities are considered. Briefly, a child with a high biologic vulnerability experiences separation from caregivers as an especially stressful experience. Over the course of repeated separation experiences, a child comes to associate distress reactivity and interoceptive cues. When the child's distress is repeatedly not alleviated through contact with the caregiver and is prolonged, the child comes to fear the separation and the associated cues and the possibility that they will occur in the future. When both biologic (eg, high distress reactivity) and psychologic (eg, insecure attachment) vulnerabilities are present, the child is considered at risk for the development of panic attacks and PD. Finally, Ollendick [106] suggests that behavioral inhibition or avoidance (eg, AG) may develop when other coping mechanisms or regulatory mechanisms (eg, secure attachment with caregiver) are absent.

As with some other anxiety disorders, there appears to be a heritability factor for PD. For example, in one study Last and colleagues [107] examined the presence of anxiety disorders in 5 to 18 year-old-children and their first- and second-degree relatives. For comparison purposes, a group of children with ADHD and a group without any form of psychopathology were included. Results indicated that the first-degree relatives of children with overanxious disorder (now generalized anxiety disorder) had higher rates of PD than relatives of children with other anxiety disorders.

Hayward and colleagues [108] found that the onset of panic attacks was best predicted by pubertal status, rather than by age. In this study of 10- to 16-year-old children, pubertal status was calculated through self-report, and structured diagnostic interviews were administered to assess for panic attacks. A multiple logistic regression was performed to examine the predictive relationships among age, pubertal status, and panic attack history. Pubertal status emerged as a significant predictor of a history of panic attacks. Furthermore, youth in each age group (≤ 11 years, 12 years, ≥ 13 years) who were in the more advanced stages of puberty were more likely to have had a history of panic attacks than same-aged peers at earlier stages of puberty. Although puberty emerged as a significant variable to consider in the onset of panic attacks, research needs to explicate the reasons for this. As the authors discuss, pubertal status is correlated with psychologic changes, increased social anxiety, as well as a host of other factors. In sum, although the evidence is somewhat mixed, it is clear that the onset of PD during childhood is extremely rare and becomes more common during mid to late adolescence.

Another study by Hayward and colleagues [94] examined the predictive relationships among female gender, negative affectivity, anxiety sensitivity, and childhood separation anxiety disorder and panic symptoms in 2365 ethnically diverse high school students. To examine whether these factors were unique to panic, the relationship between these factors and major depression was also examined. Diagnoses were made based on a structured diagnostic interview, and self-report measures were collected, with assessments taking place annually for 3 years. Results identified negative affectivity as a nonspecific risk factor for both the onset of panic attacks and depression and anxiety sensitivity as a specific risk factor for panic attacks. After adjusting for the effects of depression, neither childhood SAD nor female gender predicted full (ie, referred to as "4-symptom" attacks) panic attacks. Additional findings for gender were somewhat complicated and varied based on whether the panic attack was a limited (ie, $\leq$four symptoms) or full symptom attack. Specifically, findings indicated that females were more likely to experience full-symptom attacks, whereas males were more represented among those with limited-symptom attacks. However, when the data were adjusted for past or present major depression, female gender did not predict four-symptom panic attacks. Thus, the authors hypothesized that the finding that females are more represented than males among those with four-symptom attacks is because of the overlap with depression. Females were also more likely than males to have a lifetime history of PD but also to experience comorbid depression.

Developmental course

Although research is accumulating on the development of PD in children and adolescents, very little is known about the course of the disorder in youth. One study conducted by Biederman and colleagues [98] examined the course and correlates (comorbidity) of PD and AG in 472 consecutively referred youth, ages 4 to 18 years. Diagnoses were based on the Schedule for Affective Disorders and Schizophrenia for School-Age-Children-Epidemiologic version [109], which was administered to the mothers. Results indicated that individuals who met criteria for PD were likely to experience symptoms for an average of 3.5 years, suggesting the chronicity of PD. Unfortunately, the results were based on a retrospective rather than prospective methodology. To our knowledge, no longitudinal studies of youth with PD have been conducted.

Studies of adults with PD find that, although a significant proportion of individuals have symptom-free periods, the rate of relapse is high [110,111]. In combination with the findings that many adults with PD report an onset in mid-adolescence, one can reasonably speculate that the course for the disorder is chronic.

Treatment

Given the paucity of research available on the phenomenology of PD in children, few studies have examined the efficacy of any form of treatment of PD in youth. In adults, there is a relatively large number of reports supporting the use of cognitive-behavioral procedures and, in particular, panic control treatment (PCT) [112,113]. PCT combines traditional components of CBT (eg, psychologic education, cognitive restructuring, progressive muscle relaxation) with interoceptive exposure. In a multiple baseline design, Ollendick [114] examined the effectiveness of CBT in four adolescents, ages 13 to 17, who were diagnosed with PD with AG based on a structured diagnostic interview. Adolescents also completed measures of anxiety sensitivity, self-efficacy, and anxiety and depressive symptoms, and kept a record of their panic attacks.

Treatment included psychologic education regarding the nature of panic, progressive muscle relaxation (including cue-controlled and applied relaxation), breathing retraining, the development of positive self-statements, cognitive coping, self-instruction strategies, and exposure. Treatment duration lasted from 10 to 12 weeks and was followed by one 2-week and one 1-month maintenance session. Follow-up took place 6 months after treatment. Results at both post-treatment and follow-up indicated a significant decline in the frequency of panic attacks, agoraphobic avoidance, and for most participants, anxiety sensitivity and anxiety and depressive symptoms.

Hoffman and colleagues [115] reported on the effects of a randomized controlled study of PCT for 14- to 17-year-old adolescents (PCT-A) on self-report measures of anxiety sensitivity, anxiety, and depression. Participants were randomly assigned to active treatment or a wait-list control; those in the active treatment condition received 11 sessions of therapy. Participants completed assessments at pre- and post-treatment and at 3-month follow-up. Results indicated consistent and significant declines in anxiety sensitivity and anxiety symptoms from pre- to post-treatment, relative to the wait-list control group. Although participants in the active treatment also evidenced declines in depressive symptoms, these findings did not reach statistical significance.

With respect to the pharmacologic treatment of panic disorder in youth, there is scant literature from which to draw conclusions. There are currently no randomized clinical trials that have examined the efficacy of medications in the treatment of PD in youth or the relative efficacy of psychotherapy and pharamacotherapy. Based on a review of the literature, Birmaher and Ollendick [116] suggest that when medications are indicated, SSRIs should be used first. This seems to be a reasonable recommendation given that research to date on the use of medications to treat anxiety in youth suggests that they are safe and effective, at least in the short term [83–85,117,118].

School refusal

Symptom picture

Unlike SAD and PD, "school refusal" is not a diagnosis in the DSM-IV-R [89]. In the past, the label "school refusal" applied to all youth who consistently avoided school or endured the school day with distress, without examining the cause of the school refusal. School refusal was often used interchangeably with "school phobia," yet as research has found, not all school refusers are anxious [46,119,120]. Consequently, many researchers now argue for the examination and classification of school refusal based on the function of the behavior [121,122] and use the label school refusal to refer broadly to all youth who refuse school and who may or may not have accompanying internalizing or externalizing psychopathology [121,123].

Kearney and colleagues [87] developed a classification system for school behavior that evaluates school behavior according to whether youth refuse school for negative or positive reinforcement. The previous classification system includes youth who refuse school in an effort to avoid school-related stimuli or social or evaluative situations that cause the child distress. The latter classification system includes youth who refuse school to gain attention from significant others or to engage in activities that are deemed more pleasant than the school environment.

Given the heterogeneity of school refusal, the symptom picture for youth with this behavioral difficulty varies widely and depends in large part on whether accompanying psychopathology is present. It is possible that school refusal is part of the symptom picture of an internalizing (eg, SAD) or externalizing (eg, oppositional defiant disorder) disorder. However, it is also possible that no form of psychopathology accompanies school refusal behavior. In cases in which school refusal is part of an externalizing disorder, the symptom picture may include defiance and oppositionality. When school refusal is part of an internalizing disorder, the symptom picture also may include somatic symptoms and mood difficulties. In either case, school refusal behavior often includes pleas to parents to stay home from school and distress during the school day and has been associated with family and peer relationship difficulties [46].

Epidemiology

As noted by Elliot [124], prevalence rates for school refusal are likely to vary greatly because of a number of factors, including definitional issues and the method by which the behavior is assessed. However, recent reviews of school refusal suggest that approximately 1% and 5% of nonclinic-referred and clinic-referred children, respectively, exhibit school refusal [125–127]. Although school refusal may occur at any age, Ollendick and Mayer [128] suggest that peak onset occurs during ages 5 to 6 and 10 to 11, ages that correspond with transition times to kindergarten and middle school. King and colleagues [129] suggest that other high-risk times for the onset of school refusal occur when children move to a different community or to a new school in the same community and after major social events or holidays. Some research finds that school refusal occurs equally in males and females [126].

In an effort to examine the diagnostic correlates of the taxonomic categories of school refusal, Kearney and Albano [122] conducted a study with 143 youth ages 5 to 17 years old who presented with primary school refusal. Children and parents were administered the Anxiety Disorders Interview Schedule for Children—Child and Parent versions to assess psychopathology. Children and parents were also administered the School Refusal Assessment Scale to gauge the relative strength of one of the following four functional conditions for school refusal: (1) avoidance of school-related stimuli that provoke negative affectivity; (2) escape from school-related aversive social or evaluative situation; (3) attention from significant others; or (4) tangible reinforcement outside of school. When functional profiles occurred with equal strength, they were considered "mixed." Results indicated that SAD was the most frequent diagnosis, occurring in 22% of the sample. Approximately one third of the sample did not have any psychiatric diagnosis. When diagnoses across functions were examined, SAD was more prevalent in the attention-seeking group. Overall, anxiety disorders were more frequently associated with negative-reinforcement functions (eg, avoidance). whereas disruptive behavior disorders were more frequent in the group that refused school to gain tangible reinforcement outside of the school setting. With respect to age differences, children who refused school to avoid stimuli that provoked negative affectivity or for attention were likely to be younger. Children who refused school to pursue tangible reinforcement outside of school or to avoid social or evaluative situations were likely to be older. No significant gender differences were found across the profiles. Lastly, children who refused school to avoid stimuli that provoked negative affectivity tended to have the most severe diagnoses.

Etiology

As with most mental health disorders, researchers have not identified one etiologic pathway to school refusal. Rather, pathways to school refusal are likely to be closely tied to the function that the behavior serves and to vary across individuals. King and colleagues [129] suggest a complex etiologic pathway for school refusal that may include a biologic predisposition [127], stressful life events, or a combination thereof. One study conducted by McShane and colleagues [130] examined factors associated with the onset of school refusal behavior in a sample of children and adolescents ages 10 to 17 years. Diagnoses were determined by retrospectively examining the records of youth presenting to a psychiatric clinic. An inspection of medical records permitted an assessment of demographic and other factors that may have been related to the youths' difficulties. Results revealed several factors that were associated with the onset of school refusal, including conflict at home (43%), conflict with peers (34%), academic difficulties (31%), family separation (21%), changing school or moving home (25%), and physical illness (20%). Other studies examining present functioning provide support for the finding that family conflict and otherwise maladaptive patterns of functioning are relatively common in families of school refusers [131–133].

Developmental course

Some researchers have suggested that up to 25% of cases of school refusal remit spontaneously or are otherwise readily addressed by parents [134]. However, for the cases that do not remit, there can be both short-term and long-term implications for the child's functioning. For example, Flakierska-Praquin and colleagues [135] conducted a 20- to 29-year follow-up study of 35 school phobics. Diagnoses were based on a retrospective review of several hundred case reports of 7- to 12-year-old children who had received either in-patient or outpatient treatment at a psychiatric clinic. Importantly, the authors note that all children had a diagnosis of separation anxiety disorder, likely because of the conceptualization of school refusal at the time. Participants had a mean age of 34.3 years at follow-up. Comparison groups included a child psychiatric group that did not exhibit school refusal behavior and a general population sample. Groups were compared on an overall measure of adjustment as well as a review of records (ie, school health, psychiatric clinics, national health insurance, demographic registers, and police registers). Results indicated that the school refusal group was more likely to seek psychiatric services as adults than those from the general population. Individuals in the nonschool-refusing psychiatric group were more likely to be registered for criminal offenses than the other two groups. Although not statistically significant, information gathered from the national demographic register indicated that 14% of school refusers continued to live with their parents at follow-up, compared with 9% and 0% of individuals in the psychiatric control and general population groups, respectively. Last, school refusers had fewer children than the other two groups. Other research examining the outcome of youth with school refusal also has found an increased long-term risk of psychopathology and social and employment difficulties [136,137].

Treatment

Cognitive-behavioral therapy generally is considered the first-line treatment approach to manage school refusal [123,124,129], and studies are accumulating to support its use [138–140]. One randomized control trial compared a CBT program to a wait-list control condition using a sample of 5- to 15-year-old youth with school refusal. Based on a diagnostic interview, children exhibited diverse diagnostic profiles that included no diagnoses, anxiety disorders, externalizing disorders, and comorbid diagnoses. The CBT treatment program was modeled after the program developed by Kendall [140a] and included six sessions with the child, five sessions with the parents, and typically one session with the youth's teacher. Parent and teacher sessions involved teaching of behavioral management skills. Pre- and post-treatment assessments included child, parent, and teacher report, and clinician ratings. Results indicated that, compared with children in the wait-list control condition, children in the CBT condition attended school significantly more, showed greater improvements on self-report measures of distress (eg, fear and coping), had parents who rated significant improvements in internalizing difficulties, and were rated significantly higher on clinician ratings of functioning. No significant between-group differences were found for the teacher report. A 3- to 5-year follow-up of children in the CBT group indicated overall maintenance of the treatment gains [139].

Other research suggests the potential benefit of "prescriptive treatment" based on the functional type of school refusal [141,142]. For example, this approach suggests parent training in contingency management for youth who refuse school for attention and social skills building and anxiety management for youth who refuse school to avoid negative social evaluation. However, because of small sample sizes and lack of adequate controls in the existing work, the incremental validity of this treatment approach awaits further empirical investigation.

With respect to pharmacologic treatment, a few controlled studies have specifically examined the treatment of anxiety-based school refusal using tricyclic antidepressants [80,143]. However, as King and Bernstein [123] and

Elliott [124] note in their reviews of school refusal, the studies have yielded conflicting findings. A randomized, double blind controlled study conducted by Bernstein and colleagues [143] examined the effectiveness of CBT plus imipramine or CBT plus a placebo in the treatment of school refusing adolescents who had comorbid anxiety and depression. Following a multimethod assessment battery that included necessary medical work-ups, a diagnostic interview, self-report measures of symptoms, and clinician ratings, youth were randomized to one of the two treatment conditions. Over the course of treatment, youth participated in eight 45- to 60-minute sessions of CBT treatment and weekly pharmacotherapy visits with the psychiatrist that lasted approximately 10 to 15 minutes. Results indicated significantly greater school attendance for the CBT plus imipramine group than for the CBT plus placebo group. The CBT plus imipramine group also demonstrated significantly faster decreases in depression over the course of treatment, compared with the CBT plus placebo group. Although this study found positive effects for a TCA when combined with CBT, the overall conflicting results from studies make their use in children controversial [124]. As previously reviewed, the SSRIs have been found to be safe and effective, at least in the short term, for treating anxiety in youth [83–85]. Thus, when school refusal is accompanied by an anxiety disorder, these medications are more likely to be prescribed than are other forms of medications. Furthermore, the use of medication interventions is more likely part of a multimodal treatment program that includes a nonpharmacologic form of therapy [144].

Summary

The review of the literature suggests several areas of future research that apply to SAD, PD, and school refusal, both generally and specifically. In general, longitudinal research is needed to help explicate the etiologic pathways and developmental courses of the disorders. Although literature is accumulating on risk factors associated with the development of anxiety disorders in youth (eg, behavioral inhibition, anxiety sensitivity, and family factors) in general, future research needs to examine whether unique relationships exist between these factors and specific disorders. With respect to SAD and PD in particular, longitudinal studies designed to examine the relationship between SAD and PDAG are sorely needed. The CBT approach to treating anxiety in youth has undergone empirical scrutiny, supporting its overall efficacy. Research is needed to evaluate CBT with adolescents, and to examine the predictors and parameters of more versus less successful outcomes. Additional work is needed regarding the pharmacologic treatment of SAD, PD, and school refusal, although the preliminary research suggests that SSRIs might be helpful in treating these difficulties. Methodologically rigorous randomized trials comparing the relative efficacy of psychotherapeutic and pharmacologic treatments will be beneficial in identifying which treatments are indicated for what types of youth.

References

[1] Costello EJ, Angold A. Epidemiology. In: March JS, editor. Anxiety disorders in children and adolescents. New York: Guilford; 1995. p. 109–24.
[2] Costello EJ, Mustillo S, Erkanli A, et al. Prevalence and development of psychiatric disorders in childhood and adolescence. Arch Gen Psychiatry 2003;60:837–44.
[3] Ferdinand RF, Verhurlst FC. Psychopathology from adolescence into young adulthood: an 8-year follow-up study. Am J Psychiatry 2003;15:1586–94.
[4] Ialongo N, Edelsohn G, Werthamer-Larsson L, et al. The significance of self-reported anxious symptoms in first grade children: prediction to anxious symptoms and adaptive functioning in fifth grade. J Child Psychol Psychiatry 1995;36:427–37.
[5] Strauss CC, Lahey B, Frick P, et al. Peer social status of children with anxiety disorders. J Consult Clin Psychol 2003;1:137–41.
[6] Woodward LJ, Fergusson DM. Life course outcomes of young people with anxiety disorders in adolescence. J Am Acad Child Adolesc Psychiatry 2001;40:1086–93.
[7] Anderson JC, Williams S, McGee R, et al. DSM-III disorders in preadolescent children: prevalence in a large sample from the general population. Arch Gen Psychiatry 1987;44:69–76.
[8] Bird HR, Canino G, Rubio-Stipec M, et al. Estimates of the prevalence of childhood maladjustment in a community survey in Puerto Rico: the use of combined measures. Arch Gen Psychiatry 1988;45(12):1120–6.
[9] Costello EJ. Child psychiatric disorders and their correlates: a primary care pediatric sample. J Am Acad Child Adolesc Psychiatry 1989;28:851–5.
[10] Prior M, Sanson A, Smart D, et al. Psychological disorders and their correlates in an Australian community sample of preadolescent children. J Child Psychol Psychiatry 1999;40:563–80.
[11] Breton JJ, Bergeron L, Valla JP, et al. Quebec child mental health survey: prevalence of DSM-III-R mental health disorders. J Child Psychol Psychiatry 1999;40:375–84.
[12] Kashani JH, Orvaschel H. Anxiety disorders in mid-adolescence: a community sample. Am J Psychiatry 1988;145:960–4.
[13] Kashani JH, Orvaschel H. A community study of anxiety in children and adolescents. Am J Psychiatry 1990;147:313–8.
[14] Cohen P, Cohen J, Kasen S, et al. An epidemiological study of disorders in late childhood and adolescence. I. age and gender-specific prevalence. J Child Psychol Psychiatry 1993;34:851–67.
[15] Costello EJ, Costello AJ, Edelbrock C, et al. Psychiatric disorders in pediatric primary care: prevalence and risk factors. Arch Gen Psychiatry 1988;45:1107–16.
[16] Lewinsohn PM, Hops H, Roberts RE, et al. Adolescent psychopathology: prevalence and incidence of depression and other DSM-III-R disorders in high school students. J Abnorm Psychol 1993;102:133–44.
[17] McGee R, Feehan M, Williams S, et al. DSM-III disorders in a large sample of adolescents. J Am Acad Child Adolesc Psychiatry 1990;29:611–9.
[18] Last CG, Francis G, Hersen M, et al. Separation anxiety and school phobia: a comparison using DSM-III criteria. Am J Psychiatry 1987;144:653–7.
[19] Last CG, Perrin S, Hersen M, et al. DSM-III-R anxiety disorders in children: sociodemographic and clinical characteristics. J Am Acad Child Adolesc Psychiatry 1992;31:1070–6.
[20] Francis G, Last CG, Strauss CC. Expression of separation anxiety disorder: the roles of gender and age. Child Psychiatry Hum Dev 1987;18:82–9.
[21] Compton SN, Nelson AH, March JS. Social phobia and separation anxiety symptoms in community and clinical samples of children and adolescents. J Am Acad Child Adolesc Psychiatry 2000;39:1040–6.
[22] Ginsburg GS, Silverman WK. Phobic and anxiety disorders in Hispanic and Caucasian youth. J Anxiety Disord 1996;10:517–28.
[23] Last CG, Perrin S. Anxiety disorders in African-American and white children. J Abnorm Child Psychol 1993;21:153–64.

[24] Velez CN, Johnson J, Cohen PA. A longitudinal analysis of selected risk factors for childhood psychopathology. J Am Acad Child Adolesc Psychiatry 1989;28:861–4.

[25] Eaves LJ, Silberg JL, Meyer JM, et al. Genetics and developmental psychopathology: 2. the main effects of genes and environment on behavioral problems in the Virginia Twin Study of Adolescent Behavioral Development. J Child Psychol Psychiatry 1997;38:965–80.

[26] Topolski TD, Hewitt JK, Eaves LJ, et al. Genetic and environmental influences on child reports of manifest anxiety and symptoms of separation anxiety and overanxious disorder: a community-based twin study. Behav Genet 1997;27:15–28.

[27] Cronk NJ, Slutske WS, Madden PAF, et al. Risk for separation anxiety disorder among girls: paternal absence, socioeconomic disadvantage, and genetic vulnerability. J Abnorm Psychol 2004;113:237–47.

[28] Beidel DC, Turner SM. Shy children, phobic adults: nature and treatment of social phobia. Washington (DC): American Psychological Association; 1998.

[29] Merikangas K, Avenevoli S, Dierker L, et al. Vulnerability factors among children at risk for anxiety disorders. Biol Psychiatry 1999;46:1523–35.

[30] Weissman MM, Leckman JF, Merikangas KR, et al. Depression and anxiety disorders in parents and children: results from the Yale family study. Arch Gen Psychiatry 1984;41:845–52.

[31] Mufson L, Weissman MM, Warner V. Depression and anxiety in parents and children: a direct interview study. J Anxiety Disord 1992;6:1–13.

[32] Warner V, Mufson L, Weissman MM. Offspring at high and low risk for depression and anxiety: mechanisms of psychiatric disorder. J Am Acad Child Adolesc Psychiatry 1995;34:786–97.

[33] Capps L, Sigman M, Sena R, et al. Fear, anxiety, and perceived control in children of agoraphobic parents. J Child Psychol Psychiatry 1996;37:445–52.

[34] Biederman J, Faraone SV, Hirshfeld-Becker DR, et al. Patterns of psychopathology and dysfunction in high-risk children of parents with panic disorder and major depression. Am J Psychiatry 2001;158:49–57.

[35] Last CG, Hersen M, Kazdin AE, et al. Psychiatric illness in the mothers of anxious children. Am J Psychiatry 1987;144:1580–3.

[36] Kagan JR, Reznick JS, Snidman N. Biological bases of childhood shyness. Science 1988;240:167–71.

[37] Rosenbaum JF, Biederman J, Gersten M, et al. Behavioral inhibition in children of parents with panic disorder and agoraphobia: a controlled study. Arch Gen Psychiatry 1988;45:463–70.

[38] Biederman J, Rosenbaum JF, Bolduc-Murphy EA, et al. A 3-year follow-up of children with and without behavioral inhibition. J Am Acad Child Adolesc Psychiatry 1993;32:814–21.

[39] Biederman J, Rosenbaum JF, Hirshfeld DR, et al. Psychiatric correlates of behavioral inhibition in young children of parents with and without psychiatric disorders. Arch Gen Psychiatry 1990;47:21–6.

[40] Schwartz CE, Snidman N, Kagan J. Adolescent social anxiety as an outcome of inhibited temperament in childhood. J Am Acad Child Adolesc Psychiatry 1999;38:1008–15.

[41] Pine DS, Klein RG, Coplan JD, et al. Differential carbon dioxide sensitivity in childhood anxiety disorders and nonill comparison group. Arch Gen Psychiatry 2000;57:960–7.

[42] Pine DS, Coplan JD, Papp LA, et al. Ventilatory physiology of children and adolescents with anxiety disorders. Arch Gen Psychiatry 1998;55:123–9.

[43] Pine DS, Klein RG, Roberson-Nay R, et al. Response to 5% carbon dioxide in children and adolescents: relationship to panic disorder in parents and anxiety disorders in subjects. Arch Gen Psychiatry 2005;62(1):73–80.

[44] Dumas JE, LaFreniere PJ. Mother-child relationships as sources of support or stress: a comparison of competent, average, aggressive, and anxious dyads. Child Dev 1993;64:1732–54.

[45] Hudson JL, Rapee RM. Parent-child interactions and anxiety disorders: an observational study. Behav Res Ther 2001;39:1411–27.

[46] Last CG, Strauss CC. School refusal in anxiety-disordered children and adolescents. J Am Acad Child Adolesc Psychiatry 1990;29:31–5.

[47] Siqueland L, Kendall PC, Steinberg L. Anxiety in children: perceived family environments and observed family interaction style. J Clin Child Psychol 1996;25:225–37.

[48] Whaley SE, Pinto A, Sigman M. Characterizing interactions between anxious mothers and their children. J Consult Clin Psychol 1999;67:826–36.

[48a] Suveg C, Zeman J, Flannery-Schroeder E, et al. Emotion socialization in families of children with an anxiety disorder. J Abnorm Child Psychol 2005;33:145–55.

[49] Dumas J, LaFreniere P, Serketich W. "Balance of power": transactional analysis of control in mother-child dyads involving socially competent, aggressive, and anxious children. J Abnorm Psychol 1995;104:104–13.

[50] Hibbs ED, Hamburger SD, Kruesi MJ, et al. Factors affecting expressed emotion in parents of ill and normal children. Am J Orthopsychiatry 1993;63:103–12.

[51] Hibbs ED, Hamburger SD, Lenane M, et al. Determinants of expressed emotion in families of disturbed and normal children. J Child Psychol Psychiatry 1991;32:757–70.

[52] Lieb R, Wittchen H, Hofler M, et al. Parental psychopathology, parenting styles, and the risk of social phobia in offspring: a prospective-longitudinal community study. Arch Gen Psychiatry 2000;57:859–66.

[53] Dadds MR, Barrett PM, Rapee RM, et al. Family process and child anxiety and aggression: an observational analysis 1996;24:715–34

[54] McClure EB, Brennan P, Hammen C, et al. Parental anxiety disorders, child anxiety disorders, and the perceived parent-child relationship in and Australian high-risk sample. J Abnorm Child Psychol 2001;29:1–10.

[55] Barrett PM, Rapee RM, Dadds MR, et al. Family enhancement of cognitive style in anxious and aggressive children. J Abnorm Child Psychol 1996;37:187–203.

[56] Chorpita BF, Albano AM, Barlow DH. Cognitive processing in children: relation to anxiety and family influences. J Clin Child Psychol 1996;25:170–6.

[57] Ginsburg GS, Silverman WK, Kurtines WM. Family involvement in treating children with anxiety and phobic disorders: a look ahead. Clin Psychol Rev 1995;15:457–73.

[58] Stark KD, Humphrey LL, Crook K, et al. Perceived family environments of depressed and anxious children: child's and maternal figure's perspectives. J Abnorm Child Psychol 1990;18:527–47.

[59] Klein DF. Delineation of two drug-responsive anxiety syndromes. Psychopharmacologia 1964;17:397–408.

[60] Battaglia M, Bertella S, Politi E, et al. Age at onset of panic disorder: influence of familial liability to the disease and of childhood separation anxiety disorder. Am J Psychiatry 1995; 162:1362–4.

[61] Silove D, Manicavasagar V, O'Connell D, et al. Genetic factors in early separation anxiety: implications for the genesis of adult anxiety disorders. Acta Psychiatr Scand 1995;92:17–24.

[62] Lipsitz JD, Martin LY, Mannuzza S, et al. Childhood separation anxiety disorder in patients with adult anxiety disorders. Am J Psychiatry 1994;151:927–9.

[63] Last CG, Perrin S, Hersen M, et al. A prospective study of childhood anxiety disorders. J Am Acad Child Adolesc Psychiatry 1996;35:1502–10.

[64] Pine DS, Cohen P, Gurley D, et al. The risk for early adulthood anxiety and depressive disorders in adolescents with anxiety and depressive disorders. Arch Gen Psychiatry 1998; 55:56–64.

[65] Aschenbrand SG, Kendall PC, Webb A, et al. Is childhood separation anxiety disorder a predictor of adult panic disorder and agoraphobia? a seven-year longitudinal study. J Am Acad Child Adolesc Psychiatry 2003;42:1478–85.

[66] Kazdin A, Weisz J. Identifying and developing empirically supported child and adolescent treatments. J Consult Clin Psychol 1998;66:100–10.

[67] Ollendick TH, King NJ. Empirically supported treatments for children with phobic and anxiety disorders: current status. J Clin Child Psychol 1998;27:156–67.

[68] Kendall PC. Treating anxiety disorders in children: results of a randomized clinical trial. J Consult Clin Psychol 1994;62:200–10.

[69] Kendall PC, Flannery-Schroeder E, Panichelli-Mindell SM, et al. Therapy for youths with anxiety disorders: a second randomized clinical trial. J Consult Clin Psychol 1997;65: 366–80.

[70] Barrett PM. Evaluation of cognitive-behavioral group treatments for childhood anxiety disorders. J Clin Child Psychol 1998;27:459–68.

[71] Barrett PM, Dadds MR, Rapee RM. Family treatment of childhood anxiety: a controlled trial. J Consult Clin Psychol 1996;64:333–42.

[72] Cobham VE, Dadds MR, Spence SH. The role of parental anxiety in the treatment of childhood anxiety. J Consult Clin Psychol 1998;66:893–905.

[73] Howard B, Kendall PC. Family cognitive-behavioral therapy for anxiety-disordered children: a multiple-baseline evaluation. Cognit Ther Res 1996;20:423–43.

[74] Mendlowitz SL, Manassis K, Bradley S, et al. Cognitive-behavioral group treatments in childhood anxiety disorders: the role of parental involvement. J Am Acad Child Adolesc Psychiatry 1999;38:1223–9.

[75] Silverman WK, Kurtines WM, Ginsburg GS, et al. Contingency management, self-control, and education support in the treatment of childhood phobic disorders: a randomized clinical trial. J Consult Clin Psychol 1999;67:675–87.

[76] Silverman WK, Kurtines WM, Ginsburg GS, et al. Treating anxiety disorder in children with group cognitive behavior therapy: randomized clinical trial. J Consult Clin Psychol 1999; 67:995–1003.

[77] Flannery-Schroeder EC, Kendall PC. Group and individual cognitive-behavioral treatments for youth with anxiety-disorders: a randomized clinical trial. Cognit Ther Res 2000;24:251–78.

[78] Kendall PC, Brady E, Verduin TV. Comorbidity in childhood anxiety disorders and treatment outcome. J Am Acad Child Adolesc Psychiatry 2001;40:787–94.

[78a] Flannery-Schroeder E, Suveg C, Kendall PC, et al. Effect of comorbid externalizing disorders on child anxiety treatment outcomes. Behavior Change 2004;21:14–25.

[78b] Southam-Gerow MA, Kendall PC, Weersing VR. Examining outcome variability: correlates of treatment response in a child and adolescent anxiety clinic. J Clin Child Psychol 2001;30: 422–36.

[79] Labellarte MJ, Ginsburg GS, Walkup JT, et al. The treatment of anxiety disorders in children and adolescents. Biol Psychiatry 1999;46:1567–78.

[80] Bernstein GA, Garfinkel Borchardt CM. Comparative studies of pharmacotherapy for school refusal. J Am Acad Child Adolesc Psychiatry 1990;29:773–81.

[81] Gittelman-Klein R, Klein DF. Controlled imipramine treatment of school phobia. Arch Gen Psychiatry 1971;25:204–7.

[82] Klein RG, Koplewicz HS, Kanner A. Imipramine treatment in children with separation anxiety disorder. J Am Acad Child Adolesc Psychiatry 1992;31:21–8.

[83] Birmaher B, Waterman GS, Ryan ND, et al. Fluoxetine for childhood anxiety disorders. J Am Acad Child Adolesc Psychiatry 1994;33:993–9.

[84] Fairbanks JM, Pine DS, Tancer NK, et al. Open fluoxetine treatment of mixed anxiety disorders in children and adolescents. J Am Acad Child Adolesc Psychiatry 1997;7:17–29.

[85] RUPP Anxiety Study Group. An eight-week placebo-controlled trial of fluvoxamine for anxiety disorders in children and adolescents. N Engl J Med 2001;344:1279–85.

[86] Nelles WB, Barlow DH. Do children panic? Clin Psychol Rev 1988;8:259–72.

[87] Kearney CA, Albano AM, Eisen AR, et al. The phenomenology of panic disorder in youngsters: an empirical study of a clinical sample. J Anxiety Disord 1997;11(1):49–62.

[88] Moreau D, Weissman MM. Panic disorder in children and adolescents: a review. Am J Psychiatry 1992;149:1306–14.

[89] American Psychiatric Association. Diagnostic and statistical manual of mental disorders. 4th edition, revised. Washington (DC): American Psychiatric Association; 1994.

[90] Ollendick TH, Mattis SG, King NJ. Panic in children and adolescents: a review. J Clin Psychol Psychiatry 1994;35:113–34.

[91] Last CG, Strauss CC. Panic disorder in children and adolescents. J Anxiety Disord 1989;3: 87–95.
[92] Essau C, Conradt J, Petermann F. Frequency, comorbidity, and psychosocial impairment of anxiety disorders in German adolescents. J Anxiety Disord 2000;14(3):263–79.
[93] Hayward C, Killen JD, Taylor CB. The relationship between agoraphobia symptoms and panic disorder in a non-clinical sample of adolescents. Psychol Med 2003;33:733–8.
[94] Hayward C, Killen JD, Kraemer HC, et al. Predictors of panic attacks in adolescents. J Am Acad Child Adol Psychiatry 2000;39(2):207–14.
[95] Verhulst FC, van der Ende J, Ferdindand RF, et al. The prevalence of DSM-III-R diagnoses in a national sample of Dutch adolescents. Arch Gen Psychiatry 1997;54(4):329–36.
[96] Whitacker A, Johnson J, Shaffer D, et al. Uncommon troubles in young people: prevalence estimates of selected psychiatric disorders in a nonreferred adolescent population. Arch Gen Psychiatry 1990;47:487–96.
[97] Alessi NE, Robbins DR, Dilsaver SC. Panic and depressive disorders among psychiatrically hospitalized adolescents. Psychiatry Res 1987;20:275–83.
[98] Biederman J, Faraone SV, Marrs A, et al. Panic disorder and agoraphobia in consecutively referred children and adolescents. J Am Acad Child Adolesc Psychiatry 1997;36(2):214–23.
[99] Thyer BA, Parrish RT, Curtis GC, et al. Ages of onset of DSM-III anxiety disorders. Compr Psychiatry 1985;26:113–22.
[100] Weissman MM, Bland RC, Canino GJ, et al. The cross-national epidemiology of panic disorder. Arch Gen Psychiatry 1997;54(4):305–9.
[101] Kessler RC, McGonagle K, Zhao S, et al. Lifetime and 12-month prevalence of DMS-III-R psychiatric disorders in the United States: results from the National Comorbidity Survey. Arch Gen Psychiatry 1994;51(1):8–19.
[102] Ginsburg GS, Drake KL. Anxiety sensitivity and panic attack symptomatology among low-income African American adolescents. J Anxiety Disord 2002;16:83–96.
[103] Hirshfeld-Becker DR, Biederman J, Rosenbaum JF. Behavioral inhibition. In: Morris TL, March JS, editors. Anxiety disorders in children and adolescents. New York: Guilford Press; 2004. p. 27–58.
[104] Barlow DH. Anxiety and its disorders: the nature and treatment of anxiety and panic. New York: Guilford Press; 1988.
[105] Mattis SG, Ollendick TH. Panic in children and adolescents: a review. In: Ollendick TH, Prinz RJ, editors. Advances in clinical psychology, Volume 19. New York: Plenum Press; 1997.
[106] Ollendick TH. Panic disorder in children and adolescents: new developments, new directions. J Clin Child Psychol 1998;27(3):234–45.
[107] Last CG, Hersen M, Kazdin A, et al. Anxiety disorders in children and their families. Arch Gen Psychiatry 1991;48:928–34.
[108] Hayward C, Killen JD, Hammer LD, et al. Pubertal stage and panic attack history in sixth- and seventh-grade girls. Am J Psychiatry 1992;149(9):1239–43.
[109] Orvaschel H, Puig-Antich JH. Schedule for affective disorders and schizophrenia for school-age children, epidemiologic version. 4th edition. Pittsburgh (PA): Western Psychiatric Institute and Clinic; 1987.
[110] Goisman RM, Warshaw MG, Peterson LG. Panic, agoraphobia, and panic disorder with agoraphobia: data from a multicenter anxiety disorders study. J Nerv Ment Dis 1994;18(2):72–9.
[111] Keller MB, Yonkers KA, Warshaw MG. Remission and relapse in subjects with panic disorder and panic with agoraphobia: a prospective short interval naturalistic follow-up. J Nerv Ment Dis 1994;182(5):290–6.
[112] Barlow DH, Craske MG, Cerny JA, et al. Behavioral treatment of panic disorder. Behav Ther 1989;20:261–82.
[113] Barlow DH, Gorman JM, Shear MK, et al. Cognitive-behavioral therapy, imipramine, or their combination for panic disorder: a randomized controlled trial. JAMA 2000;283(19):2529–36.
[114] Ollendick TH. Cognitive-behavioral treatment of panic disorder with agoraphobia in adolescents: a multiple baseline design analysis. Behav Ther 1995;26:517–31.

[115] Hoffman EC, Cohen EM, Mattis SG, et al. The effect of cognitive-behavioral treatment of panic disorder in adolescence on self-report measures of anxiety and depression [poster]. Presented at the 34th Annual Convention of the Association for the Advancement of Behavior Therapy. New Orleans (LA), November 16–19, 2000.

[116] Birmaher B, Ollendick TH. Childhood onset panic disorder. In: Ollendick TH, March JS, editors. Phobic and anxiety disorders in children and adolescents: a clinician's guide to effective psychosocial and pharmacological interventions. New York: Oxford University Press; 2003. p. 110–32.

[117] Birmaher B, Alexson DA, Monk K, et al. Fluoxetine for the treatment of childhood anxiety disorders. J Am Acad Child Adolesc Psychiatry 2003;42:415–23.

[118] Renaud J, Birmaher B, Wassic SC, et al. Use of selective serotonin reuptake inhibitors for the treatment of childhood panic disorder: a pilot study. J Child Adolesc Psychopharmacol 1999;9:73–83.

[119] Evans L. Functional school refusal subtypes: anxiety, avoidance, and malingering. Psychol Sch 2000;27(2):183–91.

[120] Kearney CA, Beasley JF. The clinical treatment of school refusal behavior: a survey of referral and practice characteristics. Psychol Sch 1994;31:128–32.

[121] Kearney CA, Silverman WK. The evolution and reconciliation of taxonomic strategies for school refusal behavior. Behav Ther 1999;30:673–96.

[122] Kearney CA, Albano AM. The functional profiles of school refusal behavior: diagnostic aspects. Behav Modif 2004;28(1):147–61.

[123] King NJ, Berstein GA. School refusal in children and adolescents: a review of the past 10 years. J Am Acad Child Adolesc Psychiatry 2001;40(2):197–205.

[124] Elliott JG. Practitioner review: school refusal: issues of conceptualization, assessment, and treatment. J Child Psychol Psychiatry 1999;40(7):1001–12.

[125] Burke AE, Silverman WK. The prescriptive treatment of school refusal. Clin Psychol Rev 1987;7(4):353–62.

[126] Granell de Aldax E, Vivas E, et al. Estimating the prevalence of school refusal and school-related fears: a Venezuelan sample. J Nerv Ment Dis 1984;172:722–9.

[127] King NJ, Ollendick TH, Tonge BJ. School refusal: assessment and treatment. Boston: Allyn & Bacon; 1995.

[128] Ollendick TH, Mayer JA. School phobia. In: Turner SM, editor. Behavioural theories and treatment of anxiety. New York: Plenum Press; 1984. p. 367–406.

[129] King N, Tonge BJ, Heyne D, et al. Research on the cognitive-behavioral treatment of school refusal: a review and recommendations. Clin Psychol Rev 2000;(4):495–507.

[130] McShane G, Walter G, Rey JM. Characteristics of adolescents with school refusal. Aust N Z J Psychiatry 2001;35:822–6.

[131] Bernstein GA, Warren SL, Massie ED, et al. Family dimensions in anxious-depressed school refusers. J Anxiety Disord 1999;13:513–28.

[132] Bernstein GA, Svingen P, Garfinkel BD. School phobia: patterns of family functioning. J Am Acad Child Adolesc Psychiatry 1990;29:24–30.

[133] Kearney CA, Silverman WK. Family environment of youngsters with school refusal behavior: a synopsis with implications for assessment and treatment. Am J Fam Ther 1995;23:59–72.

[134] Kearney CA, Tillotson CA. School attendance. In: Watson D, Gresham M, editors. Handbook of child behaviour therapy. New York: Plenum Press; 1998. p. 143–61.

[135] Flakierska-Praquin N, Lindström M, Gillberg C. School phobia with separation anxiety disorder: a comparative 20- to 29-year follow-up study of 35 school refusers. Compr Psychiatry 1997;38(1):17–22.

[136] Berg I, Jackson A. Teenage school refusers grow up: a follow-up study of 168 subjects, ten years on average after in-patient treatment. Br J Psychiatry 1985;147:366–70.

[137] Buitelaar JK, van Andel H, Duyx JHM, et al. Depressive and anxiety disorders in adolescence: a follow-up study of adolescents with school refusal. Acta Paedopsychiatr 1994;56: 249–53.

[138] King NJ, Tonge BJ, Heyne D, et al. Cognitive-behavioral treatment of school-refusing children: a controlled evaluation. J Am Acad Child Adolesc Psychiatry 1998;37:395–403.

[139] King N, Tonge BJ, Heyne D, et al. Cognitive-behavioural treatment of school-refusing children: maintenance of improvement at 3- to 5-year follow-up. Scandinavian Journal of Behaviour Therapy 2001;30(2):85–9.

[140] Last CG, Hersen M, Franco N. Cognitive-behavioral treatment of school phobia. J Am Acad Child Adolesc Psychiatry 1998;37:404–11.

[140a] Kendall PC. Cognitive-behavioral therapy for anxious children: therapist manual. 2nd edition. Ardmore (PA): Workbook Publishing; 2000.

[141] Kearney CA, Pursell C, Alvarez K. Treatment of school refusal behavior in children with mixed functional profiles. Cognitive and Behavioral Practice 2001;8:3–11.

[142] Kearney CA, Silverman WK. Functionally based prescriptive and nonprescriptive treatment for children and adolescents with school refusal behavior. Behav Ther 1999;30(4):673–95.

[143] Bernstein GA, Borchardt CM, Perwien AR, et al. Imipramine plus cognitive-behavioral therapy in the treatment of school refusal. J Am Acad Child Adolesc Psychiatry 2000;39:276–83.

[144] Bernstein GA, Shaw K, American Academy of Child and Adolescent Psychiatry. Summary of the practice parameters for the assessment and treatment of children and adolescents with anxiety disorders. J Am Acad Child Adolesc Psychiatry 1997;36(11):1639–41.

ELSEVIER
SAUNDERS

Child Adolesc Psychiatric Clin N Am
14 (2005) 797–818

CHILD AND
ADOLESCENT
PSYCHIATRIC CLINICS
OF NORTH AMERICA

Childhood Social Anxiety Disorder: From Understanding to Treatment

Denise A. Chavira, PhD*, Murray B. Stein, MD, MPH, FRCPC

Anxiety and Traumatic Stress Disorders Clinic, Department of Psychiatry,
University of California San Diego, 9500 Gilman Drive (0985), La Jolla, CA 92093-0985, USA

Childhood social anxiety disorder (SAD) has been frequently characterized as "just shyness" or a behavior that the child will "grow out of"; however empirical findings suggest that its presentation is not always so benign. During the past decade, social anxiety disorder has been revealed as a condition that is highly prevalent and associated with significant impairment. To address this current status, more focus has been directed toward understanding the causes of social anxiety disorder as well as developing and examining the efficacy of various interventions. Significant strides have been made, and the stage is set for innovative studies to advance the understanding and treatment of childhood social anxiety disorder.

Definition, prevalence, and age at onset

SAD, also known as social phobia (SP), has existed in the Diagnostic and Statistical Manual of Mental Disorders (DSM) nomenclature for over 20 years. During this time, although it has undergone many revisions, the criterion of excessive fear of social or performance situations in which a person is exposed to scrutiny or possible humiliation has remained its defining feature. Using DSM, Third Edition, Revised (-III-R) criteria [1], a 3-month prevalence rate of 2.5% was reported in children age 8 to 17 years old [2]. Using a 6-month interval,

* Corresponding author.
E-mail address: dchavira@ucsd.edu (D.A. Chavira).

1056-4993/05/$ – see front matter © 2005 Elsevier Inc. All rights reserved.
doi:10.1016/j.chc.2005.05.003

prevalence rates rose to approximately 5% in youth 12 to 18 years old, with girls having modestly higher rates than boys [3,4]. More substantial changes to the social anxiety disorder criteria set occurred with the publication of DSM-IV [5], making it difficult to compare prevalence rates from past and more recent studies. Specifically, DSM-IV did away with overanxious disorder and avoidant disorder of childhood, given that many cases of these disorders were indistinguishable from social anxiety disorder [6,7]. Two large epidemiologic studies [8,9] of German adolescents have found rates of DSM-IV social anxiety disorder to be 0.5% in children and 2.0% to 4.0% in adolescents. In both studies, females had higher rates of social anxiety disorder than males. Data from the Great Smoky Mountains Study [10], a large epidemiologic and longitudinal study of childhood psychiatric disorders, which included DSM-III-R and DSM-IV criteria in the diagnostic assessment, suggest lower prevalence rates (ie, 0.3% for 9–12 year olds and 0.7% for 13–16 year olds) [10,11]. In a smaller community study [12] that used a diagnostic method similar to the aforementioned study, 3-month prevalence rates were 0.8% for 9 to 12 year olds and 1.7% for 13 to 17 year olds. Prevalence rates are variable across studies likely because of changing diagnostic criteria, study methodology, informant report, and criteria used to delimit clinical significance. Despite such variability, the considerable prevalence of social anxiety disorder remains evident.

Epidemiologic data suggest that adolescents have higher rates of social anxiety disorder than younger age groups. Essau and colleagues [8] have found an increase greater than twofold between the 12- to 13-year-old and 14- to 15-year-old groups (0.5% versus 2.0%, respectively), whereas Wittchen and colleagues [9] have found a twofold increase among the 14- to 17-year-old and 18- to 24-year-old groups (4.0% versus 8.7%, respectively). Similarly, data from the Great Smoky Mountains Study [10] indicate that disorders such as social anxiety, panic, depression. and substance abuse increase over time, whereas other disorders such as separation anxiety and attention deficit hyperactivity disorder (ADHD) decrease over time [13]. The increasing prevalence of social anxiety disorder across age groups may be understood partially as increased self-consciousness in the context of both developmental and environmental transitions (ie, puberty, dating, new schools, peer influences, and other factors).

The mean age of onset for social phobia is often reported as occurring during adolescence [14,15]; however, studies also support earlier onset, between the ages of 7 and 8 years old [11,16]. Some evidence suggests that the earlier onset group may be more likely to have the more severe, generalized type of social anxiety disorder, although findings have not been conclusive in this regard [17].

Phenomenology

Children and adolescents with social anxiety disorder may have one or more social fears. The presence of multiple social fears across both interactional and performance situations seems to be a qualitatively distinct condition compared with a single circumscribed social fear (eg, public speaking, athletic performance, writing, using public bathrooms). For this reason, subtyping systems (ie, generalized social anxiety disorder and nongeneralized social anxiety disorder) have been created. Paralleling findings from the adult literature, generalized social anxiety disorder in youth appears to be a more pervasive and disabling condition than nongeneralized social anxiety disorder [9,18,19]. Children with social anxiety disorder, likely those with the generalized type, report that they experience a distressing social situation almost every other day and that most of these situations occur in school [6]. Both children and adolescents rate "talking to peers" as one of their most feared situations [20,21]. Other commonly reported fears (ie, reported by more than 50% of children with social anxiety disorder) include reading aloud in class, musical or athletic performances, joining in a conversation, speaking to adults, starting a conversation, and writing on the blackboard [22]. Frequent physiologic responses include heart palpitations, shakiness, sweating, flushes, chills, and nausea [23]. Behavioral concomitants such as avoidance and social skills deficits also are reported [8,22,24], as are anxious or negative cognitions, although the latter seem to be less prevalent in younger children. The extent to which children and adolescents exhibit social skills or information processing deficits remains a topic of debate.

In a study by Spence and colleagues [24], 27 children with social anxiety disorder rated themselves and were rated by their parents as less socially skilled and less socially competent than a matched nonclinical group of children (ages 7–14 years old). Observers also reported significant deficits in the mean length of responses, number of peer interactions, and number of spontaneous initiations made with peers compared with nonanxious children. Similarly, Beidel and colleagues [22] have found that children with social anxiety disorder (N = 50) were rated as less skilled when reading aloud and interacting with a same-aged peer and likewise exhibited longer speech latencies than nonanxious children.

The literature on cognitive biases has been less consistent [6,25]. In the aforementioned study [24], children with social anxiety disorder were less likely than their nonanxious peers to anticipate positive social situations, but no differences occurred for negative social situations. Also, no differences were found for expectations regarding negative and positive nonsocial events. When children were asked to recall their cognitions after watching themselves on a video replay of a performance and a social interaction task, children with social anxiety disorder reported more negative expectancies about their performance on both tasks. Interestingly, although there were trends toward significance, self-evaluations of performance for both the reading and interaction tasks did not reveal significant between group differences, nor were there differences in observer ratings of actual performance on the reading task.

Using standardized information processing paradigms, additional differences have been noted. Muris and colleagues [26] presented a sample of 252 non-referred socially anxious children with ambiguous stories of social situations and instructed them to figure out as quickly as possible whether a story was scary.

Socially anxious children needed to hear fewer sentences of a story before deciding it was scary and more often perceived threat while listening to the stories than did control children. A poorer recognition of facial affect also has been found among children with social anxiety disorder. In one study [27], 15 children with social anxiety disorder and 14 control children were asked to identify emotions on slides with pictures of facial affect. Children with social anxiety disorder had poorer facial affect recognition skills than controls did and reported greater anxiety at the completion of the task. In another study, 149 second and third graders participated in a facial discrimination trial [28]; regression analyses showed that higher rates of errors were associated with higher social anxiety scores and fewer spontaneous comments.

At this point the causal directions among these variables are unknown. Traditional cognitive models support the hypothesis that cognitive processes drive social anxiety by creating distortions of self and social performance [29,30]. Behavioral models contend that individuals who are socially anxious have social skills deficits that lead to poorer outcomes and avoidant behaviors and, thus, realistic negative appraisals of social competence and outcome expectancy [31]. According to Rapee and Heimberg [30], "the negative view of how others see one's appearance or behavior may be the results of actual deficits (eg, disfigurement, social skills deficits), distorted perceptions of one's appearance or behavior as seen by others, or both." Longitudinal data are needed to clarify these findings. In the meantime, interventions are probably best served by the inclusion of both cognitive and behavioral strategies in which respective merits can be informed by dismantling designs.

Sequelae

Social anxiety disorder in youth is a risk factor for poor psychosocial outcomes. Longitudinal studies with clinical and community samples suggest that social anxiety disorder during youth is associated with later anxiety, major depression, substance abuse disorders [13,32–34], and suicide attempts [35]. Second, social anxiety disorder often persists into adulthood and often goes untreated [36], a pattern that comes at a cost to both society and the individual. Third, social anxiety disorder is associated with educational underachievement, low self-esteem, and loneliness [37–39].

On the other hand, some studies have found that social anxiety disorder can act as a protective factor for various behavioral problems. Myers and colleagues [40] have assessed social anxiety and substance abuse in a sample of 724 high school students. Using dispositional structural equation modeling, substance use was associated with a lower grade point average, male gender, white, higher levels of negative affectivity, and lower levels of social anxiety. In another study, Mason and colleagues [41] have examined behavior problems at ages 10 and 11 as predictors of adult depression, social anxiety disorder, and violence at age 21 years. Findings suggest that self-reported shyness inhibited later violence, and few child behavioral problems predicted social anxiety disorder. Additionally, some studies suggest that the presence of anxiety with ADHD may alter the symptom pattern of ADHD, resulting in inhibition of some disruptive behaviors; however these findings are not consistent [42,43].

Comorbidity

Based on epidemiologic data [8,9,34], social anxiety disorder is most frequently comorbid with depressive disorders, substance use disorders, and other anxiety disorders. In a recent cross-sectional study [19] of 190 randomly selected children (ages 8–17 years old) from a primary care setting, the generalized type of social anxiety disorder was highly comorbid with major depression, generalized anxiety disorder, specific phobias, and ADHD, whereas little comorbidity was present for the nongeneralized subtype of social anxiety disorder. As expected, rates of comorbidity, particularly with other anxiety disorders, are usually higher in treatment-seeking samples [14,44,45].

The case of selective mutism

Although selective mutism is still classified among other disorders of infancy [5], positioning selective mutism as distinct and separate from social anxiety disorder is not well supported [46]. Instead, it seems more likely that selective mutism is an early onset and severe form of social anxiety disorder [47,48]. Data supporting this position include comorbidity rates of social anxiety disorder and selective mutism ranging from 97% to 100% [48,49]. In addition, children with selective mutism are often described as shy, anxious, withdrawn, and serious [50,51], characteristics also used to define socially anxious youth. Using a self-report checklist methodology to assess the presence of social anxiety disorder and selective mutism in parents of youth with selective mutism, rates of 70% and 37% respectively were found [49].

Although data seem to favor selective mutism as a severe form of social anxiety, other investigators contend that this position may be premature [52]. In a study [52] aimed at addressing this question, 23 children with comorbid selective mutism and social anxiety disorder and 23 age-matched controls with social anxiety disorder alone were compared. Clinician and observer ratings for children with selective mutism revealed higher ratings of social distress than for children with social anxiety disorder alone. Child self-report data however did not indicate differences on measures of trait anxiety, general fears, Child Behavior Checklist (CBCL) broadband internalizing or externalizing scales [53], or on self-ratings of distress after behavioral tasks involving interactions with same-aged peers. Interestingly, children with the comorbid condition scored higher than children with social anxiety disorder alone on the CBCL delinquency subscale, but the difference was small and not in the clinically significant range.

Findings from this study are therefore mixed; informants report more anxiety and distress, yet children's self reports are not consistent with this perception.

In another comparative study, Manassis and colleagues [54] assessed a sample of 14 children with comorbid selective mutism and social anxiety disorder and nine children with social anxiety disorder alone. Anxiety rating scales, cognitive and academic tests, and assessments of language abilities using parents' reports and the child's performance on nonverbal language tests were administered. Both groups had similar levels of anxiety and academic ability, but children with comorbid selective mutism and social anxiety disorder performed less well on the task assessing the ability to discriminate one sound from another. The groups did not differ on the other assessment of phonemic awareness or on two receptive language tasks. Parents did not rate the speech, syntax, and fluency of the comorbid group as different overall in the home environment than that of the social anxiety only group. Although other studies support the presence of language impairments among children with selective mutism [55,56], presently, findings are mixed, and the directional relationship between social anxiety and speech problems is unknown.

Many issues remain unresolved with regard to the relationship of social anxiety disorder and selective mutism. Future studies, which include physiologic assessments during performance tasks, could provide objective indices of anxiety symptoms, which are likely very relevant for socially anxious children who may exhibit self-presentation biases on self-report measures [57]. Similarly, diagnostic interviews with parents of children who have selective mutism will clarify the nature of delinquent and oppositional behaviors and the extent to which these behaviors are related to situations involving speech refusal. In the present authors' clinical practice as well as that of colleagues (Lindsey Bergman, PhD, personal communication, 2004, and Elisa Shipon Blum, OD, personal communication, 2004), variations in the presentation of children with selective mutism are noted (eg, mutism with social anxiety, mutism with mild to moderate language impairments, and mutism with behavioral problems in the absence of significant social anxiety). Additional research is necessary to clarify whether these variations represent qualitatively distinct conditions. Longitudinal studies also are necessary to understand the extent to which selective mutism is a transient versus stable disorder as well as to document its natural course and potential long-term sequelae.

Relationship to shyness

Shyness, the tendency to be socially reticent, is very common [58,59]. In the short term, shy children, particularly those with "stable" or persistent shyness, are often lonely and prone to low self-esteem [37,60]. In the long term, childhood shyness and related personality characteristics may constitute risk factors for delayed milestones and the development of social anxiety disorder [61,62].

Closer scrutiny of the relationship between shyness and social anxiety disorder is therefore warranted.

Longitudinal studies of shyness

Longitudinal studies of shy children report delays in various lifetime milestones; shy boys get married and become parents later than nonshy boys, whereas shy girls are less likely to attend college than nonshy girls [63]. There also is some support for the notion that childhood shyness later transforms into anxiety disorders [64]. In a community study of approximately 2000 families followed over 15 years from infancy to early adolescence, a shy temperament in infancy or early childhood, as measured by the mother's ratings, increased the odds (approximately 2–3 times) of anxiety disorders in early or mid-adolescence. Conversely, children with adolescent anxiety problems were several-fold times more likely to have been rated as shy during childhood than adolescents who were not anxious. Still, most shy children did not develop an anxiety disorder, and most adolescents with anxiety disorders had not been especially shy. The authors concluded that childhood shyness has "modest, but clinically meaningful" predictive utility for adolescent anxiety disorders in a community sample [64].

Behavioral inhibition and related traits

Behavioral inhibition [65,66], a temperamental characteristic similar to shyness but measured through behavioral tasks in the clinical laboratory, also poses an increased risk for later social anxiety disorder. In an important follow-up study [67] of children classified at age 2 as inhibited or uninhibited, 61% of the children who were originally classified as inhibited had current social anxiety at age 13 compared with 27% who were originally classified as uninhibited [68]. Furthermore, the relationship was specific, in that childhood behavioral inhibition did not increase the odds for specific phobia, separation anxiety, or performance anxiety.

More recently, in a 21-year longitudinal study [69] of anxious or withdrawn behaviors in over 1000 youth, a link among children internalizing symptoms at age 8 and social phobia, specific phobia, panic or agoraphobia, and major depression during adolescence and young adulthood was found. This relationship was observed even after controlling for various social childhood (child abuse and conduct and attentional problems) and family factors (eg, maternal education, parental separation, family stressful life events, and parental internalizing disorders). Taken together, these studies suggest that temperamental factors such as shyness or related inhibited behaviors may act as risk factors for the development of social anxiety disorder and that such characteristics may have genetic underpinnings.

Familial-genetic influences

Familial aggregation studies

Bottom-up studies

Studies of common traits found in both children and parents provide further support for the relationship between shyness and social phobia and a possible genetic transmission of such traits. In a community study [70] of 867 preschoolers and their mothers, 108 children were rated by their mothers as being shy, and 74 were randomly selected to form a shy subgroup. This subgroup was further divided into children who were highly shy and children who were highly shy and had other problems (eg, behavioral or feeding or other problems). The control group was subdivided into children without any problems and children who were not shy but had other problems. Mothers of children with pure shyness had higher rates of affective disorders, anxiety disorders, and social anxiety disorder than the control groups did; the odds of a social anxiety disorder history was over seven times that of a combined control group. Methodologic considerations temper the conclusions that can be drawn. Specifically, mothers were classified as having social anxiety disorder even when significant impairment or distress criteria were not recognized. Nevertheless, a parallel picture emerges in clinical samples, in which children with anxiety disorders are also likely to have parents with anxiety disorders [71,72].

Top-down studies

In studies of adult probands, social anxiety disorder has been found consistently to aggregate in families, [73–75], including among their children [76]. There also is evidence to suggest that the more severe, generalized subtype of the disorder shows the strongest tendency toward familial aggregation [75,77], and one study [78] suggests that social anxiety disorder aggregates independently of other phobic disorders (ie, agoraphobia or simple phobia). These findings indicate that social anxiety disorder, particularly the generalized subtype, has a familial basis.

Twin studies

Twin studies suggest that shyness, behavioral inhibition, and social anxiety have a heritable component [79–82]. In a study [83] of childhood anxiety in 326 same-sex twin pairs (174 monozygotic and 152 dizygotic pairs), higher correlations were found for social anxiety symptoms in monozygotic than in dizygotic twin pairs. In a larger community sample [84], which included 4564 pairs of 4-year-old twins, various anxiety-related behaviors including general distress, separation anxiety, fear, obsessive-compulsive behaviors, and shyness or inhibition were assessed. Findings support some degree of genetic influence for all five behaviors; however, the contributions for general distress, separation anxiety, and fear were modest, whereas the contributions for obsessive-compulsive behaviors and shyness or inhibition (heritability estimate of 62%) were substantial. Other studies also have suggested that a portion of the familial resemblance in social anxiety is heritable [85–87], particularly for phobic disorders, including social anxiety disorder (51% heritable) [88]. It is likely that the genetic risk for social anxiety disorder is shared partially with other phobic types (eg, agoraphobia) and is partially specific [85]. Interestingly, there may be considerable overlap in the genes that influence social anxiety disorder and major depression [89], suggesting that the high comorbidity seen between these two disorders may have a strong genetic basis.

Environmental influences

Genetic influences on social anxiety account for only a portion of variance in the expressed phenotype. Adhering to a diathesis stress model, it is likely that certain environmental factors facilitate the actual expression of a clinical phobia [88]. Conditioning experiences, family environment, and parenting styles have been hypothesized as a few of these factors.

Conditioning experiences

Behavioral models suggest that fears may be acquired through classical conditioning and subsequent higher order conditioning, leading to stimulus generalization. Retrospective data from adults suggest that approximately 40% to 60% of adults can recall an event, usually referred to as a traumatic conditioning event, that precipitated the onset of their social anxiety [90,91]. For the most part, traumatic conditioning experiences have been better linked to the development of the specific nongeneralized subtype of social phobia (eg, public speaking or athletic performances) [91], whereas the generalized subtype may be more related to temperamental characteristics. Given patient reports that socially traumatic conditioning experiences have often occurred, detailed evaluation of these kinds of experiences in monozygotic twins discordant for social anxiety disorder would be a particularly informative research strategy.

Modeling

Social learning theory proposes that fears can be acquired through modeling and vicarious learning experiences [92]. The role of modeling in social anxiety has been demonstrated in experimental paradigms that usually involve presenting a child with an ambiguous story and asking the children and parent to describe what they would do in the various scenarios. In such studies, anxious children are more likely than nonanxious children to choose more avoidant solutions, which subsequently are reinforced by their parents [93]. A less direct pathway is suggested from retrospective reports (of childhood) from adults with social anxiety disorder. Compared with adults with agoraphobia, adults with social anxiety disorder recall that their parents had greater concerns about the opinions of others, seeking to isolate them as children, and de-emphasized family sociability [94,95]. Cumulatively, these learning experiences may lead to few social opportunities and limited rehearsal of social skill sets.

Family environment and parenting styles

Parenting styles also may influence the manifestation of anxiety symptoms. Anxious and controlling parenting styles may foster dependency and child insecurities about competency, which may facilitate the development of anxious beliefs about self, others, and the world. In retrospective studies, socially anxious adults recall their parents as having been more controlling (or overprotective) and less affectionate [96–99] than agoraphobic and nonphobic controls. Socially anxious youth also describe their current families as more restrictive, socially isolating, and less warm [100–102]. Using observational methodologies, which usually involve assessing parent-child interactions in free play or structured tasks, associations between greater parental control and child shyness and social anxiety have been found and effect sizes usually have been in the medium to large range [103–105].

Given the cross-sectional and often retrospective nature of these findings, causality cannot be inferred. Also, questions regarding directionality remain unanswered; for example, it may be that (1) parental behaviors influence the development of child shyness and social inhibition; (2) socially anxious youth have a way of interacting and communicating that elicits specific behaviors from parents; or (3) a combination thereof. Longitudinal studies are necessary to answer these questions. At this point, it would seem prudent that interventions be informed by such findings and incorporate family factors such as parental overcontrol or overprotection and modeling of avoidant responses as focal points in interventions. Interestingly, to date, the effects of parent-oriented interventions for child anxiety disorders and social phobia, over and above those targeted at the child have been mixed [106–108]. Additional studies investigating parent and child characteristics that may moderate treatment effects are necessary.

Assessment

There are several questionnaires specifically targeting child social anxiety symptoms. The Social Anxiety Scale-Children Revised (SASC-R) [109] and the Social Anxiety Scale-Adolescents (SAS-A) [110] are based on the conceptual model of Watson and Friend [111], who proposed that social anxiety consists of both fears of negative evaluation as well as social avoidance and distress. The SASC-R and SAS-A and their corresponding parent versions consist of 18 items and four filler items. A five-point Likert scale is used, and total scores range from 18 to 80 for the social anxiety items. A three-factor solution has been proposed, and internal consistency estimates range from 0.86 to 0.91 for fear of negative evaluation (FNE), 0.78 to 0.83 for social avoidance and distress in new situations (SAD-New), and 0.69 to 0.76 for social avoidance and distress in general (SAD-General) [110,112]. More recent estimates support Cronbach's α reliability coefficients in the range of 0.76 to 0.91 for the subscales and 0.93 for the total score [113]. Test-rest-retest estimates range from 0.63 to 0.75 for FNE, 0.61 to 0.75 for SAD-New, and 0.47 to 0.51 for SAD-General, using 2-, 4-, and 6-month intervals [114,115]. Concurrent validity has been established with other popular measures of social anxiety [116], and in a clinic sample, adolescents with social anxiety disorder reported greater SAS-A scores than adolescents with other anxiety disorders [117]. Clinical cutoffs ranging from 50 to 54 (depending on gender and age group) have been suggested to identify high socially anxious children and adolescents [110,112].

The Social Phobia and Anxiety Inventory for Children (SPAI-C) [118] is a 26-item self-report scale designed to assess the more clinical manifestations of social anxiety disorder as defined by the DSM. Items address physical, cognitive, and behavioral symptoms associated with social anxiety disorder in children between the ages of 8 and 14. The adult version, the SPAI [119], is recommended for adolescents aged 14 and older, although two items remain more appropriate for adults. The total score ranges from 0 to 52, with higher scores reflecting greater severity and frequency of social phobic symptoms. Initial factor analyses has revealed both a three-factor [118] and five-factor solution [120] (ie, assertiveness, general conversation, public performance, physical or cognitive symptoms, and behavioral avoidance). In a recent study [113] using confirmatory factor analyses, a five-factor model was supported. Internal consistency coefficients range from 0.92 to 0.95 for the total score [113,118] and 0.65 to 0.83 for the five factors [113]. Test-retest reliability across 2 weeks is 0.86 [113]. The SPAI-C is able to distinguish between children with social anxiety and those with other clinical disorders [120,121]. A cutoff of 18 suggests a possible social anxiety disorder diagnosis. Recent studies have found that both the child and adolescent versions of the SAS and the SPAI-C are moderately correlated [116], supporting the differing emphases of social anxiety in general (ie, the SAS) versus more typical clinical symptoms of social phobia (ie, the SPAI-C).

The Liebowitz Social Anxiety Scale for Children and Adolescents [122] is a new clinician administered instrument for children and adolescents (age 7–18 years old) and was modeled after the adult version of this scale (the Liebowtiz Social Anxiety Scale [LSAS]) [123]. The LSAS has been used widely in treatment outcome research for adults, and the LSAS-Children and Adults (CA) shows promise in this regard as well as for other purposes. The scale consists of 24 items (12 social interaction situations and 12 performance situations); and clinicians are asked to provide ratings of anxiety and avoidance for each item. A four-point Likert scale is used, with anxiety ratings ranging from 0 to 3 (none, mild, moderate, and severe, respectively) and avoidance ratings ranging from 0 to 3 (never, occasionally, often, and usually, respectively). Internal consistency coefficients range from $\alpha = 0.83$ to 0.97 and 1 week test- retest intraclass correlation coefficients range from 0.89 to 0.94. The LSAS-CA is significantly correlated with other measures of social anxiety and less well correlated with depression inventories. Receiver operating characteristic analyses indicate that the LSAS-CA is able to discriminate between individuals with social phobia and individuals who are healthy (using a score of 22.5) as well as those with other anxiety disorders (using a score of 29.5).

Treatment

Pharmacotherapeutic interventions

Among adults with social anxiety, pharmacologic treatments such as selective serotonin reuptake inhibitors (SSRI) have garnered much support [124–126]; however, among children and adolescents, comparatively little information is available regarding the safety and efficacy of SSRI treatment. Presently, most of the studies have been the open-label type (Table 1) [128–131], but overall, such studies support the effectiveness and safety of SSRI among children. Similarly, data emerging from double blind placebo-controlled studies for youth with anxiety disorders, among whom are included children with social anxiety disorder, also are promising, with response rates (ie, much improved or very much improved on a clinical global impression of change measure) ranging from 61% to 76% [134,135]. Interestingly, in these studies, the presence of a social anxiety disorder diagnosis has been associated with greater illness severity and a less favorable response to treatment [134,136]. Most recently, findings from a large double blind placebo-controlled study [132] of an SSRI (paroxetine) administered to 319 children with social anxiety disorder (N = 319) have emerged. In this study, approximately 75% of children were considered responders compared with 38% of those in the placebo group (see Table 1). Importantly, no children had serious side effects, and the medication was well-tolerated.

Despite better insights into the causes of childhood social phobia, the conduct of randomized controlled trials, especially for pharmacotherapy, has been impeded by many ethical and practical considerations specific to working with children. According to Caldwell and colleagues [137], there is a poor awareness and understanding among parents of randomized clinical trial procedures such as random allocation, the use of placebo, and the informed consent process. Also, concerns about risks of participation, fears of one's child being treated as an experimental subject, anxiety about unknown factors inherent in research, and concerns about researcher's priorities being primary to the child's best interests can temper the enthusiasm for participation in such trials [137]. In the absence of definitive efficacy and effectiveness data to inform prescribing practices, clinicians are guided by practice experience, and the extrapolation of efficacy and safety data from adults. The result has been the routine "off-label" application of antianxiety drugs (and other psychotropic agents [138]) with US Food and Drug Administration indications in adults, to disorders in children and adolescents [139]. Recently, the use of antidepressants in children and ado-

Table 1
Pharmacologic interventions for youth with social anxiety disorder and related conditions

Study [reference]	Disorder	Sample size (N)	Age (y)	Design	Treatment	Duration	Results
Black and Uhde, 1994 [127]	Selective mutism	16	—	Double blind placebo-controlled	Fluoxetine	12 wk	"More improved on mutism and global change but still symptomatic"
Dummit et al, 1996 [128]	Selective mutism	21	5–14	Open label	Fluoxetine	9 wk	76% had "clinical improvement" defined by dichotomized Clinical Global Impressions–Scale scores [133]
Mancini et al, 1999 [129]	SAD	7	7–18	Open label Case series, chart review	Nefazadone, Paroxetine, Sertraline	7 mo	100% showed significant improvement
Compton et al, 2001 [130]	SAD	14	10–17	Open label	Sertraline	8 wk	36% responders 29% partial responders
Chavira and Stein, 2002 [131]	SAD	12	8–16	Open label with psychoeducation	Citalopram	12 wk	41.7% much improved 41.7% very much improved
Wagner et al, 2004 [132]	SAD	319	8–16	Double blind placebo-controlled	Paroxetine	—	47.8% very much improved 29.8% much improved 38.3% placebo group responders (very much or much improved)

lescents has come under investigation by regulatory authorities (and the media) because of concerns of possible increased suicidal thinking, suicide attempts, or self-harm [132]. At this point, more research is needed to evaluate the safety profile of antidepressant medications in children with anxiety disorders. The extant research is extremely promising, with good evidence of an acceptable risk-benefit ratio, particularly when children do not respond to treatments with even lower risk (eg, counseling, behavioral therapies [BT], and cognitive behavioral therapy [CBT]). In these instances, clinicians and parents will need to weight the potential risks and benefits and make an informed decision about the use of pharmacotherapy on a case-by-case basis.

Psychosocial interventions

Studies of psychosocial treatments for social anxiety disorder also are scarce, but overall studies support the efficacy of CBT and BT programs (Table 2) [108,140–143]. CBT and BT interventions usually span 12 to 20 sessions and exist in individual and group formats. Follow-up data are promising and suggest that many of the gains from psychosocial interventions are maintained post-treatment (approximately 1 year later) [44,108,141]. Studies that have assessed the benefits of an added family component have been mixed. In the study by Spence and colleagues [108], the presence of parental involvement in an intervention for social anxiety disorder did not produce statistically significant differences ($P = .053$) between the active treatment groups. In a randomized clinical trial for children with various anxiety disorders, there were no statistically significant differences between children assigned to CBT alone versus those assigned to CBT plus seven extra sessions of parent cognitive training [107]. Other randomized CBT trials for children with anxiety disorders, however, suggest that the family component did lead to added benefits [106,144].

Presently, most of these studies rely on outcome measures assessing symptom reduction and the continued presence of diagnostic criteria. Future studies may fare well to include measures that assess functional improvement, quality of life indicators, treatment acceptability, and satisfaction ratings. Although useful treatment approaches exist, little is known about parents' perceptions of these treatments. The absence of data is surprising given that the value of such interventions may be constrained by parents' and possibly children's attitudes toward proposed treatments. In a study conducted by the present authors' research group, parents endorsed favorable attitudes toward counseling and somewhat neutral beliefs about medication [145]. Data from this study also has revealed that anxiety disorders were the most prevalent but least often treated psychiatric condition [146] among children seen by pediatricians. Among children with a current anxiety disorder, 31% had received counseling or medication treatment during their lifetime, compared with 40% of children with depression and 79% with ADHD. Other studies have suggested that pediatricians are less likely to recognize childhood mood and anxiety disorders, and educators are somewhat unfamiliar with social anxiety disorder, especially relative to ADHD

Table 2
Cognitive-behavioral and behavior interventions for youth with social anxiety disorder

Study [reference]	Sample size (N)	Age (y)	Design	Duration	Treatment groups	Results (responders)
Albano et al, 1995 [44]	5	13–15	No control group	16 sessions	Group CBT	80%
Hayward et al, 2000 [140]	35	15.5[a]	Randomized clinical trial	16 sessions	Group CBT	45%
					No treatment	4%
Beidel et al, 2000 [141]	57	8–12	Randomized clinical trial	24 sessions (12 wk)	Social effectiveness therapy for children	65%
					Test anxiety control	5%
Spence et al, 2001 [108]	50	7–14	Randomized clinical trial	12 wk + 2 booster sessions	CBT	58%
					CBT parent	87.5%
					Wait-list control	7%
Masia et al, 2001 [142]	6	13–17	No control group (school setting)	14 sessions	Group CBT	100% 50% (diagnosis free)
Gallagher et al, 2004 [143]	23	8–11	Randomized clinical trial	3 sessions (3 wk)	CBT group intervention	33% (parent report) 41.6% (child report)
					Wait-list control	0

[a] Mean age of adolescents in study.

[147,148]. Future studies investigating reasons for this gap, including the influence of attitudes and beliefs on recognition, service engagement, use, and treatment outcome are necessary. Furthermore, efforts to improve the generalizability of empirically supported treatments for child anxiety disorders are warranted. To date, investigators have begun to examine the comparative efficacy of interventions across ethnic groups [149,150], abbreviated cognitive behavioral and psychologic education treatment to improve feasibility [131,143], and the transportability of empirically supported treatments to real world settings [142]. Additional investigations of this nature will significantly improve the access to and quality of care available to children with social anxiety disorder.

Summary

During the past two decades, childhood social anxiety disorder has emerged as a prevalent and impairing disorder warranting the concern and attention of health care professionals and educators. Given evolving classification systems, additional descriptive and epidemiologic studies are warranted to understand the prevalence and impact of social anxiety disorder as well as related conditions such as selective mutism. Continued translational research efforts that attempt to identify causative factors and incorporate such findings into practice are necessary. Controlled treatment outcome studies need to test psychopharmacologic and psychosocial interventions, and the combination thereof. Furthermore, models that incorporate components to enhance transportability and acceptability will be critical for future dissemination of empirically supported treatments. Interventions that are effective, feasible and generalizable are likely to have significant impact at a time when mental health provisions for children are wanting.

References

[1] American Psychiatric Association. Diagnostic and statistical manual of mental disorders. 3rd edition, revised. Washington (DC): American Psychiatric Association; 1987.
[2] Simonoff E, Pickles A, Meyer JM, et al. The Virginia twin study of adolescent behavioral development: influences of age, sex, and impairment on rates of disorder. Arch Gen Psychiatry 1997;54:801–8.
[3] Costello EJ, Angold A, Keeler GP. Adolescent outcomes of childhood disorders: the consequences of severity and impairment. J Am Acad Child Adolesc Psychiatry 1999;38:121–8.
[4] Verhulst FC, van der Ende J, Ferdinand RF, et al. The prevalence of DSM-III-R diagnoses in a national sample of Dutch adolescents. Arch Gen Psychiatry 1997;54:329–36.
[5] American Psychiatric Association. Diagnostic and statistical manual of mental disorders. 4th edition, revised. Washington (DC): American Psychiatric Association; 1994.
[6] Beidel DC. Social phobia and overanxious disorder in school-age children. J Am Acad Child Adolesc Psychiatry 1991;30:545–52.
[7] Francis G, Last CG, Strauss CC. Avoidant disorder and social phobia in children and adolescents. J Am Acad Child Adolesc Psychiatry 1992;31:1086–9.
[8] Essau CA, Conradt J, Petermann F. Frequency and comorbidity of social phobia and social fears in adolescents. Behav Res Ther 1999;37:831–43.

[9] Wittchen H-U, Stein MB, Kessler RC. Social fears and social phobia in a community sample of adolescents and young adults: prevalence, risk factors and co-morbidity. Psychol Med 1999; 29:309–23.

[10] Costello EJ, Angold A, Burns BJ, et al. The Great Smoky Mountains Study of Youth: goals, design, methods, and the prevalence of DSM-III-R disorders. Arch Gen Psychiatry 1996;53: 1129–36.

[11] Costello EJ, Egger HL. Developmental epidemiology of anxiety disorders. In: Ollendick T, March J, editors. Phobic and anxiety disorders in children and adolescents. New York: Oxford University Press; 2004. p. 61–91.

[12] Angold A, Costello EJ, Burns BJ, et al. Effectiveness of nonresidential specialty mental health services for children and adolescents in the "real world." J Am Acad Child Adolesc Psychiatry 2000;39:154–60.

[13] Costello EJ, Mustillo S, Erkanli A, et al. Prevalence and development of psychiatric disorders in childhood and adolescence. Arch Gen Psychiatry 2003;60:837–44.

[14] Last CG, Perrin S, Hersen M, et al. DSM-III-R anxiety disorders in children: sociodemographic and clinical characteristics. J Am Acad Child Adolesc Psychiatry 1992;31:1070–6.

[15] Turner SM, Beidel DC, Dancu CV, et al. Psychopathology of social phobia and comparison to avoidant personality disorder. J Abnorm Psychol 1986;95:389–94.

[16] Schneier FR, Johnson J, Hornig CD, et al. Social phobia: comorbidity and morbidity in an epidemiological sample. Arch Gen Psychiatry 1992;49:282–8.

[17] Chavira DA, Stein MB. Phenomenology and epidemiology of social phobia. In: Stein DJ, Hollander E, editors. Textbook of anxiety disorders. Washington (DC): American Psychiatric Press, Inc.; 2001. p. 289–300.

[18] Stein MB, Chavira DA. Subtypes of social phobia and comorbidity with depression and other anxiety disorders. J Affect Disord 1998;50:S11–6.

[19] Chavira DA, Stein MB, Bailey K, et al. Comorbidity of generalized social anxiety disorder and depression in a pediatric primary care sample. J Affect Disord 2004;80:163–71.

[20] Strauss CC, Last CG. Social and simple phobias in children. J Anxiety Disord 1993;1:141–52.

[21] Hofmann SG, Albano AM, Heimberg RG, et al. Subtypes of social phobia in adolescents. Depress Anxiety 1999;9:15–8.

[22] Beidel DC, Turner SM, Morris TL. Psychopathology of childhood social phobia. J Am Acad Child Adolesc Psychiatry 1999;38:643–50.

[23] Beidel DC, Christ MG, Long PJ. Somatic complaints in anxious children. J Abnorm Child Psychol 1991;19:659–70.

[24] Spence SH, Donovan C, Brechman-Toussaint M. Social skills, social outcomes, and cognitive features of childhood social phobia. J Abnorm Psychol 1999;108:211–21.

[25] Epkins CC. Cognitive specificity and affective confounding in social anxiety and dysphoria in children. Journal of Psychopathology and Behavioral Assessment 1996;18:83–101.

[26] Muris P, Merckelbach H, Damsma E. Threat perception bias in nonreferred, socially anxious children. J Clin Child Psychol 2000;29:348–59.

[27] Simonian SJ, Beidel DC, Turner SM, et al. Recognition of facial affect by children and adolescents diagnosed with social phobia. Child Psychiatry Hum Dev 2001;32:137–45.

[28] Battaglia M, Ogliari A, Zanoni A, et al. Children's discrimination of expressions of emotions: relationship with indices of social anxiety and shyness. J Am Acad Child Adolesc Psychiatry 2004;43:358–65.

[29] Beck AT, Emery G, Greenberg RL. Anxiety disorders and phobias: a cognitive perspective. New York: Basic Books; 1985.

[30] Rapee RM, Heimberg RG. A cognitive-behavioral model of anxiety in social phobia. Behav Res Ther 1997;35:741–56.

[31] Turner SM, Beidel DC, Cooley MR, et al. A multi-component behavioral treatment for social phobia: social effectiveness therapy. Behav Res Ther 1994;32:381–90.

[32] Essau CA, Conradt J, Petermann F. Course and outcome of anxiety disorders in adolescents. J Anxiety Disord 2002;16:67–81.

[33] Pine DS, Cohen P, Gurley D, et al. The risk for early-adulthood anxiety and depressive

disorders in adolescents with anxiety and depressive disorders. Arch Gen Psychiatry 1998; 55:56–64.

[34] Stein MB, Fuetsch M, Muller N, et al. Social anxiety disorder and the risk of depression. Arch Gen Psychiatry 2001;58:251–6.

[35] Gould MS, King R, Greenwald S, et al. Psychopathology associated with suicidal ideation and attempts among children and adolescents. J Am Acad Child Adolesc Psychiatry 1998;37:915–23.

[36] Wittchen H-U, Nelson CB, Lachner G. Prevalence of mental disorders and psychosocial impairments in adolescents and young adults. Psychol Med 1998;28:109–26.

[37] Fordham K, Stevenson-Hinde J. Shyness, friendship quality, and adjustment during middle childhood. J Child Psychol Psychiatry 1999;40:757–68.

[38] Van Ameringen M, Mancini C, Farvolden P. The impact of anxiety disorders on educational achievement. J Anxiety Disord 2003;17:561–71.

[39] Woodward LJ, Fergusson DM. Life course outcomes of young people with anxiety disorders in adolescence. J Am Acad Child Adolesc Psychiatry 2001;40:1086–93.

[40] Myers MG, Aarons GA, Tomlinson K, et al. Social anxiety, negative affectivity, and substance use among high school students. Psychol Addict Behav 2003;17:277–83.

[41] Mason WA, Kosterman R, Hawkins JD, et al. Predicting depression, social phobia, and violence in early adulthood from childhood behavior problems. J Am Acad Child Adolesc Psychiatry 2004;43:307–15.

[42] Newcorn JH, Halperin JM, Jensen PS, et al. Symptom profiles in children with ADHD: effects of comorbidity and gender. J Am Acad Child Adolesc Psychiatry 2001;40:137–46.

[43] Pliszka SR, Carlson CL, Swanson JM. Anxiety disorders. In: Pliszka SR, Carlson CL, Swanson JM, editors. ADHD with comorbid disorders: clinical assessment and management. New York: Guilford Press; 1999. p. 150–62.

[44] Albano AM, Marten PA, Holt CS, et al. Cognitive-behavioral group treatment for social phobia in adolescents: a preliminary study. J Nerv Ment Dis 1995;183:649–56.

[45] Chavira DA, Stein MB. Combined psychoeducation and treatment with selective serotonin reuptake inhibitors for youth with generalized social anxiety disorder. J Child Adolesc Psychopharmacol 2002;12:47–54.

[46] Anstendig KD. Is selective mutism an anxiety disorder? rethinking its DSM-IV classification. J Anxiety Disord 1999;13:417–34.

[47] Black B, Uhde TW. Elective mutism as a variant of social phobia. J Am Acad Child Adolesc Psychiatry 1990;31:1090–4.

[48] Dummit III ES, Klein RG, Tancer NK, et al. Systematic assessment of 50 children with selective mutism. J Am Acad Child Adolesc Psychiatry 1997;36:653–60.

[49] Black B, Uhde TW. Psychiatric characteristics of children with selective mutism: a pilot study. J Am Acad Child Adolesc Psychiatry 1995;34:847–56.

[50] Steinhausen HC, Juzi C. Elective mutism: an analysis of 100 cases. J Am Acad Child Adolesc Psychiatry 1996;35:606–14.

[51] Kumpulainen K, Rasanen E, Raaska H, et al. Selective mutism among second-graders in elementary school. Eur Child Adolesc Psychiatry 1998;7:24–9.

[52] Yeganeh R, Beidel DC, Turner SM, et al. Clinical distinctions between selective mutism and social phobia: an investigation of childhood psychopathology. J Am Acad Child Adolesc Psychiatry 2003;42:1069–75.

[53] Achenbach TM, Edelbrock C. Manual for the child behavior checklist and revised child behavior profile. Burlington (VT): University of Vermont, Department of Psychiatry; 1983.

[54] Manassis K, Fung D, Tannock R, et al. Characterizing selective mutism: is it more than social anxiety? Depress Anxiety 2003;18:153–61.

[55] Kolvin I, Fundudis T. Elective mute children: psychological development and background factors. J Child Psychol Psychiatry 1981;22:219–32.

[56] Steinhausen HC, Juzi C. Elective mutism: an analysis of 100 cases. J Am Acad Child Adolesc Psychiatry 1996;35:606–14.

[57] DiBartolo PM, Albano AM, Barlow DH, et al. Cross-informant agreement in the assessment of social phobia in youth. J Abnorm Child Psychol 1998;26:213–20.

[58] Stein MB, Walker JR. Triumph over shyness: conquering shyness and social anxiety. New York: McGraw Hill; 2001.

[59] Zimbardo PG. Shyness: what it is, what to do about it. Reading (MA): Addison-Wesley; 1977.

[60] Crozier WR. Shyness and self-esteem in middle childhood. Br J Educ Psychol 1995;65:85–95.

[61] Hayward C, Killen JD, Kraemer HC, et al. Linking self-reported childhood behavioral inhibition to adolescent social phobia. J Am Acad Child Adolesc Psychiatry 1998;37:1308–16.

[62] Rosenbaum JF, Biederman J, Bolduc-Murphy EA, et al. Behavioral inhibition in childhood: a risk factor for anxiety disorders. Harv Rev Psychiatry 1993;1:2–16.

[63] Caspi A, Edler GH, Bem DJ. Moving away from the world: life course patterns of shy children. Dev Psychol 1988;24:824–31.

[64] Prior M, Smart D, Sanson A, et al. Does shy-inhibited temperament in childhood lead to anxiety problems in adolescence? J Am Acad Child Adolesc Psychiatry 2000;39:461–8.

[65] Garcia-Coll C, Kagan J, Reznick JS. Behavioral inhibition in young children. Child Dev 1984; 55:1005–19.

[66] Kagan J, Reznick JS, Snidman N. Biological basis of childhood shyness. Science 1988;240: 167–71.

[67] Kagan J. Temperamental contributions to social behavior. Am Psychol 1989;22:668–74.

[68] Schwartz CE, Snidman N, Kagan J. Adolescent social anxiety as an outcome of inhibited temperament in childhood. J Am Acad Child Adolesc Psychiatry 1999;38:1008–15.

[69] Goodwin RD, Fergusson DM, Horwood LJ. Early anxious/withdrawn behaviours predict later internalising disorders. J Child Psychol Psychiatry 2004;45:874–83.

[70] Cooper PJ, Eke M. Childhood shyness and maternal social phobia: a community study. Br J Psychiatry 1999;174:439–43.

[71] Last CG, Hersen M, Kazdin AE, et al. Anxiety disorders in children and their families. Arch Gen Psychiatry 1991;48:928–34.

[72] Martin C, Cabrol S, Bouvard MP, et al. Anxiety and depressive disorders in fathers and mothers of anxious school-refusing children. J Am Acad Child Adolesc Psychiatry 1999;38: 916–22.

[73] Fyer AJ, Mannuzza S, Chapman TF, et al. A direct-interview family study of social phobia. Arch Gen Psychiatry 1993;50:286–93.

[74] Reich JH, Yates W. Family history of psychiatric disorders in social phobia. Compr Psychiatry 1988;29:72–5.

[75] Stein MB, Chartier MJ, Hazen AL, et al. A direct-interview family study of generalized social phobia. Am J Psychiatry 1998;155:90–7.

[76] Mancini C, Van Ameringen M, Szatmari M, et al. A high-risk pilot study of the children of adults with social phobia. J Am Acad Child Adolesc Psychiatry 1996;35:1511–7.

[77] Mannuzza S, Schneier FR, Chapman TF, et al. Generalized social phobia: reliability and validity. Arch Gen Psychiatry 1995;52:230–7.

[78] Fyer AJ, Mannuzza S, Chapman TF, et al. Specificity in familial aggregation of phobic disorders. Arch Gen Psychiatry 1995;52:564–73.

[79] Daniels D, Plomin R. Origins of individual differences in infant shyness. Dev Psychol 1985; 21:118–21.

[80] Fisher L, Kagan J, Reznick JS. Genetic etiology of behavioral inhibition among 2-year-old children. Infant Behavior and Development 1994;17:405–12.

[81] Robinson JL, Kagan J, Reznick JS, et al. The heritability of inhibited and uninhibited behavior: a twin study. Dev Psychol 1992;28:1030–7.

[82] Rowe DC, Plomin R. Temperament in early childhood. J Pers Assess 1977;41:150–6.

[83] Warren SL, Schmitz S, Emde RN. Behavioral genetic analyses of self-reported anxiety at 7 years of age. J Am Acad Child Adolesc Psychiatry 1999;38:1403–8.

[84] Eley TC, Bolton D, O'Connor TG, et al. A twin study of anxiety-related behaviours in preschool children. J Child Psychol Psychiatry 2003;44:945–60.

[85] Kendler KS, Myers J, Prescott CA. Parenting and adult mood, anxiety and substance use disorders in female twins: an epidemiological, multi-informant, retrospective study. Psychol Med 2001;30:281–94.

[86] Skre I, Onstad S, Torgersen S, et al. A twin study of DSM-III-R anxiety disorders. Acta Psychiatr Scand 1993;88:85–92.

[87] Torgersen S. Genetic factors in anxiety disorders. Arch Gen Psychiatry 1983;40:1085–9.

[88] Kendler KS, Karkowski LM, Prescott CA. Fears and phobias: reliability and heritability. Psychol Med 1999;29:539–53.

[89] Nelson EC, Grant JD, Bucholz KK, et al. Social phobia in a population-based female adolescent twin sample: co-morbidity and associated suicide-related symptoms. Psychol Med 2000; 30:797–804.

[90] Ost LG. Ways of acquiring phobias and outcome of behavioral treatments. Behav Res Ther 1985;23:683–9.

[91] Stemberger RT, Turner SM, Beidel DC, et al. Social phobia: an analysis of possible developmental factors. J Abnorm Psychol 1995;104:526–31.

[92] Bandura A. Principles of behavior modification. New York: Holt, Rinehart & Winston; 1969.

[93] Barrett PM, Rapee RM, Dadds MR, et al. Family enhancement of cognitive style in anxious and aggressive children. J Abnorm Child Psychol 1996;24:187–203.

[94] Bruch MA, Heimberg RG, Berger P, et al. Social phobia and perceptions of early parental and personal characteristics. Anxiety Research 1989;2:57–65.

[95] Bruch MA, Heimberg RG. Differences in perceptions of parental and personal characteristics between generalized and nongeneralized social phobics. J Anxiety Disord 1994;8:155–68.

[96] Arrindell WA, Emmelkamp PMG, Monsma A, et al. The role of perceived parental rearing practices in the etiology of phobic disorders: a controlled study. Br J Psychiatry 1983;143: 183–7.

[97] Arrindell WA, Kwee MGT, Methorst GJ, et al. Perceived parental rearing styles of agoraphobic and socially phobic in-patients. Br J Psychiatry 1989;155:526–35.

[98] Parker G. Reported parental characteristics of agoraphobics and social phobics. Br J Psychiatry 1979;135:550–60.

[99] Parker G, Roussos J, Hadzi-Pavlovic D, et al. The development of a refined measure of dysfunctional parenting and assessment of its relevance in patients with affective disorders. Psychol Med 1997;27:1193–203.

[100] Caster J, Inderbitzen H, Hope DA. Relationship between youth and parent perceptions of family environment and social anxiety. J Anxiety Disord 1999;13:237–51.

[101] Messer SC, Beidel DC. Psychosocial correlates of childhood anxiety disorders. J Am Acad Child Adolesc Psychiatry 1994;33:975–83.

[102] Bögels SM, van Oosten A, Muris P, et al. Familial correlates of social anxiety in children and adolescents. Behav Res Ther 2001;39:273–87.

[103] Mills RSL, Rubin KH. Are behavioral and psychological control both differentially associated with childhood aggression and social withdrawal? Can J Behav Sci 1998;30:132–6.

[104] Rubin KH, Cheah CSL, Fox N. Emotional regulation parenting and display of social reticence in preschoolers. Early Educ Dev 2001;12:97–115.

[105] Stevenson-Hinde J, Glover A. Shy girls and boys: a new look. J Child Psychol Psychiatry 1996;37:181–7.

[106] Barrett PM, Dadds MR, Rapee RM. Family treatment of childhood anxiety: a controlled trial. J Consult Clin Psychol 1996;64(2):333–42.

[107] Nauta MH, Scholing A, Emmelkamp PM, et al. Cognitive-behavioral therapy for children with anxiety disorders in a clinical setting: no additional effect of a cognitive parent training. J Am Acad Child Adolesc Psychiatry 2003;42:1270–8.

[108] Spence SH, Donovan C, Brechman-Toussaint M. The treatment of childhood social phobia: the effectiveness of a social skills training-based, cognitive-behavioral intervention, with and without parental involvement. J Child Psychol Psychiatry 2001;41:713–26.

[109] La Greca AM, Dandes SK, Wick P, et al. The development of the Social Anxiety Scale for Children (SASC): reliability and concurrent validity. J Clin Child Psychol 1988;17:84–91.

[110] La Greca AM, Lopez N. Social anxiety among adolescents: linkages with peer relations and friendships. J Abnorm Child Psychol 1998;26:83–95.

[111] Watson D, Friend R. Measurement of social-evaluative anxiety. J Consult Clin Psychol 1969; 33:448–57.

[112] La Greca AM, Stone WL. Social Anxiety Scale for Children-Revised: factor structure and concurrent validity. J Clin Child Psychol 1993;22:17–27.

[113] Storch EA, Masia-Warner C, Dent HC, et al. Psychometric evaluation of the Social Anxiety Scale for Adolescents and the Social Phobia and Anxiety Inventory for Children: construct validity and normative data. J Anxiety Disord 2004;18:665–79.

[114] La Greca AM, Silverman WK, Wasserstein SB. Children's predisaster functioning as a predictor of posttraumatic stress following Hurricane Andrew. J Consult Clin Psychol 1998;66:883–92.

[115] Vernberg EM, Abwender DA, Ewell KK, et al. Social anxiety and peer relationships in early adolescence: a prospective analysis. J Clin Child Psychol 1992;21:189–96.

[116] Morris TL, Masia CL. Psychometric evaluation of the social phobia and anxiety inventory for children: concurrent validity and normative data. J Clin Child Psychol 1998;27:452–8.

[117] Ginsburg GS, La Greca AM, Silverman WK. Social anxiety in children with anxiety disorders: relation with social and emotional functioning. J Abnorm Child Psychol 1998;26:175–86.

[118] Beidel DC, Turner SM, Morris TL. A new inventory to assess childhood social anxiety and phobia: the Social Phobia and Anxiety Inventory for Children. Psychol Assess 1995;7: 73–9.

[119] Turner SM, Beidel DC, Dancu CV, et al. An empirically derived inventory to measure social fears and anxiety: the Social Phobia and Anxiety Inventory. J Consult Clin Psychol 1989; 1:35–40.

[120] Beidel DC, Turner SM, Fink CM. Assessment of childhood social phobia: construct, convergent, and discriminant validity of the Social Phobia and Anxiety Inventory for Children (SPAI-C). Psychol Assess 1996;8:235–40.

[121] Beidel DC, Turner SM, Hamlin K, et al. The Social Phobia and Anxiety Inventory for Children (SPAI-C): external and discriminative validity. Behav Ther 2000;31:75–87.

[122] Masia-Warner C, Storch EA, Pincus DB, et al. The Liebowitz social anxiety scale for children and adolescents: an initial psychometric investigation. J Am Acad Child Adolesc Psychiatry 2003;42:1076–84.

[123] Liebowitz MR. Social phobia. Mod Probl Pharmacopsychiatry 1987;22:141–73.

[124] Stein MB, Fyer AJ, Davidson JR, et al. Fluvoxamine treatment of social phobia (social anxiety disorder): a double-blind placebo-controlled study. Am J Psychiatry 1999;156:756–60.

[125] Stein MB, Liebowitz MR, Lydiard RB, et al. Paroxetine treatment of generalized social phobia (social anxiety disorders): a randomized controlled trial. JAMA 1998;280:708–13.

[126] Van Ameringen M, Mancini C, Streiner D. Sertraline in social phobia. J Affect Disord 1994; 31:141–5.

[127] Black B, Uhde TW. Treatment of elective mutism with fluoxetine: a double-blind, placebo-controlled study. J Am Acad Child Adolesc Psychiatry 1994;33:1000–6.

[128] Dummit III ES, Klein RG, Tancer NK, Asche B, Martin J. Fluoxetine treatment of children with selective mutism: an open trial. J Am Acad Child Adolesc Psychiatry 1996;35(5): 615–21.

[129] Mancini C, Van Ameringen M, Oakman JM, et al. Serotonergic agents in the treatment of social phobia in children and adolescents: a case series. Depress Anxiety 1999;10:33–9.

[130] Compton SN, Grant PJ, Chrisman AK, et al. Sertraline in children and adolescents with social anxiety disorder: an open trial. J Am Acad Child Adolesc Psychiatry 2001;40:564–71.

[131] Chavira DA, Stein MB. Combined psychoeducation and treatment with selective serotonin reuptake inhibitors for youth with generalized social anxiety disorder. J Child Adolesc Psychopharmacol 2002;12:47–54.

[132] Wagner KD, Berard R, Stein MB, et al. A multicenter, randomized, double-blind, placebo-controlled trial of paroxetine in children and adolescents with social anxiety disorder. Arch Gen Psychiatry 2004;61(11):1153–62.

[133] National Institute of Mental Health. Special feature: rating scales and assessment instruments for use in pediatric psychopharmacology research. Psychopharmacol Bull 1985;21:839.

[134] Birmaher B, Axelson DA, Monk K, et al. Fluoxetine for the treatment of childhood anxiety disorders. J Am Acad Child Adolesc Psychiatry 2003;42:415–23.

[135] Research Unit on Pediatric Psychopharmacology Anxiety Study Group. Fluvoxamine for the treatment of anxiety disorders in children and adolescents. N Engl J Med 2001;344:1279–85.

[136] Research Unit on Pediatric Psychopharmacology Anxiety Study Group. Searching for moderators and mediators of pharmacological treatment effects in children and adolescents with anxiety disorders. J Am Acad Child Adolesc Psychiatry 2003;42:13–21.

[137] Caldwell PH, Murphy SB, Butow PN, et al. Clinical trials in children. Lancet 2004;364:803–11.

[138] Zito JM, Safer DJ, DosReis S, et al. Psychotropic practice patterns for youth: a 10-year perspective. Arch Pediatr Adolesc Med 2003;157:17–25.

[139] Labellarte MJ, Ginsburg GS, Walkup JT, et al. The treatment of anxiety disorders in children and adolescents. Biol Psychiatry 1999;46:1567–78.

[140] Hayward C, Varady S, Albano AM, et al. Cognitive-behavioral group therapy for social phobia in female adolescents: results of a pilot study. J Am Acad Child Adolesc Psychiatry 2000;39: 721–6.

[141] Beidel DC, Turner SM, Morris TL. Behavioral treatment of childhood social phobia. J Consult Clin Psychol 2000;68:1072–80.

[142] Masia CL, Klein RG, Storch EA, et al. School-based behavioral treatment for social anxiety disorder in adolescents: results of a pilot study. J Am Acad Child Adolesc Psychiatry 2001; 40:780–6.

[143] Gallagher HM, Rabian BA, McCloskey MS. A brief group cognitive-behavioral intervention for social phobia in childhood. J Anxiety Disord 2004;18:459–79.

[144] Mendlowitz SL, Manassis K, Bradley S, et al. Cognitive-behavioral group treatments in childhood anxiety disorders: the role of parental involvement. J Am Acad Child Adolesc Psychiatry 1999;38:1223–9.

[145] Chavira DA, Stein MB, Bailey K, et al. Parental opinions regarding treatment for social anxiety disorder in youth. J Dev Behav Pediatr 2003;24:315–22.

[146] Chavira DA, Stein MB, Bailey K, et al. Child anxiety disorders in primary care: prevalent but untreated. Depress Anxiety 2004;20(4):155–64.

[147] Wren FJ, Scholle SH, Heo J, et al. Pediatric mood and anxiety syndromes in primary care: who gets identified? Int J Psychiatry Med 2003;33:1–16.

[148] Herbert JD, Crittenden K, Dalrymple KL. Knowledge of social anxiety disorder relative to attention deficit hyperactivity disorder among educational professionals. J Clin Child Adolesc Psychol 2004;33:366–72.

[149] Ferrell CB, Beidel DC, Turner SM. Assessment and treatment of socially phobic children: a cross cultural comparison. J Clin Child Adolesc Psychol 2004;33:260–8.

[150] Pina AA, Silverman WK, Fuentes RM, et al. Exposure-based cognitive-behavioral treatment for phobic and anxiety disorders: treatment effects and maintenance for Hispanic/Latino relative to European-American youths. J Am Acad Child Adolesc Psychiatry 2003;42:1179–87.

ELSEVIER
SAUNDERS

Child Adolesc Psychiatric Clin N Am
14 (2005) 819–843

CHILD AND
ADOLESCENT
PSYCHIATRIC CLINICS
OF NORTH AMERICA

Specific Phobia

Wendy K. Silverman, PhD, ABPP*, Jacqueline Moreno, MS

*Child Anxiety and Phobia Program, Child and Family Psychosocial Research Center,
Department of Psychology, Florida International University, University Park Campus,
11200 SW 8th Street, DM Building, Room 203, Miami, FL 33199, USA*

Although the past decade has witnessed an evolution in the way in which the psychological and psychiatric communities conceptualize the childhood anxiety disorders, conceptualization of specific phobia has changed very little. In fact, the classification of specific phobia in the Diagnostic and Statistical Manual of Mental Disorders, Fourth Edition (DSM-IV) [1] and the International Classification of Disorders (ICD-10) [2] are largely consistent with criteria for distinguishing excessive and maladaptive phobias from more "normal," nonmaladaptive fears proposed 30 years ago by Miller and colleagues [3]. These criteria state that a phobia, unlike a fear (1) is excessive (ie, out of proportion, given the situation); (2) cannot be reasoned away; (3) is beyond voluntary control; (4) leads to avoidance of the feared stimulus; (5) persists over time; (6) is maladaptive; and (7) is not age- or stage-specific. This article describes specific phobia of childhood and its clinical presentation, discusses issues related to the differential diagnosis of specific phobia, considers the issue of comorbidity among phobic and anxiety disorders and developmental trends in the manifestation of fears, summarizes the epidemiology, causes, and course of specific phobia, and presents assessment and treatment issues. Finally, a case study is offered that serves to illuminate the major topics outlined in the article.

This work was supported in part by National Institute of Mental Health grant R01MH63997-01A1 (to W.K. Silverman).

* Corresponding author.

E-mail address: silverw@fiu.edu (W.K. Silverman).

Description and clinical presentation of the disorder

In both the DSM-IV and ICD-10, specific phobias are classified as "adult" disorders, with the same criteria applied to child disorders. The only exception is the DSM-IV indication that "although adolescents and adults with this disorder recognize that their fear is excessive or unreasonable, this may not be the case with children" [1]. The DSM-IV [1] classifies specific phobia into five subtypes: (1) animal (eg, dogs or insects); (2) natural environment (eg, storms or heights); (3) blood-infection-injury (eg, injections or the sight of blood); (4) situational (eg, transportation or enclosed places); and (5) other (eg, choking or loud noises).

According to the DSM-IV and ICD-10, specific phobia is a persistent fear that is restricted to a circumscribed stimulus (object or situation), such that the stimulus is avoided whenever possible or is endured only with intense anxiety occurring immediately on exposure. The intensity of the fear typically is severe enough to lead to interference in the child's functioning in academic, social, or family activities. Generally, these criteria incorporate the description of Miller and colleagues [3] outlined above. In contrast to developmentally appropriate fears (eg, a toddler's fear of strangers), phobias are excessive and out of proportion to the demands of the situation, cannot be reasoned away, are beyond voluntary control, lead to avoidance, persist over time, and are maladaptive (ie, they interfere with activities or relationships). Examples of phobias commonly observed among children are heights, small animals, injections, darkness, loud noises, and thunder and lightning [4]. A phobic reaction may be viewed as a reaction that manifests itself along three systems: the subjective or cognitive, behavioral or motoric, and physiologic or bodily [5,6].

The existence of anticipatory fear raises the possibility that, for some children, the experience of fear has a cognitive component. A child with a phobia of dogs, for example, may have worrisome "what if" thoughts, such as "what if I see a dog at my parents' friend's home," or "at the playground." A common theme or motif is that of safety. That is, a child with specific phobias commonly believes that exposure to or confrontation with the phobic object or event will result in harm befalling him or her (eg, the dog will bite and give the child rabies or the lightening will strike and hit him or her). Such thoughts typically lead to extreme distress, and if the distress is severe, it can interfere with the child's ability to concentrate on or attend to other material.

Other cognitive components that may play a role in phobias include feelings of disgust and cognitive bias. Some studies suggest that there is an interaction between fear and disgust, which can maintain and even exacerbate phobias [7,8]. Disgust has been hypothesized as a concurrent emotion that in interaction with fear may result in increased avoidance behavior [9]. Finally, using an information-processing approach, some findings indicate that phobic children may have a cognitive bias for threatening stimuli [10]. However, several limitations with the information-processing paradigm warrant consideration [11].

In terms of the motoric or behavioral system, the most common reaction is flight or avoidance. Avoidance behavior may occur when the child is in the presence of the feared stimulus, or it may occur in anticipation of the confrontation with the feared stimulus. Examples of avoidance owing to anticipatory anxiety include a child with a phobia of dogs who avoids walking down certain streets or going to a playground because the child believes he or she may encounter a dog, or the child avoids visiting friends and relatives who own a dog. Although avoidance is the most common behavioral reaction, when avoidance is not possible, the child may run to a parent or loved one, seeking safety or comfort. Additional behaviors might include screaming, crying, freezing, or clinging. Generally, the more severe the phobia, the more extensive the avoidance behavior and, thus, the more likely it is that interference in functioning will result. In such instances, the child's avoidance behavior is disrupting not only the child's daily activities (eg, school and peer relationships) but also the functioning of the family. For example, the child's avoidance is making it difficult for the family to engage in many activities (eg, visiting friends and relatives).

In terms of the physiologic domain, children with specific phobias report a wide range of physiologic reactions on exposure to the phobic object or event. These reactions include rapid heartbeat, shakiness, stomachaches or feelings of "butterflies in the stomach," and sweating.

Differential diagnosis

The DSM-IV [1] requires that several other anxiety conditions be ruled out before assigning the diagnosis of specific phobia. According to the DSM diagnostic criteria for specific phobia, the fear of a circumscribed object or situation must not be related to the fear of separation (as in separation anxiety disorder), the fear of humiliation or embarrassment in certain social situations (as in social phobia), the fear of having a panic attack (as in panic disorder), or the fear of being in places or situations from which escape might be difficult or embarrassing or in which help might not be available (as in agoraphobia).

Although specific phobias are similar to obsessions in that they have a repetitive and ruminative quality [12], a diagnosis of specific phobia of dirt, for example, would not be given to a child who displays obsessive fears about contamination and consequently avoids situations in which he or she might become dirty. Similarly, it is necessary to distinguish between specific phobia and post-traumatic stress disorder (PTSD); for example, a diagnosis of specific phobia of hurricanes would not be assigned to a child who avoids visiting the site where his or her house stood before a destructive and devastating hurricane. That is, in PTSD, phobic avoidance of stimuli associated with trauma is present frequently but should not result in a diagnosis of specific phobia.

Finally, although not specified in the DSM or ICD classification schemes, children who exhibit school refusal behavior often are labeled as having a "school phobia." However, numerous authors [13–17] have noted that rather than being a homogeneous group, as has been assumed historically, children refuse school for a variety of reasons. Thus, although it is possible that a child who refuses school may have a specific phobia (eg, the ringing of the school bell or heights in a multistory school building), diagnostically it is important to rule out school refusal behavior caused by other conditions such as separation anxiety disorder or social phobia. Such distinctions are likely to have important implications for treatment [18].

Comorbidity

Comorbidity is common in childhood psychopathology [19]. This is true as well with regard to the childhood anxiety disorders, in which comorbid diagnoses may include additional anxiety disorders, other internalizing disorders (eg, depression), and externalizing behavior problems (eg, attention deficit and conduct disorders) [20–28]. Although estimates of comorbidity among anxiety disorders vary across studies, in general, it appears the rate may be as high as 50% [29]. Rates of comorbidity may be underestimated in many studies because of the use of pooled diagnostic groups (eg, a group of "anxious" children that includes children who present with multiple anxiety disorders, such as separation anxiety disorder, overanxious disorder, and phobic disorder).

Curtis and colleagues [30] have examined the prevalence and comorbidity of various specific phobias in a community sample of 915 individuals (ages 15 to 54 years) with a lifetime history of specific phobia. Results indicate that only 24.4% had a single phobia, 26.4% had two phobias, 23.5% had three phobias, 10.4% had four phobias, and 17.3% had more than four co-occurring phobias. Lewinsohn and colleagues [31] have examined lifetime comorbidity among anxiety disorders in a community sample of high school children (ages 14 to 19 years). Specific phobia was found to be comorbid with separation anxiety disorder (odds ratio, 4.7) and social phobia (odds ratio, 7.2). In an epidemiologic study of 36 adolescents (ages 12 to 17 years) with specific phobias, Essau and colleagues [32] report that 47.2% subjects had comorbid anxiety disorders, 36.1% had comorbid depressive disorders, 33.3% had comorbid somatoform disorders, and 8.3% had comorbid substance use disorders.

Finally, Last and colleagues [33] have reported that of 188 children referred to a childhood anxiety disorders clinic, 80 children met the diagnoses of specific phobia. Of these 80 children, 75% had a lifetime history of additional, specific anxiety disorders, 32.5% had a lifetime history of any depressive disorder, and 22.5% had a lifetime history of any behavior disorder. The most common additional specific anxiety diagnosis was separation anxiety disorder (38.8%) [18]. In a study by Silverman and colleagues [34], a report of a clinical trial for phobic disorders in youth (N = 104, ages 6 to 16 years), 87 children met the primary diagnosis of specific phobia. Of the total sample, 72% of subjects had a least one comorbid diagnosis: 19% had an additional specific phobia, 16% had separation anxiety disorder, 14% had overanxious disorder, 6% had ADHD, and the remaining 17% were distributed over eight additional diagnostic categories, with a rate of less than 5%.

Developmental trends and age of onset

As mentioned earlier, normal childhood fears are relatively common, with children typically experiencing a number of different fears during the course of development [35–38]. The literature is heavy in its coverage of the developmental trends of the fears of childhood [39–42] but is relatively light in its coverage of the developmental trends of more excessive fears and phobias experienced by relatively fewer children. Thus, the age trends observed among common nonclinical childhood fears are summarized below [36,42].

Briefly, in infancy, children show a tendency to experience fears regarding loss of support, loud noises, and unfamiliar people. In early childhood, fears of imaginary creatures, small animals, and the dark begin to predominate. Starting at approximately age 6, school fears (eg, achievement) typically emerge and persist into later childhood, when fears of a more social nature and fear of bodily injury become more evident.

In a study encompassing a cross-section of 54 elementary school children (ages 4 to 12 years), Bauer [43] has reported similar trends: there was a decrease in the frequency of fears with imaginary themes (eg, fear of ghosts and monsters and bedtime fears involving frightening dreams) from first to sixth grade and an increase in the frequency of realistic fears involving bodily injury and social concerns over the same age range. According to Bauer [43], these trends reflect the Piagetian notion that children's perceptions of reality change from more global and diffuse to more sophisticated and realistic. A predominance of social fears relative to such fears as the dark, heights, and animals seems to be characteristic of adolescent children as well [44].

With regard to excessive fears of childhood, that is, phobias, investigators have tended to focus more of their attention on age of onset, rather than developmental trends. Assessing relatively large samples of adults with phobic disorders, some studies [45,46] report similar estimates, placing the mean age of onset at approximately 20 and 16 years, respectively. Although earlier studies [47,48] have found differing ages of onset, these efforts were limited by small samples. Perhaps the most extensive and informative of the phobia-onset studies have been conducted by Öst and colleagues [49–51]. Comparing six different DSM-III groups of phobic adult patients (agoraphobics, social phobics, and four subgroups of specific phobics: animal, blood, dental, and claustrophobia, who were referred for treatment to a clinical research center), Öst [51] found a large variation in the age of onset. With the exception of claustrophobia (mean age of onset 20.18 years), patients with specific phobias had the earliest onset relative to patients with agoraphobia (approximately 28 years of age) and social phobia (approximately 16 years of age). In addition, significant differences in age of onset were found across the four specific phobic groups: animal phobia started early in childhood (approximately 7 years of age), whereas blood phobia began somewhat later (approximately 9 years of age), followed by dental phobia (approximately 12 years of age).

According to Öst [51], these findings suggest that specific phobia is not a homogeneous group but a collection of separate perhaps related disorders, which can be differentiated by the ages at which they tend to first appear. Additional support for this notion comes from Kendler and colleagues [52] who have found a similar pattern of the age of onset in a large sample of adult female patients. Specifically, animal phobia had the earliest onset (approximately 6 years old) followed by situational phobia (approximately 10 years old), social phobia (approximately 11 years old), and agoraphobia (approximately 16 years old). However, research on the age of onset has the limitation of being based on participants' retrospective reports.

Using a clinic sample of children (ages 5 to 18 years) diagnosed along DSM-III-R criteria, Last and colleagues [33] have reported that separation anxiety disorder had the earliest onset (mean 7.5 years) followed by avoidance disorder (mean 8.2 years), simple phobia (referred to as specific phobia in DSM-IV [mean 8.4 years]), overanxious disorder, (subsumed under generalized anxiety disorder in DSM-IV [mean 8.8 years]), obsessive-compulsive disorder (mean 10.8 years), social phobia (mean 11.3 years), and panic disorder (mean 14.1 years). Studying a large clinic sample of children (ages 4 to 18 years) with phobic disorders diagnosed along DSM-III-R criteria, Biederman and colleagues [53] have shown similar results: separation anxiety disorder had the earliest onset (mean 4.3 years) followed by simple phobia (mean 5.0 years), avoidant disorder (mean 5.3 years), agoraphobia (mean 5.6 years), obsessive-compulsive disorder (mean 5.7 years), overanxious disorder (mean 6.7 years), panic disorder (mean 6.8 years), and social phobia (mean 7.2 years).

Course

There is a paucity of research on the natural course of childhood specific phobia. Perhaps this is the result, in part, of the ethical problems involved in conducting this type of research (ie, abstinence from treatment would need to be encouraged, either implicitly or explicitly), coupled with the methodologic difficulties involved in conducting longitudinal research. Despite the small number of studies, there are two important studies that are cited frequently. The first is the longitudinal study on the natural history of phobia conducted by Agras and colleagues [54]. The second is the follow-up results of the treatment study conducted by Hampe and colleagues [55].

Using an epidemiologic survey, Agras and colleagues [54] have identified 30 phobic individuals (10 children under the age of 20 years old and 20 adults) with a variety of fears, including fear of illness and death, agoraphobia, animal fears, and fear of heights. These individuals were followed over a 5-year period during which none received psychiatric treatment or psychotherapy for the phobic condition. After 5 years, 100% of the children were viewed as "improved" compared with 43% of the adults. The authors interpreted the data to mean that many phobic conditions improve without any form of treatment and that child phobics improve more rapidly than their adult counterparts do [54]. Although these results appear encouraging, especially for children with phobias, Ollendick [56] points out that "improved" children in the study by Agras and colleagues were not completely free from symptoms, and the majority of children assessed at follow-up continued to exhibit symptoms of sufficient intensity to be rated between "no disability" and "maximum disability." Thus, Ollendick's reinterpretation of Agras and colleagues' findings [54] suggests that phobias or at least some of the symptoms of phobias persist over time for some children.

Hampe and colleagues [55] have examined 2-year follow-up data obtained on 62 children between the ages of 6 and 15 years who had received treatment for phobias. Overall, at the end of this 2-year period, 80% of the children no longer exhibited the phobias for which they had been treated. A much smaller percentage of children (7%) continued to display phobias. These findings indicate that for a small proportion of youngsters, phobias persist despite treatment. However, because the study by Hampe and colleagues [55] used only parent and clinician ratings and behavior checklists to assess phobic symptoms and predated the current DSM classification scheme for specific phobia, the interpretation of the findings is limited.

Retrospective studies such as those cited earlier [45,46,51] are another source by which the course of phobias may be evaluated [7]. These studies are limited, however, in that they are based on participants' retrospective reports. Nevertheless, a study by Abe [57] has reported that among 86 mothers invited for a routine medical examination, approximately 30% reported extreme fears that began during childhood or adolescence and were still present at the time of the examination. In the Öst study [51], the average age of the sample of agoraphobics, social phobics, and specific phobics was 34 years. The subjects' phobia problems began, on average, between the ages of 7 and 28 years, with the specific phobias beginning earliest. In addition, Milne and colleagues [58] have examined the frequency of clinical phobias and subclinical fears over a 3-year period in a community sample of adolescents (in grades seven, eight, and nine). Although only 11% of youths continued to meet diagnostic criteria for the same initial specific phobia, 58% of youths continued to present with subsyndromal fears (ie, they remained symptomatic but reported less impairment). In sum, these findings coupled with Ollendick's [56] reinterpretation of the data from Agras and colleagues [54] suggest that specific phobias tend to persist into adulthood for some proportion of youths.

Epidemiology

Epidemiologic studies on the rate of childhood specific phobia based on DSM or ICD defined criteria are scant. In contrast, several studies have examined the prevalence of "excessive fears or worries" or phobias in children. Prudence is warranted when examining these data, however, given the blurry and differing definitions used across studies and the different samples, different procedures, and different measures used [12]. Because of these differences, estimates of the prevalence of excessive fears or worries or phobias have varied, ranging from 1.7% to 16% [59,60]. Despite the different samples and methodologies used, a consistent rate of approximately 7% to 9% has been reported in a number of studies [61–65].

According to the DSM-IV, the prevalence rates of specific phobias vary with culture and ethnicity depending on the type of phobia [1]. Using samples of children, several studies have demonstrated prevalence rates of 2.4% to 3.6% in New Zealand [66,67], 2.6% in Puerto Rico [68], 2.6% in Switzerland [69], and 3.5% in Germany [32]. Using a sample of 3021 individuals (ages 14 to 24 years) in Munich, Wittchen and colleagues [70] have reported a lifetime prevalence of specific phobia of 2.3% and a 12-month prevalence of 1.8%. Prevalence rates also appear to vary with gender, depending on the type of phobia (eg, 75%–90% of animal, natural environment, and situation-type phobics are females, and 55%–70% of blood-injection-injury–type phobics are females) [1]. Several studies indicate that the prevalence of specific phobia and fear is higher in females than males [20,32,62,64,71–73].

Regarding ethnicity, research using clinical samples indicates no differences in rates of specific phobias between Euro-American and Hispanic-American [74] and Euro-American and African-American [75] youths. Ingman and colleagues [76] have found that children (ages 8 to 17 years) from Nigeria (n = 310) and Kenya (n = 551) reported higher rates of specific fears than children from the United States, Australia, and China. Using a community sample of 975 Japanese and 862 German children (ages 8 to 12 years), Essau and colleagues [73] have found that Japanese children reported more symptoms related to physical injury fears than German children did. In addition, using a community sample of 3200 Hellenic children in Greece (ages 8 to 12 years), Mellon and colleagues [72] have found Hellenic children reported higher rates of fear scores than American, Australian, Chinese, and British children but not Nigerian children. Whether prevalence rates of specific phobia vary with age, ethnicity, and socioeconomic status in children is unclear. Additional epidemiologic studies using community and clinical samples are needed to clarify this issue. Such studies should examine prevalence rates among diverse child groups and include samples that comprise a range of ages and socioeconomic groups.

Causes

A number of factors play a role in the acquisition of specific phobia [24,56,77,78]. With respect to genetic factors, studying adult pairs of same-sex twins, Torgersen [79] has found evidence that monozygotic twins are more similar than dizygotic twins in the strength and nature of their phobic fears.

Furthermore, these similarities appear to be unrelated to similarities in environmental situations, suggesting that at least a proportion of excessive fears are determined by genetic factors alone, with little or no environmental influence. These results corroborate findings reported by other investigators [80,81] who, using similar twin samples to study the causes of phobias, concluded that genetic factors contribute significantly to the onset of phobic fears.

A number of studies have established the familial aggregation of DSM-III phobias and phobia-like symptoms [82–87]. In a study that focused exclusively on specific phobias [83], probands diagnosed with specific phobia as well as their first-degree relatives were interviewed with the Kiddie-Schedule for Affective Disorders and Schizophrenia in School-Age Children (K-SADS) [88]. A total of 119 first-degree relatives of a "normal" proband group (n = 38) served as the comparison group. Relatives of probands with specific phobia exhibited specific phobia themselves (31%), more than the relatives of the normal proband group (11%). In addition, 15% of the children (27% of daughters and 6% of sons) of the specific phobic probands were diagnosed with specific phobia, compared with 8% of the children of the normal probands. Based on these findings, the authors conclude that specific phobia is a highly familial disorder that breeds true.

Additional support for the importance of genetic factors in the transmission of phobias comes from a univariate genetic analysis conducted by Kendler and colleagues [52] on 2163 adult female twins. Results indicated that specific phobias (specifically, animal and situational) have the lowest rate of heritability among the phobic disorders and are likely to be more influenced by specific environmental influences than other phobic disorders. Thus, the role of environmental factors in the transmission of specific phobias should not be overlooked. The earlier findings of Silverman and colleagues [89] provide further support that specific phobias (and other anxiety disorders) "run in families." In this study as well, however, it was not possible to disentangle the effects of genetic versus environmental factors.

In terms of the environmental factors that may be important in the causes of specific phobia, several learning theories have been proposed. Perhaps most influential among these has been the model proposed by Rachman [90], in which phobias are acquired through direct (ie, conditioning) or indirect (ie, vicarious exposure or the transmission of information or instruction) acquisition. Research conducted with adult phobic patients suggests that direct conditioning plays a major role [48,49]. For example, the work of Öst and colleague [49] indicates that adult phobia-disordered patients attribute their phobias more to direct conditioning than to indirect experiences (although among adults with simple phobias of small animals and dental procedures, attributions about acquisition were more evenly distributed across Rachman's other pathways.)

Some studies provide support for the pathways proposed by Rachman [90] in the development of phobias in children. Ollendick and colleagues [91] administered a questionnaire designed to assess the pathways for 10 highly prevalent fears (eg, nuclear war, fire or getting burned, and other fears) to 1092 Australian and American school children (ages 9 to 14 years). Results indicate that vicarious and instructional factors were most influential (56% and 89%, respectively). These factors, however, were combined frequently with direct conditioning experiences. Merckelbach and colleagues [92] interviewed 22 spider-phobic girls (age 9 to 14 years) and their parents (a majority were mothers) about the origins of the child's fear. Results indicate that although 45.5% of children and 54.5% of parents reported the child had "always been afraid," 40.9% of children and 36.4% of parents reported conditioning events. In another study, Merckelbach and Muris [93] interviewed 26 spider-phobic girls (mean age 12.6 ± 2.6 years) and 26 nonphobic control girls (mean age 12.4 ± 2.5 years) and their parents (majority mothers) about the origins of the child's fear. Results indicate that phobic girls reported significantly more conditioning events than nonphobic girls (42.3% and 7.7%, respectively), and phobic girls reported more modeling experiences mediated by their mothers than nonphobic girls (64.5% and 38.5%, respectively). In addition, agreement between child and parent was 65.4% for conditioning and 50% for the option "always been afraid." Finally, King and colleagues [94] surveyed parents of 30 children who had dog phobia (16 girls and 14 boys, mean age 5.95 years). Results show that the majority of parents endorsed modeling as the most important influence in the acquisition of their child's dog phobia (53.34%) followed by direct conditioning events (26.7%), unknown origins (13.34%), and instruction or information (6.7%).

Additional support for Rachman's model [90] may be found in studies examining the role of negative life events and fear information in the development of fears in children. Ollendick and colleagues [95] have examined the relationships among negative life events, negative attributional style, avoidant coping, and fear level in 99 children (ages 8 to 16 years) who had survived residential fires. Results indicate that although negative life events, negative attributional style, and avoidant coping predicted fear level, mothers' educational level moderated the relationships between negative life events and fear level. Specifically, negative life events predicted fear level in children whose mothers had low education, and negative attributional style and avoidant coping predicted fear level in children whose mothers had high education. Muris and colleagues [96] have examined the relationship between negative information and fear level in 285 children (ages 4 to 12 years) by giving either positive or negative information about a "beast." Results indicate that children who received negative information about the beast reported increased fear levels of the beast during post and follow-up (immediately after receiving the information and one week after), and children who received positive information about the beast reported decreased fear levels of the beast during post and follow-up. In addition, fear levels of the beast appeared to generalize during post and follow-up: children who received negative information reported increased fear levels of dogs and predators, and children who received positive information about the beast reported decreased fear levels of dogs and predators. Finally, Field and Lawson [97] have examined the relationships among the type of information given about an animal, a self-reported measure of fear, and behavioral avoidance in 59 children (ages 6 to 9 years). Results indicate that negative information significantly increased fear levels on self-reported measures and behavioral avoidance; positive information significantly decreased fear levels on self-reported measures and behavioral avoidance. No significant changes on self-reported measures or behavioral avoidance were found for children who received no information.

Despite research interest generated by direct conditioning models and Rachman's proposed pathways [90], these studies have been criticized as being inadequate to fully explain the many types of fears and phobias [98], and a nonassociative model of phobic cause has been proposed [99–101]. According to the nonassociative model, some specific fears (ie, heights, water, animals, strangers) are evolutionary relevant and can occur without critical learning experiences (direct and indirect). That is, such fears have an innate survival mechanism passed on from our ancestors, which would result in fear responses in the course of normal maturational development and experiences. Phobias are seen as a result of either an enhanced genetic fear response to a particular situation or object or a deficit in the mechanisms responsible for adapting to fear responses, such as habituation.

Although the nonassociative model has generated some findings and interest among researchers in evaluating different models of phobic cause, this model also has received criticism [102–104]. Briefly, the nonassociative model has been criticized because some developmental fears are innate but are usually transient and do not develop into a phobia; the definition of conditioning used in the studies is outmoded and does not take into account current learning definitions; the failure of phobic subjects to identify a specific stimulus or responding that they were "always afraid" was interpreted as a basis for a "nonassociative" model; and the failure to fully acknowledge limitations associated with both retrospective and prospective studies.

Overall, it is unlikely that there is any one factor (or pathway) that accounts for the development of such problems in youngsters; therefore, searching for the single factor (or pathway) is not likely to be fruitful [4,56]. Essentially, what is needed is the formulation of several models that indicate how these and other factors interrelate, thereby leading to the development of specific phobia. Such models might then be tested with longitudinal designs and with more complex analytic procedures.

Assessment

A phobia is a complex multichannel response pattern of behavior consisting of at least three different but interrelated systems: the cognitive-subjective, the behavioral, and the physiologic [5,6]. The most prominent assessment instrument used by clinical child psychologists and psychiatrists is the structured or semistructured diagnostic interview. In addition to providing the most direct assessment of the subjective-cognitive domain and eliciting information necessary for diagnosis, the interview is useful for assessing the other two domains (eg, "Does your heart beat fast when you see a dog?" and "Do you try as hard as you can to stay away from parties?"). Several structured interviews for children and parallel parent versions have been developed [105,106]. The Anxiety Disorders Interview Schedule for DSM-IV: Child and Parent Versions (ADIS-C/P) [107], which are semistructured diagnostic interviews, were designed specifically for the diagnosis of specific phobia and other anxiety disorders in children and have been studied extensively for their reliability and validity [108–111]. They also are the most used widely interviews in childhood phobic and anxiety disorders research.

The specific phobia section of the ADIS-C contains a list of objects and events (eg, dark, dogs, and high places) to which the child rates his or her level of fear and avoidance using a nine-point (0–8) "Feelings Thermometer." The Feelings Thermometer simplifies the rating task for children and removes some of the variability attributed to language skills that occur when young children respond to questionnaires [112]. For items that elicit a fear rating of 4 or more, the child also is asked to rate the degree of interference (in terms of school, friends, family, and personal distress). Questions addressing the onset, course, and cause of each specific phobia also are included in the ADIS-C.

There also are several child self-rating scales to assess the phobic child's subjective-cognitive domain. The Revised Children's Manifest Anxiety Scale (RCMAS) [113] and the State-Trait Anxiety Inventory for Children (STAIC) [114] are used widely to measure global anxiety levels. The Childhood Anxiety Sensitivity Index (CASI) [115] is an 18-item questionnaire that assesses the degree to which bodily signs of anxiety (eg, heart beating fast) is frightening to the child. Administering the Childhood Anxiety Sensitivity Index might be useful to gauge how much the phobic symptom per se is distressing to the child and not merely the phobic stimulus.

Although the measures mentioned above are used widely and provide useful information on childhood anxiety symptoms, they do not assess specific symptoms of DSM-IV phobic disorders [116,117]. There are several childhood self-rating scales that do so, which were developed after the publication of the DSM-IV. The Multidimensional Anxiety Scale for Children (MASC) [118] is a 39-item questionnaire that assesses anxiety symptoms and yields a total anxiety disorder index and four main factor scores: social anxiety, physical symptoms, harm/avoidance, and separation/panic. The Spence Children's Anxiety Scale (SCAS) [119] is a 38-item questionnaire based on DSM-IV anxiety symptoms that yields six subscales: separation anxiety disorder, social phobia, obsessive-compulsive disorder, panic/agoraphobia disorder, generalized anxiety disorder, and physical injury fears (phobias). The original Screen for Child Anxiety Related Emotional Disorders (SCARED) [120] is a 38-item questionnaire based on DSM-IV symptoms that yields five subscales: separation anxiety disorder, social phobia, panic disorder, generalized anxiety disorder, and school phobia. The Screen for Child Anxiety Related Emotional Disorders – Revised (SCARED-R) [121] is a 66-item questionnaire based on DSM-IV symptoms that yields nine subscales: separation anxiety disorder, social phobia, obsessive-compulsive disorder, panic disorder, generalized anxiety disorder, traumatic stress disorder, and three types of specific phobias (blood-injection-injury, animal, and environmental). Finally, there is the widely used Fear Survey Schedule for Children, Revised (FSSC-R) [37]. An 80-item fear inventory, the FSSC-R assesses a broad range of fears in children and can help assess stimulus generalization. The FSSC-R contains five factors: fear of danger and death, fear of failure and criticism, fear of the unknown, fear of small animals, and medical fears.

Because parents frequently view their child's problem differently than the child [122], obtaining diagnostic and assessment data from the child's parents also is useful. Thus, parents may be administered the parent version of the ADIS (ADIS-P), which yields a diagnosis based on the parent report (as well as a composite diagnosis based on combining the child and parent interview data). In addition, with the exception of the SCARED parent version, questionnaires specifically designed to assess parents' views about specific phobia in children have not been developed. The current authors therefore have modified several of the child self-report measures (eg, the FSSC-R and the RCMAS) to make them appropriate for parents to complete. For example, using both the child and parent versions of the FSSC-R, Weems and colleagues [123] have compared 120 children (ages 6 to 17 years) with specific phobias of the dark, animals, shots or doctors, and social phobia. Results indicate that specific FSSC-R factors and items were successfully discriminated among the phobic subtypes.

Treatment

The treatment approach with the strongest research evidence is an exposure-based treatment using cognitive and behavioral treatments [24,34,124]. Usually exposure or having the child face the feared stimulus is conducted in a graded or step-by-step fashion. The present authors prefer to have child participants perform gradual exposures as delineated along the "steps of a fear hierarchy." The use of the hierarchy provides an opportunity for the child to gradually gain confidence (and reduce fear) when in the presence of the phobic stimulus, as he or she successfully completes each step of the hierarchy. The fear hierarchy for a child with a phobia of dogs might be (1) seeing pictures of dogs in magazines; (2) going to a pet shop and looking at a dog through the window; (3) going to a pet shop and petting a small puppy that is being held by somebody; (4) petting a larger size dog that is on a leash; and (5) petting yet a larger dog that is running loose [125].

Although breaking the exposure exercises into small steps through the fear hierarchy makes the task of exposure easier for the children, some youths still find it difficult to perform these exercises, even the relatively easy exercises. Merely instructing them to "just do it," is insufficient. To help facilitate children's confrontation with the feared stimulus, several cognitive and behavioral strategies might be used, including (1) contingency management procedures, (2) modeling, (3) systematic desensitization, and (4) cognitive or self-control procedures. The key features of each strategy are highlighted below and indicate the types of phobias that have been successfully reduced through each strategy.

Briefly, contingency management procedures, based on the principles of operant conditioning, stress the importance of the causal relationship between stimuli and behavior [36]. Using a transfer of control approach [126], the present authors rely on external agents of change (ie, parents and therapists) to rearrange the environment to ensure that positive consequences follow exposure to the fear stimulus and that positive consequences do not follow avoidance of the fear stimulus (ie, extinction). To ensure positive consequences follow exposure, the parent and child sign a written contract each week that states "if the child does [a specified exposure task] then [a specified reward] is provided by the parent." To ensure extinction follows avoidance, the parent is trained in basic principles of child management; the principle of extinction is a major focus of training.

Contingency management has been used most frequently to treat children with so-called school phobia. However, these children are highly heterogeneous and may include children with specific phobias relating to the school setting. Other types of specific phobias for which contingency management has been successfully used are heights [127], small animals [128–130], the dark [131,132], water [133], and claustrophobia [134].

Modeling procedures involve the child's learning to be less fearful by observing others handling the feared object or situation. The models observed may be actual or "live" models or observed on films or videotapes, or they may be "symbolic" models. The modeling procedures have been experimentally tested extensively [135], although the focus has been primarily on dental and medical fears, not clinical phobias [136,137]. In addition to these situational fears, modeling procedures have been found effective in reducing children's fears of small animals [138–140], water [141], heights [142], and test-taking [143].

Formally introduced by Wolpe [144], systematic desensitization involves the following three phases: (1) teaching the child an antagonistic response (eg, relaxation); (2) constructing a fear hierarchy; and (3) pairing the antagonistic response to each item on the hierarchy. Some of the types of phobias that have been successfully treated with systematic desensitization include darkness [145,146], loud noises [147,148], test-taking [149,150], water [151,152], heights [153], and needles [154].

Finally, self-control procedures stress cognitive processes to behavior change, with each child directly involved in regulating his or her own behavior. In the present authors' work with phobic children, we focus on teaching specific thinking styles and on applying these styles when confronted with a particular feared stimulus. We use the acronym STOP ("Scared?," "Thoughts," "Other thoughts [or things I can do]," and "Praise") to teach this skill. Generally, self-control procedures have been effective in reducing children's nighttime fears [155,156], fears of darkness [157], public speaking [158,159], and bowel movement phobia [160].

We now turn to a brief review of the studies that provide empirical support for exposure-based cognitive behavioral treatment procedures for reducing specific phobias in children. Overall, although variations (eg, the degree of parental involvement or individual versus group format) may exist, randomized clinical trials have demonstrated efficacy. In Silverman and colleagues [34], the efficacy of an exposure-based contingency management treatment condition and an exposure-based cognitive self-control treatment condition relative to an education support control condition were evaluated for treating children (ages 6 to 16 years) with phobic disorders. Results demonstrate that children in both the exposure-based contingency management and exposure-based cognitive self-control conditions showed improvement after treatment, and the treatment gains were maintained at 3-, 6-, and 12-month follow-ups. Interestingly, children in the education support control condition also showed comparable improvements at the post-treatment and 3-, 6-, and 12-months follow-ups on most of the measures, highlighting the importance of conducting further research on the mechanisms of change in exposure-based cognitive behavioral treatment programs. In addition, using the sample of subjects who participated in the studies by Silverman and colleagues [34] and [161] (which contained children with anxiety disorders but not specific phobia), Pina and colleagues [162] have compared the efficacy of cognitive-behavioral treatment between Euro-American and Hispanic-Latino youths (ages 6 to 16 years). Results show that both Euro-American and Hispanic-Latino youths demonstrated positive and statistically equivalent treatment gains and maintenance.

Dewis and colleagues [163] have examined the efficacy of computer-aided vicarious exposure versus in vivo exposure in children (ages 10 to 17 years) with spider phobia. Results indicate in vivo exposures were significantly more efficacious than computer-aided vicarious exposure and a wait list. Öst and colleagues [164] have examined the efficacy of a one-session exposure treatment with the subject alone, a one-session exposure treatment with a parent present, and a wait-list control in children (ages 7 to 17 years) with specific phobia (animal or miscellaneous category). Results indicate that both treatment conditions produced significantly better improvements than the wait-list condition at post-treatment and one-year follow-up.

Finally, Muris and colleagues [165] have examined the efficacy of eye movement desensitization and reprocessing (EMDR) versus exposure in children (ages 8 to 17 years) with spider phobia. Results indicate that although EMDR demonstrated improvement on self-report measure of spider fear, in vivo exposures produced significant improvements on both self-report measures and behavioral avoidance.

Although there is growing evidence demonstrating the efficacy of exposure-based cognitive-behavioral treatment for reducing childhood specific phobia, further research using randomized clinical trials composed of children from multiple ethnic and socioeconomic backgrounds is needed. In addition, further research in the area is needed to determine the main mechanisms of therapeutic change. The present authors are currently conducting an NIMH-funded study on this issue.

Case report

This case report is a summary of a case that was published recently in a child psychiatry journal.[1] The child's name has been changed to ensure confidentiality.

Presenting problem

Carlos, a 9-year-old Hispanic-American boy, presented with his mother to the Child Anxiety and Phobia Program (CAPP) at Florida International University, Miami, with an avoidance of buttons. The phobia began when the boy was 5 years old, in kindergarten, during an art project that involved buttons. He described the situation in which he ran out of buttons to paste on his poster board and was asked to come to the front of the class to retrieve more buttons from a large bowl on his teacher's desk. When he reached for the bowl, his hand slipped, and all the buttons in the bowl fell on him. He described this experience as distressful, and since then both he and his mother reported that his avoidance of buttons continually increased. At first, his avoidance of buttons did not present many difficulties, but as time progressed, it became more difficult for him to handle buttons. This led to several areas of interference for the boy and his family, such as not being able to dress himself and difficulty concentrating in school caused by excessive preoccupation with not touching his school uniform or anything that his buttoned shirt touched.

Diagnostic work-up and differential diagnosis

Carlos and his mother were administered their respective versions of the ADIS-C and ADIS-P [108]. In addition, Carlos completed a number of self-rating scales, including the FSSC-R, the RCMAS, the MASC, and the CASI. The mother completed parent versions of the FSSC-R and the RCMAS, along with other measures.

When Carlos and his mother presented to CAPP, the duration of his phobia was 4 years. Both reported that during this 4-year period, he did not experience significant stressors or events that could be related to the phobia's onset. Moreover, the symptom presentation did not meet criteria for DSM-IV obsessive-compulsive disorder because the types of symptoms reported by the child and the mother did not include recurrent and persistent thoughts, impulses, or images that may be intrusive, as observed in obsessive-compulsive disorder. Rather, his marked and persistent avoidance of buttons was cued by the presence

---

[1] *Portions excerpted from* Saavedra LM, Silverman WK. Case study: disgust and a specific phobia of buttons. J Am Acad Child Adolesc Psychiatry 2002;41(11):1376–9; copyright Lippincott Williams & Wilkins, with permission.

and anticipation of buttons, as observed in specific phobia. Both Carlos and his mother indicated an interference rating of "8" on the 0- to 8-point "Feelings Thermometer."

Based on the mother and child interview data, a composite DSM-IV diagnosis of specific phobia of buttons was assigned. This was the only diagnosis assigned on either the composite, child, or parent interview.

Treatment

The child was treated using an exposure-based treatment involving cognitive and behavioral procedures [130]. The treatment involved using contingency management in which the mother provided positive reinforcement contingent on the child's successful completion of gradual or graded in vivo exposures to buttons. By session four, despite the success observed in the boy's approach behaviors (eg, the boy was now wearing or handling these specific buttons), his subjective ratings of distress increased dramatically. Further probing revealed that the boy found buttons disgusting on contact with his body. He also expressed that buttons emitted unpleasant odors. The following sessions consisted of incorporating disgust-related imagery exposures and cognitions, which involved exploring with the boy the various things about buttons that he found disgusting (eg, "buttons are gross") and using specific self-control or cognitive strategies. Disgust-related imagery exposures and cognitions appeared to be successful in reducing the boy's subjective ratings of distress.

On completion of the treatment, Carlos reported minimal distress about buttons, and he now was wearing clear plastic buttons on his school uniform shirt, previously rated as most distressful, on a daily basis. Readministration of the ADIS-C/P revealed further that Carlos no longer met criteria for specific phobia of buttons. Both Carlos and his mother gave an interference rating of "2" on the "Feelings Thermometer." Follow-up assessments revealed that Carlos's progress was maintained at 12 months post-treatment.

Summary

Compared with the study of clinically significant childhood phobias, far greater attention has been paid to the study of less severe, "normal" fears. Moreover, those studies conducted on childhood phobias are limited in a number of ways, such as their use of imprecise terminology (eg, "excessive fears and worries") and their reliance on retrospective data and so on. Despite such limitations, in this article we have highlighted those areas we believe to be central in a review of the disorder.

In terms of clinical presentation, although the focus of a specific phobia varies across individuals (eg, small animals and loud noises), the response pattern tends to be manifested along three systems: the behavioral, the cognitive, and the physiologic. Fear may become a "problem," (ie, a phobia) as evidenced by children's responses along one or more of these systems. For example, a child may present with excessive avoidance (ie, the behavioral system) or with excessive catastrophic thinking (ie, the cognitive system). Accurate identification of the specific feared stimulus also is critical for proper differential diagnosis, given DSM-IV requirements that several other anxiety conditions (eg, social phobia, obsessive-compulsive disorder) be ruled out before assigning a diagnosis of specific phobia.

Despite the growing attention to the issue of comorbidity, additional research using general clinic samples (not just children referred to anxiety specialty clinics) is necessary. This would help clarify the patterns of comorbidity associated with the disorder. Although largely based on retrospective data, studies examining the age of onset indicate that specific phobia has the earliest onset of the phobic disorders. In addition, there is some evidence that among the various types of specific phobia, fear of animals may appear earlier than most other fears. Overall, findings in the area of developmental trends suggest specific phobia may be a collection of separate but related disorders. In terms of the course of the disorder, the conclusions that can be drawn are tenuous, caused by the paucity of research in this area. The limited evidence suggests a tendency of some types of phobias to improve over time without treatment, although the findings suggest that some phobic symptoms persist, if untreated.

Epidemiologic research has placed the rate of specific phobia in children in the general population at approximately 7% to 9%, and slightly higher among clinic-referred samples. In addition, findings suggest that females tend to report more fears than males. Although some studies have begun to examine the impact of ethnicity, no conclusive data can be drawn on the impact of ethnicity, age, or socioeconomic status on prevalence. The discussion of causes in this article focuses on familial and learning factors, with an emphasis on the notion that phobias are overdetermined and multidetermined. Also emphasized is the need for further research to clarify individual differences in the acquisition of phobias.

Consistent with the view of specific phobia as manifesting itself along three systems, assessment must address the cognitive, behavioral, and physiologic systems through the use of diagnostic interviews and self-rating scales. Each of these methods of assessment, however, has advantages and disadvantages. Cognizance of these advantages and disadvantages is important from both a clinical and research perspective.

Although there may be various strategies for treating specific phobia in children, exposure to the feared stimulus is viewed generally as an important part of any successful treatment program. There is evidence of the efficacy of an exposure-based cognitive behavioral treatment that couples adjunctive strategies, such as contingency management, modeling, systematic desensitization, or self-control training. Additional research examining potential factors, such as child's age, gender, ethnicity, and socioeconomic status, which may affect treatment outcome, is needed. Overall, to the extent that this article kindles the initiation of this type of treatment research, as well as the other avenues of research highlighted throughout, then a major aim of the article, as well as of the entire volume, will have been attained.

References

[1] American Psychiatric Association. Diagnostic and statistical manual of mental disorders. 4th edition. Washington (DC): American Psychiatric Association; 1994.

[2] World Health Organization. The international classification of diseases (10th rev.). Geneva (Switzerland): World Health Organization; 1992.

[3] Miller LC, Barrett CL, Hampe E. Phobias of childhood in a prescientific era. In: Davids A, editor. Child personality and psychopathology: current topics. New York: John Wiley & Sons; 1974. p. 89–134.

[4] Silverman WK, Rabian B. Specific phobia. In: Ollendick TH, King NJ, Yule W, editors. International handbook of phobic and anxiety disorders in children and adolescents. New York: Plenum Press; 1994. p. 87–109.

[5] Lang PJ. Fear reduction and fear behavior: problems in treating a construct. In: Shlien JM, editor. Research in psychotherapy. Washington (DC): American Psychiatric Association; 1968. p. 90–102.

[6] Lang PJ. Fear imagery: an information processing analysis. Behav Ther 1977;8:862–6.

[7] Wood SR, Teachman BA. Intersection of disgust an fear: normative and pathological views. Clinical Psychology: Science and Practice 2000;7(3):291–311.

[8] Saavedra LM, Silverman WK. Case study: disgust and a specific phobia of buttons. J Am Acad Child Adolesc Psychiatry 2002;41(11):1376–9.

[9] Phillips ML, Senior C, Fahy T, et al. Disgust: The forgotten emotion of psychiatry. Br J Psychiatry 1998;172:373–5.

[10] Kindt M, Brosschot JF. Cognitive bias in spider-phobic children: comparison of a pictorial and a linguistic spider stroop. Journal of Psychopathology and Behavioral Assessment 1999; 21(3):207–20.

[11] Vasey MW, Dalgleish T, Silverman WK. Research on information-processing factors in child and adolescent psychopathology: A critical commentary. J Clin Child Adolesc Psychol 2003; 32:81–93.

[12] Silverman WK, Nelles WB. Simple phobia in childhood. In: Hersen M, Last C, editors. Handbook of child and adult psychopathology: a longitudinal perspective. New York: Pergamon Press; 1991. p. 183–93.

[13] Atkinson L, Quarrington B, Cyr JJ, et al. Differential classification in school refusal. Br J Psychiatry 1985;155:191–5.

[14] Bernestein GA, Garfinkel BD. School phobia: the overlap of affective and anxiety disorders. J Am Acad Child Adolesc Psychiatry 1986;2:235–41.

[15] Burke AE, Silverman WK. Prescribed treatment for school refusal. Clin Psychol Rev 1987;7: 353–62.

[16] Last CG, Francis G. School phobia. In: Lahey BB, Kazdin AE, editors. Advances in clinical/ child psychology, Volume 11. New York: Plenum Press; 1988. p. 193–222.

[17] Ollendick TH, Mayer JA. School phobia. In: Turner SM, editor. Behavioral theories and treatment of anxiety. New York: Plenum Press; 1984. p. 367–411.

[18] Kearney CA, Silverman WK. A preliminary analysis of a functional model of assessment and treatment for school refusal behavior. Behav Modif 1990;14:340–66.

[19] Saavedra LM, Silverman WK. Classification of anxiety disorders in children: what a difference two decades make. Int Rev Psychiatry 2002;14:87–101.

[20] Anderson JC, Williams S, McGee R, et al. DSM-III disorders in preadolescent children. Arch Gen Psychiatry 1987;44:69–76.

[21] Strauss CC, Last CG, Hersen M, et al. Association between anxiety and depression in children and adolescents. J Abnorm Child Psychol 1988;16:57–68.

[22] Francis G, Strauss CC, Last CG. Social anxiety in school phobic adolescents. Paper presented at the 21st Annual Meeting of the Association for Advancement of Behavior Therapy. Boston, November 12–15, 1987.

[23] Brady U, Kendall PC. Comorbidity of anxiety and depression in children and adolescents. Psychol Bull 1992;111:244–55.

[24] King NJ, Muris P, Ollendick TH. Specific phobia. In: Morris TL, March JS, editors. Anxiety disorders in children and adolescents. 2nd edition. New York: Guilford Press; 2004. p. 263–79.

[25] Curry JF, March JS, Hervey AS. Comorbidity of childhood and adolescent anxiety disorders. In: Ollendick TH, March JS, editors. Phobic and anxiety disorders in children and adolescents: a clinician's guide to effective psychosocial and pharmacological interventions. New York: Oxford Univiversity Press; 2004. p. 116–40.

[26] Starcevic V, Bogojevic G. Comorbidity of panic disorder with agoraphobia and specific phobia: relationship with the subtypes of specific phobia. Compr Psychiatry 1997;38(6):315–20.

[27] Seligman LD, Ollendick TH. Comorbidity of anxiety and depression in children and adolescents: an integrative review. Clin Child Fam Psychol Rev 1998;1(2):125–44.

[28] Ollendick TH, Seligman LD, Goza AB, et al. Anxiety and depression in children and adolescents: a factor-analytic examination of the tripartite model. J Child Fam Stud 2003;12(2): 157–70.

[29] Beidel DC, Turner SM. Comorbidity of test anxiety and other anxiety disorders in children. J Abnorm Child Psychol 1988;16:275–87.

[30] Curtis GC, Magee WJ, Eaton WW, et al. Specific fears and phobias: epidemiology and classification. Br J Psychiatry 1998;173:212–7.

[31] Lewinsohn PM, Zinbarg R, Seeley JR, et al. Lifetime comorbidity among anxiety disorders and between anxiety disorders and other mental disorders in adolescents. J Anxiety Disord 1997;11(4):377–94.

[32] Essau CA, Conradt J, Peterman F. Frequency, comorbidity, and psychosocial impairment of specific phobia in adolescents. J Clin Child Psychol 2000;29:221–31.

[33] Last CG, Perrin S, Hersen M, et al. DSM- III-R anxiety disorders in children: sociodemographic and clinical characteristics. J Am Acad Child Adolesc Psychiatry 1992;31:1070–6.

[34] Silverman WK, Kurtines WM, Ginsburg GS, et al. Contingency management, self-control, and education support in the treatment of childhood phobic disorders: a randomized clinical trial. J Consult Clin Psychol 1999;67:675–87.

[35] Lapouse R, Monk M. Fears and worries in a representative sample of children. Am J Orthopsychiatry 1959;29:803–18.

[36] Morris RJ, Kratochwill TR. Treating children's fears and phobias: a behavioral approach. Elmsford (NY): Pergamon Press; 1983.

[37] Ollendick TH. Reliability and validity of the revised fear survey schedule for children (FSSC-R). Behav Res Ther 1983;21:685–92.

[38] Ollendick TH, Vasey MW. Developmental theory and the practice of clinical child psychology. J Clin Child Psych 1999;28:457–66.

[39] Croake J, Knox F. The changing nature of children's fears. Child Study J 1973;3:91–105.

[40] Eme R, Schmidt D. The stability of children's fears. Child Dev 1978;49:1277–9.

[41] Muris P, Merckelbach H, Gadet B, et al. Fears, worries, and scary dreams in 4- to 12-year-old children: their content, developmental patterns, and origins. J Clin Child Psychol 2000;29: 43–52.

[42] Gullone E. The development of normal fear: a century of research. Clin Psychol Rev 2000;20:429–51.

[43] Bauer DH. An exploratory study of developmental changes in children's fears. J Child Psychol Psychiatry 1976;17:69–74.

[44] McGee R, Feehan M, Williams S, et al. DSM-III disorders from age 11 to age 15 years. J Am Acad Child Adolesc Psychiatry 1992;31:50–9.

[45] Sheehan DV, Sheehan KE, Minichiello WE. Age of onset of phobic disorders: a reevaluation. Compr Psychiatry 1981;22:544–53.

[46] Thyer BA, Parrish RT, Curtis EC, et al. Ages of onset of DSM-III anxiety disorders. Compr Psychiartry 1985;26:113–22.

[47] Marks IM, Gelder MG. Different ages of onset in varieties of phobia. Am J Psychiatry 1996;123:218–21.

[48] Liddell A, Lyons M. Thunderstorm phobias. Behav Res Ther 1978;16:306–8.

[49] Öst LG, Hugdahl K. Acquisition of agoraphobia, mode of onset and anxiety response patterns. Behav Res Ther 1983;21:623–31.

[50] Öst LG. Ways of acquiring phobias and outcome of behavioral treatments. Behav Res Ther 1985;23:683–9.

[51] Öst LG. Age of onset in different phobias. J Abnorm Psychol 1987;96:123–45.

[52] Kendler KS, Neale MC, Kessler RC, et al. The genetic epidemiology of phobias in women. Arch Gen Psychiatry 1992;49:273–81.

[53] Biederman J, Faraone SV, Marrs A, et al. Panic disorder and agoraphobia in consecutively referred children and adolescents. J Am Acad Child Adolesc Psychiatry 1997;36:214–23.

[54] Agras WS, Chapin HN, Oliveau DC. The natural history of phobia. Arch Gen Psychiatry 1972;26:315–7.

[55] Hampe E, Noble M, Miller LC, et al. Phobic children at two years post-treatment. J Abnorm Psychol 1973;82:446–53.

[56] Ollendick TH. Fear reduction techniques with children. In: Hersen M, Miller P, Eisler R, editors. Progress in behavior modification, Volume 8. New York: Academic Press; 1979. p. 127–68.

[57] Abe K. Phobias and nervous symptoms in childhood and maturity: persistence and associations. Br J Psychiatry 1972;120:275–83.

[58] Milne JM, Garrison CZ, Addy CL, et al. Frequency of phobic disorders in a community sample of young adolescents. J Am Acad Child Adolesc Psychiatry 1995;34(9):1202–10.

[59] Kennedy WA. School phobia: rapid treatment of fifty cases. J Abnorm Psychol 1965;70:285–9.

[60] Werry JS, Quay HC. The prevalence of behavior symptoms in younger elementary school children. Am J Orthopsychiatry 1971;41:136–43.

[61] Agras WS, Sylvester D, Oliveau DC. The epidemiology of common fears and phobia. Compr Psychiatry 1969;10:151–6.

[62] Graziano AM, DeGiovanni IS. The clinical significance of childhood phobias: a note on the proportion of child-clinical referrals for the treatment of children's fears. Behav Res Ther 1979;17:108–12.

[63] Rutter M, Tizard J, Whitmore K. Education, health, and behavior. New York: John Wiley & Sons; 1970.

[64] Silverman WK, Kearney CA. Listening to our clinical partners: informing researchers about children's fears and phobias. J Behav Ther Exp Psychiatry 1992;23:71–6.

[65] Öst LG, Treffers PDA. Onset, course, and outcome for anxiety disorders in children. In: Silverman WK, Treffers PDA, editors. Anxiety disorders in children and adolescents: research, assessment and intervention. New York: Cambridge University Press; 2001. p. 293–312.

[66] Anderson JC, Williams S, McGee R, et al. DSM-III disorders in preadolescent children. Arch Gen Psychiatry 1987;44:69–76.

[67] McGee R, Feehan M, Williams S, et al. DSM-III disorders in a large sample of adolescents. J Am Acad Child Adolesc Psychiatry 1990;29:611–9.

[68] Bird HR, Canino G, Rubio-Stipec M, et al. Estimates of the prevalence of childhood maladjustment in a community survey in Puerto Rico. Arch Gen Psychiatry 1988;45:1120–6.

[69] Steinhausen HC, Metzke CW, Meier M, et al. Prevalence of child and adolescent psychiatric disorders: the Zurich epidemiological study. Acta Psychiatr Scand 1998;98:262–71.

[70] Wittchen H, Nelson CB, Lachner G. Prevalence of mental disorders and psychosocial impairments in adolescents and young adults. Psychol Med 1998;28(1):109–26.

[71] Ollendick TH, King NJ, Muris P. Fears and phobias in children: phenomenology, epidemiology, and aetiology. Child and Adolescent Mental Health 2002;7(3):98–106.

[72] Mellon R, Koliadis EA, Paraskevopoulos TD. Normative development of fears in Greece: self-reports on the Hellenic fear survey schedule for children. J Anxiety Disord 2004;18:233–54.

[73] Essau CA, Sakano Y, Ishikawa S, et al. Anxiety symptoms in Japanese and German children. Behav Res Ther 2004;42(5):601–12.

[74] Ginsburg GS, Silverman WK. Phobic and anxiety disorders in Hispanic and Caucasian youth. J Anxiety Disord 1996;10(6):517–28.

[75] Last CG, Perrin S. Anxiety disorders in African-American and white children. J Abnorm Child Psychol 1993;21(2):153–64.

[76] Ingman KA, Ollendick TH, Akande A. Cross-cultural aspects of fears in African children and adolescents. Behav Res Ther 1999;37(4):337–45.

[77] Antony MM, Barlow DH. Specific phobias. In: Barlow DH, editor. Anxiety and its disorders: the nature and treatment of anxiety and panic. 2nd edition. New York: Guilford Press; 2002. p. 380–417.

[78] Muris P, Merckelbach H. The etiology of childhood specific phobia: a multifactorial model. In: Vasey MW, Dadds MR, editors. The developmental psychopathology of anxiety. New York: Oxford University Press; 2001. p. 355–85.

[79] Torgersen S. The nature and origin of common phobic fears. Br J Psychiatry 1979;134:343–51.

[80] Slater E, Shields J. Genetic aspects of anxiety. In: Lader MJ, editor. Studies of anxiety. London: Royal Medico-Psychological Association; 1969. p. 62–71.

[81] Young JPR, Fenton GW, Lader MJ. The inheritance of neurotic traits: a twin study of the Middlesex Hospital questionnaire. Br J Psychiatry 1971;119:393–8.

[82] Burglass D, Clarke J, Henderson AS, et al. A study of agoraphobic housewives. Psychol Med 1977;7:73–86.

[83] Fyer AJ, Mannuzza S, Gallops MS, et al. Familial transmission of simple phobias and fears: a preliminary report. Arch Gen Psychiatry 1990;47:252–6.

[84] Moran C, Andrews G. The familial occurrence of agoraphobia. Br J Psychiatry 1985;146: 262–7.

[85] Noyes R, Crowe RR, Harris EL, et al. Relationship between panic disorder and agoraphobia. Arch Gen Psychiatry 1986;43:227–32.

[86] Reich J, Yates W. Family history of psychiatric disorders in social phobia. Compr Psychiatry 1988;29:72–5.

[87] Solyom L, Beck P, Solyom C, et al. Some etiological factors in phobic neurosis. Can Psychiatr Assoc J 1974;19:69–78.

[88] Endicott J, Spitzer RL. A diagnostic interview: the schedule for affective disorders and schizophrenia. Arch Gen Psychiatry 1978;35:837–44.

[89] Silverman WK, Cerny JA, Nelles WB, et al. Behavior problems in children of parents with anxiety disorders. J Am Acad Child Adolesc Psychiatry 1988;27:779–84.

[90] Rachman S. The conditioning theory of fear acquisition: a critical examination. Behav Res Ther 1977;15:375–87.

[91] Ollendick TH, King N, Hamilton DI. Origins of childhood fears: an evaluation of Rachman's theory of fear acquisition. Behav Res Ther 1991;29:117–23.

[92] Merckelbach H, Muris P, Schouten E. Pathways to fear in spider phobic children. Behav Res Ther 1996;34(11):935–8.

[93] Merckelbach H, Muris P. The etiology of childhood spider phobia. Behav Res Ther 1997; 35(11):1031–43.

[94] King NJ, Clowes-Hollins V, Ollendick TH. The etiology of childhood dog phobia. Behav Res Ther 1997;35(1):77.

[95] Ollendick TH, Langley AK, Jones RT, et al. Fear in children and adolescents: relations with negative life events, attributional style, and avoidant coping. J Child Psychol Psychiatry 2001;42:1029–34.

[96] Muris P, Bodden D, Merckelbach H, et al. Fear of the beast: a prospective study on the effects of negative information on childhood fear. Behav Res Ther 2003;41:195–208.

[97] Field AP, Lawson J. Fear information and the development of fears during childhood: effects on implicit fear responses and behavioural avoidance. Behav Res Ther 2003;41:1277–93.

[98] Davey GCL. Classical conditioning and the acquisition of human fears and phobias: a review and synthesis of the literature. Advances in Behavior Research and Therapy 1992;14:29–66.

[99] Menzies RG, Clarke JC. The etiology of phobias: a non-associative account. Clin Psychol Rev 1995;15:23–48.

[100] Poulton R, Menzies RG. Non-associative fear acquisition: a review of the evidence from retrospective and longitudinal research. Behav Res Ther 2002;40:127–49.

[101] Poulton R, Menzies RG. Fears born and bred: toward a more inclusive theory of fear acquisition. Behav Res Ther 2002;40:197–208.

[102] Muris P, Merckelbach H, de Jong PJ, et al. The etiology of specific fears and phobias in children: a critique of the non-associative account. Behav Res Ther 2002;40:185–95.

[103] Davey GCL. "Nonspecific" rather than "nonassociative" pathways to phobias: a commentary on Poulton and Menzies. Behav Res Ther 2002;40:151–8.

[104] Mineka S, Ohman A. Born to fear: non-associative vs associative factors in the etiology of phobias. Behav Res Ther 2002;40:173–84.

[105] Shaffer D, Fisher P, Lucas CP, et al. NIMH diagnostic interview schedule for children version IV (NIMH DISC-IV): description, differences from previous versions, and reliability of some common diagnosis. J Am Acad Child Adolesc Psychiatry 2000;39(1):28–38.

[106] Puig-Antich J, Chambers W. The schedule for affective disorders and schizophrenia for school-aged children. New York: New York State Psychiatric Institute; 1978.

[107] Silverman WK, Albano AM. The anxiety disorders interview schedule for children for DSM-IV: (child and parent versions). San Antonio (TX): Psychological Corporation; 1996.

[108] Silverman WK, Eisen AR. Age differences in the reliability of parent and child reports of child anxious symptomatology using a structured interview. J Am Acad Child Adolesc Psychiatry 1992;31:117–24.

[109] Silverman WK, Saavedra LM, Pina AA. Test-retest reliability of anxiety symptoms and diagnoses using the anxiety disorders interview schedule for DSM-IV: child and parent versions. J Am Acad Child Adolesc Psychiatry 2001;40:937–44.

[110] Rapee RM, Barrett PM, Dadds MR, et al. Reliability of the DSM-III-R childhood anxiety disorders using structured interview: inter-rater and parent-child agreement. J Am Acad Child Adolesc Psychiatry 1994;33:984–92.

[111] Wood JJ, Piacentini JC, Bergman RL, et al. Concurrent validity of the anxiety disorders section of the anxiety disorders interview schedule for DSM-IV: child and parent versions. J Clin Child Adolesc Psychol 2002;32(3):335–42.

[112] Barrios BA, Hartmann DB, Shigetomi C. Fears and anxieties in children. In: Mash EJ, Terdal LG, editors. Behavioral assessment of childhood disorders. New York: Guilford Press; 1981. p. 259–304.

[113] Reynolds CR, Richmond BO. What I think and feel: a revised measure of children's manifest anxiety. J Abnorm Child Psychol 1978;6:271–80.

[114] Spielberger CD. Manual for the state-trait anxiety inventory for children. Palo Alto (CA): Consulting Psychologists Press; 1973.

[115] Silverman WK, Fleisig W, Rabian B, et al. Childhood anxiety sensitivity index. J Clin Child Psychol 1991;20:162–8.

[116] Muris P, Merckelbach H, Ollendick TH, et al. Three traditional and three new childhood anxiety questionnaires: their reliability and validity in a normal adolescent sample. Behav Res Ther 2002;40:753–72.

[117] Seligman LD, Ollendick TH, Langley AK, et al. The utility of measures of child and adolescent anxiety: a meta-analytic review of the revised children's manifest anxiety scale, the state-trait anxiety inventory for children, and the child behavior checklist. J Clin Child Adolesc Psychol 2004;33(3):557–65.

[118] March JS, Parker J, Sullivan K, et al. The multidimensional anxiety scale for children (MASC): factor structure, reliability, and validity. J Am Acad Child Adolesc Psychiatry 1997;36:554–65.

[119] Spence SH. A measure of anxiety symptoms among children. Behav Res Ther 1998;36:545–66.

[120] Birmaher B, Khetarpal S, Brent D, et al. The screen for child anxiety related emotional

disorders (SCARED): scale construction and psychometric characteristics. J Am Acad Child Adolesc Psychiatry 1997;36:545–53.

[121] Muris P, Merckelbach H, Schmidt H, et al. The revised version of the screen for child anxiety related emotional disorders (SCARED-R): factor structure in normal children. Pers Individ Dif 1999;26:99–112.

[122] Klein RG. Parent-child agreement in clinical assessment of anxiety and other psychopathology: a review. J Anxiety Disord 1991;15:187–98.

[123] Weems CF, Silverman WK, Saavedra LS, et al. The discrimination of children's phobias using the revised fear survey schedule for children. J Child Psychol Psychiatry 1999;40:941–52.

[124] Ollendick TH, King NJ. Empirically supported treatments for children with phobic and anxiety disorders: current status. J Clin Child Psychol 1998;27(2):156–67.

[125] Silverman WK, Eisen AR. Phobic disorders. In: Ammerman RT, Last CG, Hersen M, editors. Handbook of prescriptive treatments for children and adolescents. Needham Heights (MA): Allyn & Bacon; 1993. p. 189–201.

[126] Silverman WK, Kurtines WM. Short-term treatment for children with phobic and anxiety problems: a pragmatic view. Crisis Intervention 1999;5:119–31.

[127] Holmes FB. An experimental investigation of a method of overcoming children's fears. Child Dev 1936;7:6–30.

[128] Obler M, Terwilliger RF. Pilot study on the effectiveness of systematic desensitization with neurologically impaired children with phobic disorders. J Consult Clin Psychol 1970;34:314–8.

[129] Öst LG. One-session group treatment of spider phobia. Behav Res Ther 1996;34(9):707–15.

[130] Öst LG, Ferebee I, Furmark T. One-session group therapy of spider phobia: direct versus indirect treatments. Behav Res Ther 1997;35(8):721–32.

[131] Leitenberg H, Callahan EJ. Reinforced practice and reduction of different kinds of fears in adults and children. Behav Res Ther 1973;11:19–30.

[132] Sheslow DV, Bondy AS, Nelson RO. A comparison of graduated exposure, verbal coping skills, and their combination in the treatment of children's fear of the dark. Child and Family Behavior Therapy 1983;4:33–45.

[133] Menzies RG, Clarke JC. A comparison of in vivo and vicarious exposure in the treatment of childhood water phobia. Behav Res Ther 1993;31:9–15.

[134] Öst LG, Alm T, Brandberg M, et al. One vs five sessions of exposure and five sessions of cognitive therapy in the treatment of claustrophobia. Behav Res Ther 2001;39:167–83.

[135] Barrios BA, O'Dell SL. Fears and anxieties. In: Mash EJ, Barkley RA, editors. Treatment of childhood disorders. New York: Guilford Press; 1989. p. 167–221.

[136] Melamed BG, Hawes R, Heiby E, et al. Use of filmed modeling to reduce uncooperative behavior of children during dental treatment. J Dent Res 1975;54:797–801.

[137] Melamed BG, Siegel LJ. Reduction of anxiety in children facing hospitalization and surgery by way of filmed modeling. J Consult Clin Psychol 1975;43:511–2.

[138] Bandura A, Blanchard EB, Ritter B. Relative efficacy of desensitization and modeling approaches for inducing behavioral, affective, and attitudinal changes. J Pers Soc Psychol 1969; 13:173–99.

[139] Bandura A, Menlove FL. Factors determining vicarious extinction of avoidance behavior through symbolic modeling. J Pers Soc Psychol 1968;8:99–108.

[140] Hill JH, Liebert RM, Mott DEW. Vicarious extinction of avoidance behavior through films: an initial test. Psychol Rep 1968;22:192.

[141] Lewis S. A comparison of behavior therapy techniques in the reduction of fearful avoidance behavior. Behav Ther 1974;5:648–55.

[142] Ritter B. Treatment of acrophobia with contact desensitization. Behav Res Ther 1969;7:41–5.

[143] Mann RA. The behavior-therapeutic use of contingency contracting to control an adult behavior problem: weight control. J Appl Behav Anal 1972;5:99–109.

[144] Wolpe J. Psychotherapy by reciprocal inhibition. Stanford (CA): Stanford University Press; 1958.

[145] Jackson HJ, King NJ. The emotive imagery treatment of a child's trauma-induced phobia. J Behav Ther Exp Psychiatry 1981;12:325–8.

[146] Kelley CK. Play desensitization of fear of darkness in preschool children. Behav Res Ther 1976;14:79–81.

[147] Tasto DL. Systematic desensitization, muscle relaxation and visual imagery in the counter-conditioning of a four-year-old phobic child. Behav Res Ther 1969;7:409–11.

[148] Wish P, Hasazi J, Jurgela A. Automated direct deconditioning of a childhood phobia. J Behav Ther Exp Psychiatry 1973;4:279–83.

[149] Barabasz AF. Classroom teachers as paraprofessional therapists in group systematic desensitization of test anxiety. Psychiatry 1975;38:388–92.

[150] Mann J, Rosenthal TL. Vicarious and direct counterconditioning of test anxiety through individual and group desensitization. Behav Res Ther 1969;7:359–67.

[151] Bentler PM. An infant's phobia treated with reciprocal inhibition therapy. J Child Psychol Psychiatry 1962;3:185–9.

[152] Ultee CA, Griffioen D, Schellekens J. The reduction of anxiety in children: a comparison of the effects of "systematic desentization in vitro" and "systematic desensitization in vivo." Behav Res Ther 1982;20:61–7.

[153] Croghan L, Musante GJ. The elimination of a boy's high-building phobia by in vivo desensitization and game playing. J Behav Ther Exp Psychiatry 1975;6:87–8.

[154] Rainwater N, Sweet AA, Elliott L, et al. Systematic desensitization in the treatment of needle phobias for children with diabetes. Child and Family Behavior Therapy 1989;10:19–31.

[155] Graziano AM, Mooney KC. Family self-control instruction for children's nighttime fear reduction. J Consult Clin Psychol 1980;48:206–13.

[156] Graziano AM, Mooney KC, Huber C, et al. Self-control instruction for children's fear reductions. J Behav Ther Exp Psychiatry 1979;10:221–7.

[157] Kanfer FH, Karoly P, Newman A. Reduction of children's fear of the dark by competence-related and situational threat-related verbal cues. J Consult Clin Psychol 1975;43:251–8.

[158] Cradock C, Cotler S, Jason LA. Primary prevention: immunization of children for speech anxiety. Cognit Ther Res 1978;2:389–96.

[159] Fox JE, Houston BK. Efficacy of self-instructional training for reducing children's anxiety in an evaluative situation. Cognit Ther Res 1981;19:509–15.

[160] Eisen AR, Silverman WK. Treatment of an adolescent with bowel movement phobia using self-control therapy. J Behav Ther Exp Psychiatry 1991;22:45–51.

[161] Silverman WK, Kurtines MW, Ginsburg GS, et al. Treating anxiety disorders in children with group cognitive-behavioral therapy: a randomized clinical trial. J Consult Clin Psychol 1999; 67(6):995–1003.

[162] Pina AA, Silverman WK, Fuentes RM, et al. Exposure-based cognitive-behavioral treatment for phobic and anxiety disorders: treatment effects and maintenance for Hispanic/Latino relative to European-American youths. J Am Acad Child Adolesc Psychiatry 2003;42(10):1179–87.

[163] Dewis LM, Kirkby KC, Martin F, et al. Computer-aided vicarious exposure versus live graded exposure for spider phobia in children. J Behav Ther Exp Psychiatry 2001;32:17–27.

[164] Öst LG, Svensson L, Hellstrom K, et al. One-session treatment of specific phobias in youths: a randomized clinical trial. J Consult Clin Psychol 2001;69(5):814–24.

[165] Muris P, Merckelbach H, Holdrinet I, et al. Treating phobic children: effects of EMDR versus exposure. J Consult Clin Psychol 1998;66(1):193–8.

ELSEVIER
SAUNDERS

Child Adolesc Psychiatric Clin N Am
14 (2005) 845–861

CHILD AND
ADOLESCENT
PSYCHIATRIC CLINICS
OF NORTH AMERICA

Evaluation and Treatment of Anxiety Disorders in the General Pediatric Population: A Clinician's Guide

Heidi J. Lyneham, PhD*, Ronald M. Rapee, PhD

Department of Psychology, Macquarie University, Sydney, New South Wales 2109, Australia

Anxiety disorders have been consistently recognized as one of the most common mental health problems experienced during childhood. Nonclinical levels of fear and worry have been found in up to 70% of children and adolescents [1]. Estimates of the prevalence of anxiety disorders have varied from 10% to 15% when clinical symptoms alone are examined [2,3] and from 4% to 7% of children and adolescents when criteria that necessitates the presence of significant distress or interference as a result of the symptoms are applied [2,4]. When applying these strict criteria, gender differences in prevalence rates are not evident; however, females are shown to predominate in studies of anxiety symptoms. The prevalence of anxiety disorders also has been shown to increase with age. In children and adolescents, comorbidity between the anxiety disorders and with other disorders is extensive. In children and adolescents who have a principal anxiety disorder, approximately 50% have additional anxiety disorders, 5% have mood disorders, and 20% have externalizing disorders [5,6].

Differentiating clinical anxiety from normal developmental experiences with fear and worry can be difficult, with clear developmental shifts occurring in children who have anxiety disorders and those who do not. In young children, fears are most often concrete and specific, such as fears of separation, strangers, loud noises, and injury [7,8]. As children progress through later childhood and adolescence, social, evaluative, and abstract worries become more common [9]. This progression is evident in the prevalence of specific anxiety disorders. For example, the prevalence of separation anxiety disorder decreases with age [10] as does the number and severity of specific fears [11,12]. In contrast, the prevalence

---

* Corresponding author.
E-mail address: heidi.lyneham@psy.mq.edu.au (H.J. Lyneham).

1056-4993/05/$ – see front matter © 2005 Elsevier Inc. All rights reserved.
doi:10.1016/j.chc.2005.05.002

rates for generalized anxiety disorder, social phobia, and panic disorder increase with age [13–15]. These changes in presentation are believed to relate to a child's cognitive development. For example, relationships have been found between the Piagetian-rated cognitive level and a child's ability to identify potential negative outcomes and their experience of personal worry [16]. Children's experience of embarrassment also shows developmental changes; young children rely on audience feedback to determine the strength of their performance, and older children show evidence of self-evaluation as they experience embarrassment, irrespective of audience feedback [17].

The general belief that a child is "going through a phase" and "will grow out of it" when they experience severe anxiety is unsupported. Research into the natural course of anxiety disorders that begin in childhood has shown that the disorders persist over time, although children often move through different categories of anxiety, with evidence for increasing specificity during adolescence through to adulthood [18–20]. Negative consequences have been identified in both the short and long term. In the short term, children who have anxiety disorders have been found to have increased levels of depression, lower self-esteem, difficulties with attention and concentration, lower than expected achievement, impaired peer relationships, and poor social behavior [21,22]. In the long term, these disorders are linked to higher risk for later depression, substance use, and conduct problems [23,24] and are associated with the increased use of medical and psychiatric services [24], a slow transition to independent living [25], and an increased risk for suicidal ideation and attempts [26].

Despite the high rates of anxiety disorders in the community, levels of psychiatric service use have been found to be highly discrepant. Less than half of all children who are identified as having any mental health problem do access services [2,27,28]. Children with anxious or withdrawn behavior, particularly, are less likely to access help than are children who exhibit aggressive, oppositional, or hyperactive behavior. Parents play the primary role in identifying the need for assistance with mental health issues; however, approximately 40% to 50% of parents fail to identify their child's mental health disorder, with anxiety disorders being particularly poorly recognized [29,30]. Additionally, research has found that externalizing problems in children are more referable than internalizing problems, particularly for children experiencing both types of disorder [31,32]. As a consequence of poor recognition and subsequent referral, a large number of anxious children and adolescents miss out on appropriate treatment that may improve immediate quality of life and reduce the risk of negative long-term consequences.

It is interesting to consider the reasons parents hold for seeking help for their anxious child. There does not appear to be any descriptive research specific to anxiety. However, in the present authors' university-based child and adolescent anxiety clinic, 504 parents have contacted the clinic to request assessment with view to receiving treatment in the past year. In 40% of these cases, the parent's themselves have initiated the referral through researching options available to them. Other sources of recommendation come from school counselors (17%), other mental health services (15%), general practitioners or pediatricians (12%), word of mouth (10%), psychiatrists (4%), and teachers (3%). Common reasons for seeking help include sleep difficulties, anxiety in new situations that leads to refusal to participate, lack of friends, self-criticism, problems separating from parents, school refusal or distress, a constant need for reassurance, visible sadness, chronically expressed worry, repetitive stomach aches or nausea, bullying, and shyness. Peak referral times occur within the first and second month of the school year and also at the beginning of the second school term. Aside from symptoms of withdrawal, the main reasons for seeking help appear to relate to concrete, observable symptoms that affect family or school.

Diagnostic evaluation of anxiety

A satisfactory evaluation process needs to resolve several issues, including the differential diagnosis, particularly given the high rates of comorbidity, the severity of symptoms relative to appropriate peers, and the impact of the symptoms on functioning. For the purpose of planning treatment, it is also essential to conduct an assessment (often referred to as functional assessment) of factors that maintain symptoms. The variety of questions to be answered leads to a need for a multimethod approach to evaluation. Over the past decade, there have been significant improvements in the scientific and clinical value of diagnostic interviews that facilitate differential diagnosis and in questionnaire measures of childhood anxiety disorders that enable peer comparison [33]. These newer measures have been shown to relate closely to the experience of impairment [34] and are sensitive to treatment effects [35,36]. Structured approaches to the assessment of maintenance factors also have become available.

The complexity and dependence of a young person's world leads to the need for multi-informant approaches to evaluation. This need is confirmed by research that indicates that young people may underreport certain types of symptoms because of social desirability [37,38] and that reports from parents can be influenced by their perception of behavior; for example, separation anxiety may be portrayed as oppositional behavior if the cause is believed to be deliberate defiance [39]. In addition, there is strong evidence that parents cannot comment accurately on the internal experiences of a young person [40]. Minimum standard practice involves the use of separate interview and self-report questionnaires with a child or adolescent and their primary caregivers. Additional information gathered from teachers, peers, and other individuals who are significant in the young person's life can be of particular use in determining the severity of symptoms, the impact, and maintenance factors.

Assessment tools

Several reliable and validated structured and semistructured diagnostic interviews are available for use with children and adolescents [41]. The Anxiety

Disorders Interview Schedule for Children (ADIS-C) [42] is unique in that it provides in-depth assessment of individual anxiety disorders as well as differential diagnoses for other common childhood difficulties. The ADIS-C is a semistructured diagnostic tool with separate interviews for the young person (from 6 years) and his or her parents. The administration of this interview takes 1 to 3 hours, depending on the number of disorders that need to be examined in depth. It is recommended that the young person be interviewed first to prevent contamination of the interview with information from the parents. Research indicates that the ADIS-C tool has fair to excellent reliability and validity compared with other self-report anxiety measures [43–45], with findings that also indicate that the interview can successfully distinguish between different forms of anxiety [46,47].

Although early self-report measures of anxiety were designed to assess the general construct of anxiety (eg, the Revised Children's Manifest Anxiety Scale) [48] or the breadth of feared situations (eg, the Fear Survey Schedule for Children-Revised) [49], modern measures have been designed to gauge the severity of symptoms specific to individual disorders or types of anxiety. Examples of these measures include the Spence Children's Anxiety Scales [50,51], the Screen for Child Anxiety Related Emotional Disorders [52,53] and the Multidimensional Anxiety Scale for Children [54]. These newer measures reliably distinguish between clinically anxious and nonclinical children and between anxious children and those with other types of disorders. These measures also have been shown to have limited validity in differentiating between the different anxiety disorders, although there has been some difficulty with differentiation because of the high comorbidity of anxiety disorders and the overlap of symptoms within these disorders [41]. Each of the measures have self-report and parent-report versions that can be completed in 15 to 30 minutes. The self-report measures are suitable for children from the age of 8 years old; however, younger children may require assistance with reading the questions. Normative data are available for the measures, facilitating comparison with appropriate peer groups, with both gender and age having an effect on expected scores. The questionnaires also have shown sensitivity in a variety of cultural settings without major deterioration of psychometrics [55].

In cases in which the target of an evaluation is under the age of 8 years old, it is necessary to adjust assessment tools. Diagnostic interviews for this age typically target parents alone. The present authors successfully use the parent version of the ADIS-C with parents of children as young as 3 years old, using appropriate situational modifications. Recently, a puppet-based interview has been developed for use with children 4 to 8 years old that allows the exploration of the child's self-perception and a view of their symptoms [56]. Questionnaire measures of anxiety that address situations specifically encountered by preschoolers have been developed for parents [8] and for children as young as 4 years old through a pictorial-based questionnaire with a simple visual response scale [57]. An additional useful tool for this age group can be the assessment of behavioral inhibition, a risk factor for anxiety [58]. A typical assessment involves introducing a child, with and without its mother, to unfamiliar rooms, objects, adults, and peers. The child's reactions then are rated on constructs such as approach behaviors, proximity to the mother, and time spent interacting [59].

In addition to assessing disorder-specific symptoms, a thorough assessment of resulting impairment is necessary to determine whether the symptoms amount to a disorder and if so what the severity of that disorder is. Diagnostic interviews based on Diagnostic and Statistical Manual of Mental Disorders, Fourth Edition, (DSM-IV) criteria such as the ADIS-C incorporate an assessment of impairment through questioning about interference in various aspects of a child's life [42]. This information is then used by the clinician to rate the severity of each disorder and often is used as a substitute for more formal measurement. More recently, self-report and parent report questionnaire measures of impairment have been developed. The Child and Adolescent Social and Adaptive Functioning Scale allows children 10 to 17 years old to rate their current functioning at school, with peers, within their families, and with self-care [60]. The Child Anxiety Impact Scale is a parent report of their child's functioning in school, home and family, and social domains, with questions that specifically target performance likely to be affected by anxiety [61]. The initial reliability and validity of these measures is promising with appropriate relationships, with internalizing symptom measures in clinical [61] and community [60] populations. These measures can assist clinicians to rate the impairment for diagnostic purposes as well as to determine improvement during treatment.

Practical issues

The efficacious assessment of children has always been complicated by differences that seem inherent between the different informants that are in a position to comment on a child's emotions, behavior, and functioning. Poor agreement has been shown to affect self-report and interview measures in relation to the existence of a disorder and the presence and severity of anxiety symptoms [37,62]. Parent–child agreement tends to be higher for symptoms that are concrete, observable, severe, socially acceptable and nonschool based [37]. Findings indicate that parents report more behavioral symptoms, whereas their children tend to report subjective symptoms, with parents being particularly poor reporters of children's inner feelings and experiences [40].

Given these high levels of informant disagreement, several recommendations have been made on how to combine the information to arrive at an accurate evaluation. The most common recommendation is to use an "or" rule, that is, to count a "yes" from any informant as evidence for a diagnosis or symptom [37]. In addition, it has also been recommended that clinicians judge who "should" know or "will" be willing to report against each type of symptom when valuing the information provided from informants [63]. There is evidence that agreement between a parent report and the final diagnosis is greater for diagnostic interviews with primary school-aged children [44,64], questioning the necessity of completing this component of evaluation with children under the age of 11. If the interview component is withdrawn, it remains important to gather information from self-report measures to gauge the child's internal symptoms such as worry content and to assess the impact of these symptoms from the child's perspective because this can be used to facilitate motivation during treatment phases.

Maintaining factors in child and adolescent anxiety

Research on anxiety disorders in children and adolescents have implicated four primary factors that potentially maintain the disorder individually or in combination. These factors are targeted within the highly successful cognitive-behavioral treatment (CBT) approach favored in the empirical literature [65]. A fundamental maintaining factor in child anxiety disorders is avoidance of feared situations. By minimizing direct and prolonged contact with feared situations, anxious children have no opportunity to learn that the situation is in fact harmless [66]. Avoidance also limits opportunities to participate in important developmental events and can prevent the mastery of developmental challenges, increasing the persistence of anxiety over time [67]. For example, difficulties such as crossing a road to avoid a neighbor's dog, school refusal, seeking reassurance, and use of safety behaviors (such as phoning a parent during the school day) are all behaviors that constitute avoidance and may help to maintain anxiety.

The way in which anxious children process information is another factor that may promote maintenance of anxiety disorders. Experimental studies have shown that anxious children have a negative interpretative bias, identifying threat and hostility in neutral and ambiguous situations [68–70]. Studies also have shown that anxious children underestimate the likelihood of future positive events, overestimate the likelihood of future negative events [71], and make frequent cognitive errors such as overgeneralization, catastrophizing, and personalization [72]. In addition to these cognitive biases, there is some evidence (albeit mixed) that anxious children show attentional biases toward threatening words [73] and pictures [74].

Research that has focused on protective factors against stress and anxiety also points to the importance of a child's coping skills. A reliance on avoidant or emotion-focused coping strategies results in poorer psychologic adjustment than the use of problem-focused coping strategies [75]. Additionally, a child's ability to access available social support influences their experience of emotional and behavioral problems [76]. Developmental issues appear to have an impact on the use of these coping strategies. At a young age, children's coping aims to change the aversive stimuli (by running away or verbally protesting), but as they mature, coping approaches reflect acceptance that the situation cannot be changed and begin to focus on methods of reducing the degree of aversiveness or distress (for example through positive self-talk or relaxation) [77]. In contrast, anxious children tend to rely more on the use of avoidance, distraction, and dependence on others to manage their distress [78].

Another factor that may be important in the maintenance of child anxiety is the interaction between parent and child [79]. Lower warmth, less autonomy, and increased parental catastrophizing occur more frequently among mothers of anxious children. In addition, experimental studies have shown that parents of clinically anxious children tend to support their child's avoidance behavior. For example, after a family discussion of hypothetical, ambiguous situations, anxious children are more likely to provide avoidant solutions as their parents support and agree with these solutions in preference to approach options [80]. Parents of anxious children also provide more help during stressful situations than is needed [81,82] and have lower expectations regarding their child's performance in a number of everyday life domains [83]. These parenting behaviors can be identified in both anxious and nonanxious parents and are believed to develop as a result of the child's reactive or anxious temperament, which shapes the parents' behavior [84,85]. This overprotective parenting style has the potential to reduce a child's exposure to novelty, may inhibit development of coping strategies, decrease a child's sense of control of their world, and teach a child that he or she is incapable of handling challenging situations on their own [85,86].

During a child's initial evaluation, it is useful to assess these maintaining factors and other areas that may need to be targeted during treatment. Although there are no tools that comprehensively assess factors relevant to anxiety disordered children, several tools, can assist to determine the severity of particular categories of symptoms. For example, the Children's Automatic Thoughts Scale [87] provides a self-report measure of negative thinking that is typical in anxiety, depression, and anger problems; and the Parental Expectancies Scale [83] provides a measure of parent expectations of their child in life domains such as academics and socialization. These measures can be used to identify the severity of particular maintaining factors so that they can be monitored during treatment. One additional measure is the School Refusal Assessment Scale [88]. This scale can assist in determining the maintaining factors of school refusal that may relate to various types of anxiety or preference for nonschool activities.

Another useful approach for any child with an anxiety disorder is to identify specific recent situations in which anxiety has caused great distress for the child and to use these descriptions to increase understanding of antecedents, consequences, and modifying cues for high anxiety. It is important to gain an understanding of each situation from both the parent's and child's view because the salient information for each can differ dramatically. This task also can be set as a monitoring exercise that parents and (older) children complete between therapy sessions by recording experiences immediately after an anxious event. The information gathered can be used to identify factors that are likely to encourage future expression of anxiety, which in turn assists in treatment planning.

Cognitive-behavioral approaches to treatment

Various manualized approaches to child anxiety based on cognitive behavioral therapy have been developed that address the maintaining factors described above. In common across these programs are treatment components of graded exposure to address avoidance, cognitive restructuring to address interpretive and attentional biases, and skills training that can include relaxation, problem solving, social skills, and assertiveness or stress management techniques to improve problem-focused coping skills [89,90]. The degree to which the maintaining role of parents is addressed varies widely, depending on the program. When parents are given an equal role in the treatment process, parent-directed treatment components include education regarding child skills, cognitive restructuring targeted at parental expectancies and beliefs, behavioral management, or facilitating family communication [89,91]. An integral component of the manualized treatments is the incorporation of home practice to encourage consolidation and generalization of newly learned skills [92].

The efficacy of manualized CBT has been shown consistently in individual and group settings [65] and in a variety of cultural settings [93,94]. After 10 to 16 sessions, 64% to 84% of children are considered to be treatment successes (defined as anxiety diagnosis-free or a return to the normative range on self-report questionnaires), with further improvements occurring in the following 12 months [35,95,96] and maintaining for the significant majority of children for up to 7 years [97,98]. Manualized programs typically provide detailed therapist guidelines and client materials. They are not, however, so proscriptive as to preclude therapist flexibility [99]. Instead, they provide modular tools that can be tailored to the needs of a client by adapting presentation order, introducing alternate material, or emphasizing one skill type over another.

Developmental considerations

Developmental considerations within the treatment context first influence the degree of parent involvement recommended. For preschool children, treatment that targets the parents alone, using an education program based on CBT principles, has been shown to be effective in reducing anxiety disorders [100]. As yet, no research has been published on programs that directly include anxious preschool children. For primary school children, research on family based CBT, in which equal treatment time is dedicated to the parents and children, has been shown to produce superior outcomes [96]. The additional benefit of including parents equally in treatment has not been as clear for adolescents. Clinically, however, parents still have a significant influence on the adolescent's life through lowered expectations, facilitation of avoidance, and modeling of cognitive biases. As a consequence, although equal involvement in treatment may not be necessary, encouraging a supportive role, psychologic education on how to reduce the facilitation of avoidance, and addressing parental expectations that have impact on the adolescent are often essential for a successful outcome.

An additional developmental consideration with the cognitive behavioral approach is the ability of younger children to learn, apply, and benefit from cognitive techniques. Cognitive restructuring, for example, requires a child to self-reflect, shift perspective, infer causality, reason, and process new information [101]. These skills generally develop by middle to late childhood; however, performance on the skills is highly dependant on the linguistic presentation of the task and the familiarity of the context. Modifications to questions posed can dramatically decrease the age at which a child can perform cognitive tasks. For example, by changing the context from past to future focus, children as young as 3 years old are capable of hypothetical thinking [102]. Reasoning also can be improved by providing psychologic information in a simple, understandable form [103] by providing appropriate instruction on what is required [101] and by avoiding information that may conflict with their practical world knowledge [104]. Given clear, simple instructions in the use of concrete and active skills based on familiar material from their everyday lives, young children may benefit clinically from cognitive procedures [101]. The success of the approach is likely dependent on the skill of the delivering therapist to be creative with the language used and presentation of the skills as activity-based processes with explicit links to the behavioral components.

Predictors of treatment outcome and practical considerations

Along with the increase in treatment outcome studies has come the question of what factors affect the success or failure of treatment, particularly given that no study has shown a 100% recovery rate. No relationship to outcome has been found for gender, ethnicity, age, income, principal anxiety disorder, total number of diagnoses, treatment format, child's perception of therapist relationship, or the therapist's perception of parent involvement [95,105–108]. Several studies, however, have indicated that parental psychopathology can have a negative impact on treatment outcome [107,108]. Young children in particular seem more vulnerable to poor outcome as a result of a parent's psychopathology because they rely heavily on the parent's ability to facilitate learning of skills [108]. This impact may be moderated by the type of treatment techniques targeted at the parents. For example, in families in which an anxious child resides with an anxious parent, better outcomes for the child have been achieved on post-treatment diagnostic status when the parent participated in sessions targeting management of their own anxiety [91].

The impact of comorbidity on outcome in cases of principal anxiety disorders appears to be minimal. Comorbid anxiety disorders and comorbidity with externalizing disorders do not appear to affect outcome [5,6,108]. Depressive symptoms however have been linked to poorer outcome [108]. Mannassis and Monga [109] suggest three key principles in approaching therapy for cases in which a nonanxiety disorder is comorbid with an anxiety disorder. First, they stress the importance of assessing and prioritizing symptoms based on those that are causing the greatest impairment, with both the parent's and young person's opinions influencing the choice of priorities. Second, they point to the importance of reducing general life stress by increasing the structure within the young persons' life and decreasing parental frustration. Finally, they stress the need to communicate clearly with families about the potential complexity of treatment and the aims and expectations of the therapeutic tasks that will be attempted. In many cases, clear communication with the young person's school also is likely to assist in the progress of treatment.

In the present authors' work with comorbid disorders, treatment for a principal diagnosis of anxiety often has been found to produce improvement in both internalizing and externalizing symptoms. On the practical side, however, treating anxious children who have comorbid externalizing disorders can be challenging. Mild to moderate oppositional behavior and even hyperactivity can be catered within a group treatment format with little change to the standard, manualized approach. However, in more severe cases, an individual family approach may be needed. In the treatment of attention deficit hyperactivity disorder, it is known that increasing structure, addressing learning and behavior problems, and ensuring ongoing communication between home and school are all advantageous [109] and that these approaches can be added to the anxiety management skills whenever necessary. Another common issue faced by clinicians working with anxious adolescents is concurrent alcohol or drug use that is aimed at self-medication. Within the skills section of manualized programs, it is possible to introduce psychologic education regarding the risks of interactions between different forms of drugs and how drugs can worsen anxiety. After the child has undergone education, an emphasis on finding alternative coping strategies for dealing with anxious feelings, with the ultimate aim of reducing substance use, becomes a priority [109].

From a clinical perspective, several other factors have the potential to affect the treatment process. Parent anxiety and expectations can undermine the implementation of exposure hierarchies. A parent who is anxious about similar tasks may model avoidance and catastrophizing in addition to providing mixed messages about the need for their child to perform tasks independently. For other parents, perfectionistic expectations can provide an avenue to criticize a child working on graded steps or to prevent them from experiencing and coping with failure. In both cases, in vivo exposure with the therapist guiding the parent on what to do and say and cognitive restructuring targeted at the parent regarding their expectations can be of benefit.

A potential factor that may affect the child's treatment progress is their insight and willingness to address issues, which, particularly at younger ages, is not causing interference from the child's perspective (eg, a separation anxious child may not see the inability to stay with a baby sitter as a problem). Although this issue tends to decrease as a child becomes more aware of peer expectation and performance, targeted rewards for effort (rather than success) in learning and applying skills can be of benefit. However, in some cases it is necessary to target the child by working with parents on changing what they will expect and how they react to (or support) the child's anxiety.

A final clinical issue is the necessary extent of school involvement. For some forms of anxiety, particularly social avoidance, the primary location for exposure will be during the school day. To effectively provide opportunities to complete an exposure step, to record progress, and to provide immediate feedback and rewards, the involvement and support of school staff can be crucial. Involvement of teachers in setting appropriate tasks, providing them with educational materials on how to react to anxiety (eg, limiting reassurance), and minimizing the time they need to commit on a daily basis can all improve the chance of successful treatment.

Innovative developments in treatment

After the success of treatment studies in university settings, recent research has moved to investigating the use of manualized CBT in community settings and additionally to methods of disseminating treatment using less therapist involvement. Results from a recent study [110] that implemented a manualized CBT program for child anxiety in two regional mental health centers and a study [111] that implemented the program in disadvantaged schools have indicated that manualized anxiety treatment transports well, with similar rates of treatment responders in community settings. Three recent randomized control trials at the present authors' clinic have studied in detail the ways of improving the dissemination of treatment for child anxiety. All of these studies have used parent- and child-friendly bibliotherapy materials that contain the standard manualized CBT program used in individual and group therapy. The first study examined the outcome of pure bibliotherapy in children aged 7 to 12 years old in comparison with a therapist-led family group program and a wait-list control. Results indicated that although untreated children did not change over time and the majority of children who participated in the therapist led program improved, bibliotherapy produced favorable outcomes for a significant minority of children (Rapee et al, manuscript under review, 2005).

Building on this result, and with the hope of improving access to specialized services in rural communities, a second study using the bibliotherapy materials supplemented with therapist contact using technology was conducted (Lyneham and Rapee, manuscript under review, 2005). Contact was facilitated by telephone or e-mail, with 3 to 5 hours of the therapist's time devoted to contact with the client across a 12-week treatment program. This therapist time was used to help families to apply skills that they had self-taught to a child's idiosyncratic fears and worries. Outcomes for children who participated in the telephone-supplemented bibliotherapy were equivalent to those achieved using traditional individual and group formats. E-mail support was effective for a smaller group of children but was still superior to results seen in the pure bibliotherapy study. The present authors' final study, which is currently in progress, is examining the use of bibliotherapy supplemented by a small number of parent group sessions that aim to help families apply skills introduced in the materials. Early results show promise, with the majority of families reporting significant improvements in their child's anxiety and general functioning.

Although we have not yet had the opportunity to study specific predictors of outcome in the bibliotherapy approach, several clinical factors appear to have an impact on treatment success. In a model that relies on parents to deliver treatment to their child, it is necessary that the underlying parent–child relationship be respectful and cooperative. For families in our studies in which the child has refused to work with the parent or in which parents have been unable to contain their critical responses to the child's thoughts and feelings, treatment was unsuccessful or resulted in early termination. Increased therapist contact appeared to assist in preventing early termination of treatment, because frustration and difficulties could be addressed; however, there were cases in which the parent-as-therapist approach was not appropriate, and individual child–therapist and parent–therapist treatment would be appropriate. A second issue was the significant commitment of parent time required to implement the program (although this is no more than the time that is required to travel to and attend weekly sessions with a therapist and the typical home tasks set for practice between sessions). By addressing this issue openly and setting appropriate expectations before beginning treatment, parents were able to make an informed decision. Bibliotherapy materials potentially provide clinicians the opportunity to deliver treatment in a time-efficient way, focusing clinician time on the application of skills rather than on education in the skills and are a promising future direction for clinicians in general pediatric settings.

Summary

There have been significant advances in the assessment and treatment of child and adolescent anxiety disorders over the past 10 years. These advances provide clinicians with psychometrically sound diagnostic interviews, and self-report measures of symptoms and maintenance factors. Manualized cognitive behavioral treatment packages address the four major maintenance factors with significant success across a variety of populations and are sufficiently flexible to incorporate additional treatment components for comorbid presentations. Recent research on alternative methods of presenting treatment have significant potential for improving access to specialized services for isolated families and to improve the value of therapist's time.

References

[1] Muris P, Meesters C, Merckelbach H, et al. Worry in normal children. J Am Acad Child Adolesc Psychiatry 1998;37(7):703–10.
[2] Canino G, Shrout PE, Rubio-Stipec M, et al. The DSM-IV Rates of child and adolescent disorders in Puerto Rico. Arch Gen Psychiatry 2004;61(1):85–93.

[3] Verhulst FC, van der Ende J, Ferdinand RF, et al. The prevalence of DSM-III-R diagnoses in a national sample of Dutch adolescents. Arch Gen Psychiatry 1997;54(4):329–36.

[4] Ford T, Goodman R, Meltzer H. The British child and adolescent mental health survey 1999: the prevalence of DSM-IV disorders. J Am Acad Child Adolesc Psychiatry 2003;42(10): 1203–11.

[5] Rapee R. The influence of comorbidity on treatment outcome for children and adolescents with anxiety disorders. Behav Res Ther 2003;41(1):105–12.

[6] Kendall PC, Brady EU, Verduin TL. Comorbidity in childhood anxiety disorders and treatment outcome. J Am Acad Child Adolesc Psychiatry 2001;40(7):787–94.

[7] Gullone E, King NJ, Tonge B, et al. The Fear Survey Schedule for Children–II (FSSC-II): validity data as a treatment outcome measure. Aust Psychol 2000;35(3):238–43.

[8] Spence SH, Rapee R, McDonald C, et al. The structure of anxiety symptoms among preschoolers. Behav Res Ther 2001;39(11):1293–316.

[9] Weiss DD, Last CG. Developmental variations in the prevalence and manifestations of anxiety disorders. In: Vasey MW, Dadds MR, editors. The developmental psychopathology of anxiety. New York: Oxford University Press; 2001. p. 27–42.

[10] Velez CN, Johnson J, Cohen P. A longitudinal analysis of selected risk factors for childhood psychopathology. J Am Acad Child Adolesc Psychiatry 1989;28(6):861–4.

[11] Ollendick TH, King NJ, Frary RB. Fears in children and adolescents: reliability and generalizability across gender, age and nationality. Behav Res Ther 1989;27(1):19–26.

[12] Spence SH, McCathie H. The stability of fears in children: a two-year prospective study: a research note. J Child Psychol Psychiatry 1993;34(4):579–85.

[13] Last CG, Strauss CC. Panic disorder in children and adolescents. J Anxiety Disord 1989;3(2): 87–95.

[14] Strauss CC, Last CG. Social and simple phobias in children. J Anxiety Disord 1993;7(2): 141–52.

[15] Cohen P, Cohen J, Brook J. An epidemiological study of disorders in late childhood and adolescence: II. persistance of disorders. J Child Psychol Psychiatry 1993;34(6):869–77.

[16] Muris P, Merckelbach H, Meesters C, et al. Cognitive development and worry in normal children. Cognit Ther Res 2002;26(6):775–85.

[17] Bennett M, Gillingham K. The role of self-focused attention in children's attributions of social emotions to the self. J Genet Psychol 1991;152:303–9.

[18] Last CG, Perrin S, Hersen M, et al. A prospective study of childhood anxiety disorders. J Am Acad Child Adolesc Psychiatry 1996;35(11):1502–10.

[19] Hofstra MB, van der Ende J, Verhulst FC. Child and adolescent problems predict DSM-IV disorders in adulthood: a 14-year follow-up of a Dutch epidemiological sample. J Am Acad Child Adolesc Psychiatry 2002;41(2):182–9.

[20] Hofstra MB, Van der Ende J, Verhulst FC. Continuity and change of psychopathology from childhood into adulthood: a 14-year follow-up study. J Am Acad Child Adolesc Psychiatry 2000;39(7):850–8.

[21] Ialongo N, Edelsohn G, Werthamer-Larsson L, et al. Social and cognitive impairment in first-grade children with anxious and depressive symptoms. J Clin Child Adolesc Psychol 1996; 25(1):15–24.

[22] Strauss CC, Frame CL, Forehand R. Psychosocial impairment associated with anxiety in children. J Clin Child Adolesc Psychol 1987;16(3):235–9.

[23] Parker G, Wilhelm K, Mitchell P, et al. The influence of anxiety as a risk to early onset depression. J Affect Disord 1999;52(1–3):11–7.

[24] Weissman MM, Wolk S, Wickramaratne P, et al. Children with prepubertal-onset major depressive disorder and anxiety grown up. Arch Gen Psychiatry 1999;56(9):794–801.

[25] Last CG, Hansen C, Franco N. Anxious children in adulthood: a prospective study of adjustment. J Am Acad Child Adolesc Psychiatry 1997;36(5):645–52.

[26] Rudd M, Joiner Jr TE, Rumzek H. Childhood diagnoses and later risk for multiple suicide attempts. Suicide Life Threat Behav 2004;34(2):113–25.

[27] Sawyer MG, Arney FM, Baghurst PA, et al. The mental health of young people in Australia: key findings from the Child and Adolescent Component of the National Survey of Mental Health and Well-Being. Aust N Z J Psychiatry 2001;35(6):806–14.

[28] Farmer EM, Stangl DK, Burns BJ, et al. Use, persistence, and intensity: patterns of care for children's mental health across one year. Community Ment Health J 1999;35(1):31–46.

[29] Zubrick SR, Silburn SR, Garton A, et al. Western Australian Child Health Survey: developing health and well-being in the nineties. Perth (Australia): Australian Bureau of Statistics and the Institute for Child Health Research; 1995.

[30] Teagle SE. Parental problem recognition and child mental health service use. Ment Health Serv Res 2002;4(4):257–66.

[31] Weiss B, Jackson EW, Suesser K. Effect of co-occurrence on the referability of internalizing and externalizing problem behavior in adolescents. J Clin Child Adolesc Psychol 1997;26(2):198–204.

[32] Weisz JR, Weiss B. Studying the "referability" of child clinical problems. J Consult Clin Psychol 1991;59(2):266–73.

[33] Langley AK, Bergman R, Piacentini JC. Assessment of childhood anxiety. Int Rev Psychiatry 2002;14(2):102–13.

[34] Essau CA, Muris P, Ederer EM. Reliability and validity of the Spence Children's Anxiety Scale and the Screen for child anxiety related emotional disorders in German children. J Behav Ther Exp Psychiatry 2002;33(1):1–18.

[35] Silverman WK, Kurtines WM, Ginsburg GS, et al. Treating anxiety disorders in children with group cognitive-behavioral therapy: a randomized clinical trial. J Consult Clin Psychol 1999;67(6):995–1003.

[36] Muris P, Merckelbach H, Gadet B, et al. Sensitivity for treatment effects of the screen for child anxiety related emotional disorders. Journal of Psychopathology and Behavioral Assessment 1999;21(4):323–35.

[37] Comer JS, Kendall PC. A symptom-level examination of parent-child agreement in the diagnosis of anxious youths. J Am Acad Child Adolesc Psychiatry 2004;43(7):878–86.

[38] DiBartolo PM, Albano AM, Barlow DH, et al. Cross-informant agreement in the assessment of social phobia in youth. J Abnorm Child Psychol 1998;26(3):213–20.

[39] Foley D, Rutter M, Pickles A, et al. Informant disagreement for separation anxiety disorder. J Am Acad Child Adolesc Psychiatry 2004;43(4):452–60.

[40] Herjanic B, Reich W. Development of a structured psychiatric interview for children: agreement between child and parent on individual symptoms. J Abnorm Child Psychol 1982;10(3):307–24.

[41] Schniering CA, Hudson JL, Rapee RM. Issues in the diagnosis and assessment of anxiety disorders in children and adolescents. Clin Psychol Rev 2000;20(4):453–78.

[42] Silverman WK, Albano AM. The Anxiety Disorders Interview Schedule for Children for DSM-IV: child and parent versions. San Antonio (TX): Psychological Corporation; 1996.

[43] Silverman WK, Saavedra LM, Pina AA. Test-retest reliability of anxiety symptoms and diagnoses with anxiety disorders interview schedule for DSM-IV: child and parent versions. J Am Acad Child Adolesc Psychiatry 2001;40(8):937–44.

[44] Rapee RM, Barrett PM, Dadds MR, et al. Reliability of the DSM-III-R childhood anxiety disorders using structured interview: interrater and parent-child agreement. J Am Acad Child Adolesc Psychiatry 1994;33(7):984–92.

[45] Silverman WK, Nelles WB. The Anxiety Disorders Interview Schedule for Children. J Am Acad Child Adolesc Psychiatry 1988;27(6):772–8.

[46] Wood JJ, Piacentini JC, Bergman R, et al. Concurrent validity of the anxiety disorders section of the Anxiety Disorders Interview Schedule for DSM-IV: child and parent versions. J Clin Child Adolesc Psychol 2002;31(3):335–42.

[47] Tracey SA, Chorpita BF, Douban J, et al. Empirical evaluation of DSM-IV generalized anxiety disorder criteria in children and adolescents. J Clin Child Adolesc Psychol 1997;26(4):404–14.

[48] Reynolds CR, Richmond BO. What I think and feel: a revised measure of children's manifest anxiety. J Abnorm Child Psychol 1978;6(2):271–80.

[49] Ollendick TH. Reliability and validity of the revised Fear Survey Schedule for Children (FSSC-R). Behav Res Ther 1983;21(6):685–92.

[50] Spence SH. A measure of anxiety symptoms among children. Behav Res Ther 1998;36(5): 545–66.

[51] Nauta MH, Scholing A, Rapee RM, et al. A parent-report measure of children's anxiety: psychometric properties and comparison with child-report in a clinic and normal sample. Behav Res Ther 2004;42(7):813–39.

[52] Muris P, Merckelbach H, Schmidt H, et al. The revised version of the Screen for Child Anxiety Related Emotional Disorders (SCARED-R): factor structure in normal children. Pers Individ Dif 1999;26(1):99–112.

[53] Muris P, Dreessen L, Bogels S, et al. A questionnaire for screening a broad range of DSM-defined anxiety disorder symptoms in clinically referred children and adolescents. J Child Psychol Psychiatry 2004;45(4):813–20.

[54] March JS, Parker JD, Sullivan K, et al. The Multidimensional Anxiety Scale for Children (MASC): factor structure, reliability, and validity. J Am Acad Child Adolesc Psychiatry 1997; 36(4):554–65.

[55] Muris P, Schmidt H, Engelbrecht P, et al. DSM-IV-defined anxiety disorder symptoms in South African children. J Am Acad Child Adolesc Psychiatry 2002;41(11):1360–8.

[56] Measelle JR, Ablow JC, Cowan PA, et al. Assessing young children's views of their academic, social, and emotional lives: an evaluation of the self-perception scales of the Berkeley puppet interview. Child Dev 1998;69(6):1556–76.

[57] Muris P, Meesters C, Mayer B, et al. The Koala Fear Questionnaire: a standardized self-report scale for assessing fears and fearfulness in pre-school and primary school children. Behav Res Ther 2003;41(5):597–617.

[58] Biederman J, Rosenbaum JF, Hirshfeld DR, et al. Psychiatric correlates of behavioral inhibition in young children of parents with and without psychiatric disorders. Arch Gen Psychiatry 1990;47(1):21–6.

[59] Morris TL, Hirshfeld-Becker DR, Henin A, et al. Developmentally sensitive assessment of social anxiety. Cognitive and Behavioral Practice 2004;11(1):13–28.

[60] Price CS, Spence SH, Sheffield J, et al. The development and psychometric properties of a measure of social and adaptive functioning for children and adolescents. J Clin Child Adolesc Psychol 2002;31(1):111–22.

[61] Langley AK, Bergman R, McCracken J, et al. Impairment in childhood anxiety disorders: preliminary examination of the Child Anxiety Impact Scale-Parent Version. J Child Adolesc Psychopharmacol 2004;14(1):105–14.

[62] Nauta MH, Scholing A, Rapee RM, et al. A parent-report measure of children's anxiety: psychometric properties and comparison with child-report in a clinic and normal sample. Behav Res Ther 2004;42(7):813–39.

[63] Jensen PS, Rubio-Stipec M, Canino G, et al. Parent and child contributions to diagnosis of mental disorder: are both informants always necessary? J Am Acad Child Adolesc Psychiatry 1999;38(12):1569–79.

[64] Lyneham HJ, Rapee RM. Agreement between telephone and in-person delivery of a structured interview for anxiety disorders in children. J Am Acad Child Adolesc Psychiatry 2005;44(3): 274–82.

[65] Compton SN, March JS, Brent D, et al. Cognitive-behavioral psychotherapy for anxiety and depressive disorders in children and adolescents: an evidence-based medicine review. J Am Acad Child Adolesc Psychiatry 2004;43(8):930–59.

[66] Vasey MW, Dadds MR. An introduction to the developmental psychopathology of anxiety. In: Vasey MW, Dadds MR, editors. The developmental psychopathology of anxiety. New York: Oxford University Press; 2001. p. 3–26.

[67] Vasey MW, Ollendick TH. Anxiety. In: Lewis M, Sameroff A, editors. Handbook of developmental psychopathology. 2nd edition. New York: Plenum Press; 2000. p. 511–29.

[68] Barrett PM, Rapee RM, Dadds MM, et al. Family enhancement of cognitive style in anxious and aggressive children. J Abnorm Child Psychol 1996;24(2):187–203.

[69] Chorpita BF, Albano AM, Barlow DH. Cognitive processing in children: relation to anxiety and family influences. J Clin Child Adolesc Psychol 1996;25(2):170–6.

[70] Bell-Dolan DJ. Social cue interpretation of anxious children. J Clin Child Adolesc Psychol 1995;24:1–10.

[71] Spence SH, Donovan C, Brechman-Toussaint M. Social skills, social outcomes, and cognitive features of childhood social phobia. J Abnorm Psychol 1999;108(2):211–21.

[72] Weems CF, Berman SL, Silverman WK, et al. Cognitive errors in youth with anxiety disorders: the linkages between negative cognitive errors and anxious symptoms. Cognit Ther Res 2001; 25(5):559–75.

[73] Vasey MW, Daleiden EL, Williams LL, et al. Biased Attention in childhood anxiety disorders: a preliminary study. J Abnorm Child Psychol 1995;23:267–79.

[74] Martin M, Jones GV. Integral bias in cognitive processes of emotionally linked pictures. Br J Psychol 1995;86:419–35.

[75] Field L, Prinz RJ. Coping and adjustment during childhood and adolescence. Clin Psychol Rev 1997;17(8):937–76.

[76] Compas BE. Coping with stress during childhood and adolescence. Psychol Bull 1987;101: 393–403.

[77] Band EB, Weisz JR. How to feel better when it feels bad: children's perspectives on coping with everyday stress. Dev Psychol 1988;24:247–53.

[78] Manassis K, Hudson JL, Webb A, et al. Beyond behavioral inhibition: etiological factors in childhood anxiety. Cognitive and Behavioral Practice 2004;11(1):3–12.

[79] Rapee RM. Potential role of childrearing practices in the development of anxiety and depression. Clin Psychol Rev 1997;17(1):47–67.

[80] Dadds MR, Marrett PM, Rapee RM. Family process and child anxiety and aggression: an observational analysis. J Abnorm Child Psychol 1996;24(6):715–34.

[81] Hudson JL, Rapee RM. Parent-child interactions and anxiety disorders: an observational study. Behav Res Ther 2001;39(12):1411–27.

[82] Siqueland L, Kendall PC, Steinberg L. Anxiety in children: perceived family environments and observed family interaction. J Clin Child Adolesc Psychol 1996;25(2):225–37.

[83] Eisen AR, Spasaro SA, Brien LK, et al. Parental expectancies and childhood anxiety disorders: psychometric properties of the Parental Expectancies Scale. J Anxiety Disord 2004; 18(2):89–109.

[84] Moore PS, Whaley SE, Sigman M. Interactions between mothers and children: impacts of maternal and child anxiety. J Abnorm Psychol 2004;113(3):471–6.

[85] Hudson JL, Rapee RM. From temperament to disorder: an etiological model of generalized anxiety disorder. In: Heimberg RG, Turk CC, Menin DS, editors. Generalized anxiety disorder: advances in research and practice. New York: Guildford Press; 2004. p. 51–74.

[86] Chorpita BF, Barlow DH. The development of anxiety: the role of control in the early environment. Psychol Bull 1998;124(1):3–21.

[87] Schniering CA, Rapee RM. Development and validation of a measure of children's automatic thoughts: the Children's Automatic Thoughts Scale. Behav Res Ther 2002;40(9):1091–109.

[88] Kearney CA. Identifying the function of school refusal behavior: a revision of the School Refusal Assessment Scale. Journal of Psychopathology and Behavioral Assessment 2002; 24(4):235–45.

[89] Rapee RM, Wignall A, Hudson JL, et al. Treating anxious children and adolescents: an evidence-based approach. Oakland (CA): New Harbinger; 2000.

[90] Velting ON, Setzer NJ, Albano AM. Update on and advances in assessment and cognitive-behavioral treatment of anxiety disorders in children and adolescents. Prof Psychol Res Pr 2004;35(1):42–54.

[91] Cobham VE, Dadds MR, Spence SH. The role of parental anxiety in the treatment of childhood anxiety. J Consult Clin Psychol 1998;66(6):893–905.

[92] Hudson JL, Kendall PC. Showing you can do it: homework in therapy for children and adolescents with anxiety disorders. J Clin Psychol 2002;58(5):525–34.

[93] Toren P, Wolmer L, Rosental B, et al. Case series: brief parent-child group therapy for

childhood anxiety disorders using a manual-based cognitive-behavioral technique. J Am Acad Child Adolesc Psychiatry 2000;39(10):1309–12.

[94] Pina AA, Silverman WK, Fuentes RM, et al. Exposure-based cognitive-behavioral treatment for phobic and anxiety disorders: treatment effects and maintenance for Hispanic/Latino relative to European-American youths. J Am Acad Child Adolesc Psychiatry 2003;42(10):1179–87.

[95] Kendall PC, Flannery-Schroeder E, Panichelli-Mindel SM, et al. Therapy for youths with anxiety disorders: a second randomized clincal trial. J Consult Clin Psychol 1997;65(3): 366–80.

[96] Barrett PM, Dadds MR, Rapee RM. Family treatment of childhood anxiety: a controlled trial. J Consult Clin Psychol 1996;64(2):333–42.

[97] Barrett PM, Duffy AL, Dadds MR, et al. Cognitive-behavioral treatment of anxiety disorders in children: long-term (6-year) follow-up. J Consult Clin Psychol 2001;69(1):135–41.

[98] Kendall PC, Safford S, Flannery-Schroeder E, et al. Child anxiety treatment: outcomes in adolescence and impact on substance use and depression at 7.4-year follow-up. J Consult Clin Psychol 2004;72(2):276–87.

[99] Kendall PC, Chu BC. Retrospective self-reports of therapist flexibility in a manual-based treatment for youths with anxiety disorders. J Clin Child Adolesc Psychol 2000;29(2):209–20.

[100] Rapee RM, Kennedy SJ, Ingram M, et al. Prevention and early intervention of anxiety disorders in inhibited preschool children. J Consult Clin Psychol 2005;73(3):488–97.

[101] Grave J, Blissett J. Is cognitive behavior therapy developmentally appropriate for young children? a critical review of the evidence. Clin Psychol Rev 2004;24:399–420.

[102] Robinson EJ, Beck S. What is difficult about counterfactual reasoning?. In: Mitchell P, Riggs KJ, editors. Children's reasoning and the mind. Hove (UK): Psychology Press; 2000. p. 101–19.

[103] Miller PH. Children's reasoning about the causes of human behavior. J Exp Child Psychol 1985;39:343–62.

[104] Hawkins J, Pea RD, Glick J, et al. Merds that laugh don't like mushrooms: evidence for deductive reasoning by preschoolers. Dev Psychol 1984;20:584–94.

[105] Kendall PC. Treating anxiety disorders in children: results of a randomized clinical trial. J Consult Clin Psychol 1994;62(1):100–10.

[106] Treadwell KR, Flannery-Schroeder EC, Kendall PC. Ethnicity and gender in relation to adaptive functioning, diagnostic status, and treatment outcome in children from an anxiety clinic. J Anxiety Disord 1995;9(5):373–84.

[107] Rapee RM. Group treatment of children with anxiety disorders: outcome and predictors of treatment response. Aust J Psychol 2000;52(3):125–30.

[108] Berman SL, Weems CF, Silverman WK, et al. Predictors of outcome in exposure-based cognitive and behavioral treatments for phobic and anxiety disorders in children. Behav Ther 2000;31(4):713–31.

[109] Manassis K, Monga S. A therapeutic approach to children and adolescents with anxiety disorders and associated comorbid conditions. J Am Acad Child Adolesc Psychiatry 2001;40(1): 115–7.

[110] Nauta MH, Scholing A, Emmelkamp PM, et al. Cognitive-behavioral therapy for children with anxiety disorders in a clinical setting: no additional effect of a cognitive parent training. J Am Acad Child Adolesc Psychiatry 2003;42(11):1270–8.

[111] Mifsud C, Rapee RM. Early intervention for childhood anxiety in a school setting. Outcomes for an economically disadvantaged population. J Am Acad Child Adolesc Psychiatry, in press.

ELSEVIER
SAUNDERS

Child Adolesc Psychiatric Clin N Am
14 (2005) 863–876

CHILD AND
ADOLESCENT
PSYCHIATRIC CLINICS
OF NORTH AMERICA

Cognitive-Behavior Therapy for Childhood Anxiety Disorders

Tami Roblek, PhD[a,b], John Piacentini, PhD, ABPP[b],*

[a]School of Medicine, University of California Los Angeles, 300 Medical Plaza, Room 1227,
Los Angeles, CA 90095, USA
[b]Neuropsychiatric Institute, University of California Los Angeles, 760 Westwood Plaza,
Room 68-251, Los Angeles, CA 90024, USA

Anxiety disorders affect between 12% and 20% of youngsters worldwide and are the most common class of mental health problems in this age group [1,2]. Although long considered developmentally normative and relatively innocuous, childhood anxiety disorders have been associated with significant impairment in psychosocial functioning [3–5] and have been shown to run a chronic and fluctuating course into adulthood [5–8].

The current practice in the field of anxiety treatment research has been to group three conditions, social anxiety disorder (or social phobia [SoP]), separation anxiety disorder (SAD), and generalized anxiety disorder (GAD), together and to consider them as distinctly different from other Diagnostic and Statistical Manual of Mental Disorders, 4th edition (DSM-IV) [9] anxiety disorders such as panic disorder, obsessive-compulsive disorder (OCD), post-traumatic stress disorder (PTSD), and simple phobia. These three disorders have been found to be similar in terms of underlying etiologic construct, response to treatment, comorbidities, familial associations with adult anxiety and depression, and are highly comorbid [5,10–14].

Cognitive-behavior therapy (CBT) techniques such as exposure and cognitive restructuring are commonly used in the treatment of most anxiety disorders; however, OCD [15,16], panic disorder [17], and PTSD [18] require different

This work was supported in part by National Research Service Award grant F32 MH67324 (to T. Roblek) and National Institute of Mental Health grant U01 MH64088 (to J. Piacentini).

* Corresponding author.

E-mail address: jpiacentini@mednet.ucla.edu (J. Piacentini).

components, distinct from the three core disorders noted above. In addition, most child anxiety CBT trials to date have collectively considered social phobia, separation anxiety disorder, and generalized anxiety disorder [19–21]; thus, the treatment of these three disorders will be the main focus of this article.

Etiologic models of anxiety

The development of anxiety is likely a highly complex, iterative, and multifactorial process involving an array of individual, familial, and psychosocial risk factors [22]. Although a complete review is beyond the scope of this chapter, theories of the causes that are most relevant to cognitive-behavior therapy are described briefly.

Ethologic model

The ethologic model of anxiety as proposed by Barlow [23] suggests that fear and anxiety are natural and normal emotional responses that serve an adaptive function by increasing preparedness and avoidance of harm when an individual is confronted by a perceived danger. Anxiety serves to prepare the organism for "fight or flight." Within this model, maladaptive anxiety is conceived of as a response to danger in the absence of any actual threat or a response that is excessive compared with what is reasonable for that particular threat or danger. At this point, anxiety ceases to be adaptive and results in problematic behaviors and interference in daily functioning. Many CBT interventions base the psychoeducational component of treatment on the ethologic model of anxiety. This model allows for a powerful and comprehensive framework for the individual in which to understand the basis for cognitive restructuring and facilitating compliance with the heightened distress of exposures.

Tripartite model

The tripartite model further expands the ethologic model by incorporating physiologic, cognitive, and behavioral components. These components are considered independent, but they interact constantly with each another [24,25]. The physiologic component includes the autonomic reactions of anxiety, including rapid heart rate, sweating, muscular tension, and increased respiration. The cognitive component includes anxious thoughts, worry, or self-statements involving danger. The behavioral component involves avoidance and escape behaviors and performance disruptions (ie, not able to perform in public). According to this model, maladaptive anxiety occurs as a result of distortions in one or more of these components. These components then interact to further heighten the anxiety response.

Temperament

Kagan and colleagues [26] have identified one aspect of temperament, behavioral inhibition, as a vulnerability factor for the development of anxiety disorders. Behavioral inhibition is characterized by withdrawal, cessation of speech, comfort seeking, suppression of ongoing behavior, and elevated autonomic arousal in the presence of unfamiliar or novel stimuli. Ten to fifteen percent of white children in the United States have been found to display these behaviors [27]. Anxiety disorders have been linked to behavioral inhibition. Biederman and colleagues [28,29] and Rosenbaum and colleagues [30] have found an increased risk of anxiety disorders among behaviorally inhibited children compared with noninhibited children. However, only a minority of behaviorally inhibited children develop anxiety disorders [28,31].

Familial factors

A familial aggregation of anxiety disorders has been well documented [32,33]. Turner and colleagues [34] have found that children of anxious parents are seven times more likely than children of nonanxious parents to develop an anxiety disorder. Additionally, Last and colleagues [14] have reported that parents of anxious children are more likely than parents of nonanxious children to meet criteria for an anxiety disorder. Although genetics appears to account for a proportion of familial transmission of anxiety disorders, family environment and parenting practices also have been shown to be important. Findings from studies on families of anxious youngsters highlight maladaptive levels of control, conflict, and independence compared with families of nonanxious youth [35–37].

Treatment of childhood anxiety disorders

The earliest empirically based treatments for anxiety and fears consisted of behavioral techniques, including systematic desensitization, modeling, and contingency management. Although the literature suggests these interventions can be effective for treating a variety of simple fears and specific phobias [38], the more complex symptoms of many current DSM-IV anxiety disorders, including generalized anxiety disorder, social anxiety disorder, and separation anxiety disorder, suggest the need for more comprehensive treatment protocols involving both cognitive and behavioral techniques [39].

Cognitive-behavior therapy

The multicomponent treatment protocols developed for childhood anxiety over the past decade were originally based on adult treatments [23,40], reformulated to better address the developmental characteristics of children and adolescents [19,20]. Velting and colleagues [41] point out that, although there are no official guidelines for treating anxiety disorders in children, cognitive-behavior therapy is an accepted and common thread underlying most effective treatment protocols.

Individual cognitive-behavior therapy

Kendall [20] was the first to conduct a systematic, controlled trial of cognitive-behavior therapy with children diagnosed with generalized anxiety disorder, separation anxiety disorder, and social phobia. This treatment program consists of 16 to 20 sessions (Coping Cat program), in which the first eight sessions focus on skill building, and the second eight sessions focus on exposure practice. This CBT protocol consists of six essential components: psychoeducation, physiologic management, cognitive restructuring, problem solving, exposure, and relapse prevention. In the skill-building phase, the FEAR (feeling frightened, expecting bad things to happen, actions/attitudes that will help, review and reward) acronym is presented to the patient, and four areas are targeted: (1) the identification of anxious feelings and physiologic reactions; (2) the identification and active challenging of anxious cognitions; (3) the development of a coping plan based on problem solving skills; and (4) the evaluation of coping responses and self-reward strategies. Specific strategies used in these skill-building sessions include relaxation techniques, diaphragmatic breathing, cognitive restructuring, and rewards for attempts at engaging in coping behaviors [42].

In the exposure and relapse-prevention phase of the treatment, the FEAR plan is applied in a systematic, graduated, and controlled way to a series of items on a hierarchy over the remainder of the 8 weeks of treatment. Behavioral strategies of modeling and reinforced practice are implemented to reinforce the in vivo exposures. In-session exposures and home-based "Show that I Can" tasks are key to anxiety mastery and successful fear reduction.

Kendall [20] conducted two randomized controlled clinical trials investigating the effectiveness of the Coping Cat program with children with overanxious disorder, separation anxiety or avoidant disorder. In the initial trial, Kendall compared a 16-week course of CBT to an 8-week wait-list control (WLC) condition. Kendall reported significant improvement for the CBT group across child and parent ratings of symptoms as well as behavioral observations of child anxiety compared with the wait-list condition. At post-treatment, 64% of the CBT group did not meet diagnostic criteria for an anxiety disorder compared with 5% in the wait-list condition. Treatment gains were maintained at 1-year follow-up. In a follow-up study, Kendall and Southam-Gerow [43] reported the maintenance of treatment gains over 2 to 5 years as reported by child and parent ratings and diagnostic interviews. A second larger randomized clinical trial completed by Kendall and colleagues [21] found results similar to the first study. Seventy-one percent of the children in the CBT group no longer met criteria for their primary anxiety disorder at post-treatment compared with 5.8% of the children in the wait-list condition. Treatment gains were evidenced at 1-year follow-up on both self- and parent-report measures and diagnostic interviews. In a more recent study, Kendall and colleagues [44] investigated the durability of treatment gains associated with the completion of CBT with the original sample of participants [21] 7.4 years post-treatment. Results indicated that at long-term follow-up, the primary anxiety disorder was no longer primary for 92% of the youth. The maintenance of gains was evident on youth and parent-report measures, as well. The studies of Kendall and colleagues suggest a strong support for the acute and long-term efficacy of CBT for childhood anxiety.

In examining the efficacy of in an individual and group format CBT for minority populations, Pina and colleagues [45] reported on data from a previous clinical trial [46,47]. Results indicated that Hispanic-Latino youths responded similarly and favorably to CBT as European-American youths. Treatment gains were evidenced by changes in diagnostic status, child-and parent-report, and clinically significant improvement.

Family cognitive-behavior therapy

Much research has investigated family context in the development and maintenance of childhood anxiety disorders. Kendall [20] and other investigators have suggested that the inclusion of family in the treatment of childhood anxiety may further serve to enhance and elongate treatment gains. Family involvement has been recommended [19] and increasingly recognized as an important component in the successful treatment of children with anxiety disorders. The importance of family involvement in treatment has been bolstered by findings linking parental anxiety [32,48] and problematic family interactions [19,49–51] to childhood anxiety disorders. To date, most of the investigated interventions involving parents are short term (approximately 4–12 sessions) and co-occur with individual child CBT.

Barrett and colleagues [19] and Gruner and colleagues [49] have conducted randomized clinical trials investigating parent training in the treatment of children with diagnosed anxiety. The treatment conditions included CBT, CBT plus family anxiety management (FAM) training (CBT-FAM), and a wait-list control. The CBT and CBT- FAM group received a shortened version of Kendall's Coping Cat program [20]. FAM consisted of teaching parents contingency management strategies, management of parent anxiety and communication, and problem-solving skills. Results indicated that both of the active treatments (CBT and CBT-FAM) were superior to the wait-list control condition and that gains were maintained across 6- and 12-month follow-ups. Additionally, the family training condition evidenced significantly more improvement across diagnostic status and self- and parent-report measures compared with the CBT condition alone. Specifically, 57% of the children in the CBT condition no longer met anxiety disorder criteria after treatment, compared with 84% of the children in the CBT-FAM. It is important to note that treatment condition interacted significantly with gender and age, such that females and younger children appeared to benefit most from the added family component. Overall, these studies lend credence to the importance of a structured intervention for parents in improving the treatment outcome for children with anxiety disorders.

In a later study, Barrett and colleagues [52] reassessed treatment gains at 5 to 7 years post-treatment of the youth studied earlier [19]. Although the diagnostic interviews were based only on child reports, results showed that at long-term follow-up, 85% of the treated youth no longer met diagnostic criteria for any anxiety disorder. The treatment gains across other clinicians' ratings and child and parent reports were maintained over the 5 to 7 years; however, group differences between the CBT-FAM and CBT alone conditions had largely disappeared.

A further study by Howard and Kendall [53] investigated a family-focused CBT program using a multiple baseline design with six children diagnosed with anxiety. Of the six youth involved in the treatment, four showed significant gains in parent-, child-, and teacher-report measures and showed no child anxiety diagnoses at post-treatment.

Cobham and colleagues [54] examined the differential value of parental involvement in treatment as a function of parental anxiety status. Sixty-seven children diagnosed with an anxiety disorder (SAD, overanxious disorder [OAD], GAD, SoP, and specific phobia) were grouped according to child-anxiety-only or child-plus-parent anxiety (ie, in which the child and one or both parents were anxious). The children were then randomly assigned to a child-focused CBT condition or to a child-focused CBT-plus-parental-anxiety-management condition (CBT-PAM). In the child-focused CBT condition, 82% of the child-anxiety-only group no longer met diagnostic criteria for an anxiety disorder compared with 39% of the child-plus-parent anxiety group. In the CBT-PAM condition, 80% of the child-anxiety-only group was diagnosis-free compared with 77% of the child-plus-parent anxiety group. These results suggest that children without anxious parents respond more favorably to child-focused CBT compared with children who have one or both anxious parents. Additionally, adding PAM increased the efficacy of child-focused CBT for those children with anxious parents but not for those without. Treatment gains were maintained at 6- and 12-month follow-up.

Spence and colleagues [55] extended the research on the efficacy of CBT and investigated parental involvement in the group treatment of social phobia. Fifty children were randomly assigned to one of three conditions: parent involved (PI), parent not involved (PNI), and WLC. Results indicated that 87.5% and 58% of the children in the PI and PNI conditions, respectively, were diagnosis-free at post-treatment compared with 7% in the WLC. Although the difference between the PI and PNI conditions failed to reach significance, a trend was evident for more children in the PI condition to be diagnosis-free compared with the PNI condition. Similar improvements on social skills, clinical severity ratings, self-reported anxiety, and symptoms of social anxiety were found for the PI and PNI conditions and were significantly better than the wait-list condition. Treatment effects were maintained at 12-month follow-up.

Interestingly, Spence and colleagues noted that involving parents in treatment may be more beneficial when the treatment is delivered individually rather than in a group format.

Nauta and colleagues [56] compared CBT (a Dutch version of Coping Cat) to CBT plus cognitive parent training (CPT) and a wait-list control condition. Results showed that active treatment was more effective than a wait-list condition (in which 54% and 10% of children were diagnosis-free, respectively, at post-treatment), although no added benefit was found for the CPT condition. Nauta and colleagues noted that this finding was surprising and postulated that this result might have been the result of an insufficient number of parent sessions provided or the use of separate therapists for the child intervention and parent training.

Silverman and colleagues [57,58] have underscored the need for parental involvement in child anxiety treatment. These investigators developed a treatment that emphasizes "transfer of control." They suggest that effective change involves more than a focus on parental anxiety. For example, although parents and children are informed about anxiety reduction techniques, parents learn contingency management strategies to help manage and support their child's approach to feared stimuli and encourage exposures while discouraging avoidance behaviors with positive reinforcement. The transfer of control from therapist to parent to child posits facilitating long-term treatment gains and maintenance and allows the child to develop a sense of responsibility for his or her own treatment as parental control and involvement decrease. Although multicomponent CBT protocols for childhood anxiety typically include one or more of these techniques (eg, contingency management and self-control training), the specific contribution of the transfer of control package remains to be tested.

Overall, it appears that some level of parental involvement in treatment has positive effects on the child's outcome, especially in families with at least one anxious parent. However, the durability of these positive effects remains somewhat questionable, and additional research is necessary to clarify existing research findings and delineate guidelines for maximizing the efficacy of adjunctive family intervention.

Group cognitive-behavior therapy

Evidence exists for the efficacy of individual child CBT in treating anxiety disorders; however, recent research has suggested that group CBT (GCBT) may be efficacious as well [59]. Silverman and colleagues [46] have suggested that group CBT with a parental involvement component might enhance treatment outcome because the group would allow for an additional avenue for the transfer of control by providing feedback and augmenting skill development and practice. In a controlled clinical trial in which group CBT was compared with a wait-list control condition, group CBT showed a significant improvement in the recovery rate (64% of children in GCBT and 13% in wait-list condition no longer met criteria for primary anxiety disorder), clinician severity ratings, and child- and parent-completed measures compared with the wait-list condition immediately at post-treatment and at 3-, 6-, and 12-month follow-up.

Toren and colleagues [60] examined a 10-session parent-child group treatment. This study differed from the study by Barrett [59] in that parents were not trained in cognitive-behavior techniques and were seen as facilitators of treatment rather than cotherapists. Seventy percent and 91% of the children were diagnosis-free at post-treatment and 36-month follow-up, respectively. The investigators concluded that including parents in treatment in a group format may allow for long-term maintenance of treatment effects.

Flannery-Schroeder and Kendall [61] compared individual CBT (ICBT) with group CBT and a wait-list control. The authors theorized that the GCBT would have significant advantages over the ICBT in social competence, social anxiety, friendships, and social activities, given that the group format involved significant peer interaction compared with the individual format. Diagnostically, compared with the wait-list condition (8%), 73% of the ICBT and 50% of the GCBT did not meet criteria for their primary anxiety disorder at post-treatment. Significant improvement was evidenced in the ICBT and GCBT on parent and child reports of anxious distress and coping relative to the wait-list condition. Contrary to the investigators' expectations, no significant advantages were found for the GCBT condition on social functioning relative to the ICBT condition. It was hypothesized that this finding might be because very few children were diagnosed with social concerns at the onset of treatment. Treatment gains were maintained at 3-month follow-up.

Manassis and colleagues [62] conducted a study examining the benefits of group CBT over individual CBT in children with anxiety disorders. These investigators have suggested that different children would respond differentially to one or the other treatment depending on diagnosis. Specifically, children with social anxiety would respond preferentially to a group format; children with hyperactivity would respond to an individual format; and those with phobic disorders (including separation anxiety disorder) would respond to an individual format better than those with GAD do. Unexpectedly, outcomes for the differential treatments did not show differences by diagnosis.

As pointed out by Ollendick and King [38], no studies have included an active comparison showing that CBT is more effective than another treatment. To address this issue, Muris and colleagues [63] investigated group CBT in comparison with an educational disclosure (ED) intervention and a no-treatment control condition in the treatment of childhood anxiety disorders. CBT was found to be superior to both comparison conditions on all outcome measures. Additionally, the ED and no-treatment conditions were similar in that they both showed no significant changes on any of the symptoms of anxiety and depression. Silverman and colleagues [47] compared the efficacy of contingency management or self-control paired with exposure to an education support condition in children with phobic disorders. Findings have indicated that exposure with either contingency management or self-control is equally effective across parent, child, and clinician ratings. Contrary to investigator prediction, children in the education condition also demonstrated significant treatment response. Interestingly, this condition did not include an exposure component, which has long been believed to be an important active ingredient in treating any of the anxiety disorders. Last and colleagues [64] also found similar results for an education support condition in treating children with school phobia. These findings may indicate a blurring between the "active" and education conditions as a result of cognitive-behavior components being included in the education conditions, making the results difficult to interpret.

Additional treatment considerations

Comorbidity and treatment outcome

The effects of comorbidity on treatment outcome have only recently been investigated in the area of childhood anxiety. The prevalence of comorbidity for anxiety and depression in children has been estimated to be between 15.9% and 61.9% [65], and anxious children usually present for treatment with more than one diagnosis. Findings have revealed that children with comorbid conditions usually are older and exhibit more severe symptoms [66]. These findings have contributed to the assumption that the presence of comorbid conditions has a negative affect on treatment. In discussing comorbidity in the context of treatment, Kendall and colleagues [42] have suggested ways to adapt manualized treatment components for children with comorbid anxiety and depression. They suggest that the symptom pattern of the individual should be emphasized rather than the diagnostic category.

Kendall and colleagues [67] examined psychiatric comorbidity on treatment outcome in children with anxiety disorders. Children were examined in three groups: those with a primary anxiety disorder, those with two or more anxiety disorders, and those with comorbid externalizing disorders. Results have shown that comorbidity at pretreatment is not associated with treatment outcome or maintenance of treatment gains. Specifically, 68.4% of children with no co-morbid diagnosis and 70.6% of children with a comorbid diagnosis were free of their primary diagnosis at post-treatment. The rate of comorbidity changed from pretreatment to post-treatment, with 79% of children showing a comorbid diagnosis at pretreatment and only 47% at post-treatment. These findings suggest that cognitive-behavior treatment is effective for anxious children with and without comorbid diagnoses. Rapee [68] has shown similar results in a study of 165 anxious children with and without comorbid diagnoses. However given the relatively strict eligibility requirements characterizing most clinical efficacy trials, the severity and scope of the comorbid conditions examined in the studies of Kendall and colleagues and Rapee likely do not fully reflect the comorbidity patterns seen in typical clinical settings. Additional research into this important topic is clearly warranted.

Developmental considerations

Most cognitive-behavior interventions for childhood anxiety disorders have been modified from adult interventions to include developmentally sensitive components relevant for a younger population. In working with youth, clinicians need to be aware of differences between youths' recognition and understanding of different emotional states, cognitive abilities, present versus future orientation, motivation, reliance on family, peers, and school systems and their adult counterparts [39].

A major limitation of CBT for anxious children is the difficulty many young children have in engaging in abstract or metacognitive thought (ie, thinking about thinking). Most youth do not develop strong abstract thinking skills until adolescence, making it difficult to modify anxious cognitions and biases that underlie anxious symptoms. In an effort to address these limited cognitive capabilities in CBT treatment, target cognitions and abstract concepts are made more concrete. For example, in Kendall's Coping Cat protocol [20], "thought bubbles" are used to identify anxious cognitions and their association with anxious feelings and avoidant or maladaptive behaviors. The therapist's modeling of anxious and adaptive coping thoughts and related emotional states and behaviors during role-play scenarios and exposure exercises and the inclusion of stories and metaphors are all used to enhance the youth's understanding of treatment constructs. A further cognitive limitation in working with children is their tendency to be present-oriented and to have a difficult time understanding the long-term benefits of a treatment procedure that may produce distress in the immediate situation (ie, exposures). In addition, motivation and treatment compliance may be questionable as a result of parent- or teacher-initiated referral for treatment. That is, the child may not identify their symptoms as problematic. Most CBT programs include a reward program administered in-session and at home to address these issues.

To enhance the child's identification and discrimination of emotional states and their relation to anxious symptoms, self-drawings and pictures from magazines can be used. While teaching them about the physical correlates of anxiety, Kendall [20] recommends having the youth draw their own bodies and locating where and what type of physical symptoms are most prevalent for them. This exercise allows the child to get a better sense of their particular profile of somatic symptoms and to use them as cues to begin the active steps of coping.

Most CBT includes a psychoeducational component in which the youth is provided with information on the nature and components of anxiety. This aspect of treatment depends on the child's cognitive development and needs to be tailored to the individual in a way that is relevant and appropriate. Providing analogies to explain difficult concepts (eg, a false fire alarm at school is likened to an anxiety response) is helpful and allows the youth a better understanding of the reasons behind a particular treatment procedure (ie, exposures).

Cognitive-behavior therapy and therapist flexibility

Recently, with the growth of manualized CBT treatment, questions have been posed as to the pros and cons of a manual-guided therapy, especially as it relates to the therapist's flexibility and the effect it may have on treatment outcome. Kendall and Chu [69] examined this issue by administering a retrospective self-rating form to 18 therapists who had previously administered CBT to children with anxiety disorders. Analyses have revealed no significant associations between therapist flexibility and treatment outcome. The investigators have noted that their findings are in contrast to previous findings in the literature [70,71], suggesting that as treatment is individually tailored to meet individual client demands, treatment outcome and maintenance should improve.

Summary

Although the focus of clinical and research interest has increased over the past decade, treatment development research for child and adolescent anxiety disorders continues to lag behind many other childhood disorders. Nevertheless, some advances have been made, perhaps most notably, the establishment of cognitive-behavior therapy as an efficacious and durable treatment for these conditions. CBT has demonstrated acute efficacy in individual, group, family, and school-based formats, with follow-up studies that provide impressive evidence for the durability of treatment gains up to 7 years posttreatment [44].

Despite the progress to date, additional research, some of which is ongoing, is needed to address key outstanding issues. These issues include the use of more stringent (ie, non-wait-list) comparison groups, studies examining the portability of CBT from academic to community treatment settings, and better delineation of possible treatment mechanisms and predictors of outcome, including the impact of comorbidity on response. Given the recent documentation of selective serotonin reuptake inhibitor medication as an efficacious treatment for child anxiety (eg, the RUPP Anxiety Study Group [72]), clinical trials examining the comparative and combined efficacy of CBT and medication are needed, as is research delineating guidelines for sequencing these treatments. The National Institute of Mental Health Child/Adolescent Anxiety Multisite Treatment Study comparing the efficacy of CBT, SSRI medication, CBT plus SSRI, and pill placebo is underway and will provide answers to many of these outstanding research questions.

References

[1] Pine D. Child-adult anxiety disorders. J Am Acad Child Adolesc Psychiatry 1994;33:280–1.
[2] Shaffer D, Fisher P, Dulcan MK, et al. The NIMH Diagnostic Interview Schedule for Children: version 2.3 (DISC 2.3): description, acceptability, prevalence rates, and performance in the MECA study. J Am Acad Child Adolesc Psychiatry 1996;49:865–77.
[3] Ialongo N, Edelsohn G, Werthamer-Larsson L, et al. The significance of self-reported anxious symptoms in first-grade children. J Abnorm Child Psychol 1994;22:441–55.
[4] Langley A, Bergman RL, McCracken J, et al. Impairment in childhood anxiety disorders: preliminary examination of the Child Anxiety Impact Scale-Parent Version. J Child Adolesc Psychopharmacol 2004;14:105–14.
[5] Klein RG. Anxiety disorders. In: Rutter M, Taylor E, Hersov L, editors. Child and adolescent psychiatry: modern approaches. London: Blackwell Scientific; 1995. p. 351–74.
[6] Costello E, Angold A. Epidemiology. In: March JS, editor. Anxiety disorders in children and adolescents. New York: Guilford Press; 1995. p. 109–24.
[7] Ferdinand R, Verhulst F. Psychopathology from adolescence into young adulthood: an 8-year follow-up study. Am J Psychiatry 1995;152:586–94.
[8] Pine D, et al. The risk for early-adulthood anxiety and depressive disorders in adolescents with anxiety and depressive disorders. Arch Gen Psychiatry 1998;55:56–64.
[9] American Psychiatric Association. Diagnostic and statistical manual of mental disorders. 4th edition. Washington (DC): American Psychiatric Association; 1994.
[10] Albano AM, Chorpita BF, Barlow DH. Anxiety disorders. In: Mash E, Barkley RA, editors. Child psychopathology. New York: Guilford Press; 1996. p. 196–241.
[11] Barlow DH. Anxiety and its disorders: the nature and treatment of anxiety and panic. 2nd edition. New York: Guilford Publications; 2002.
[12] Breslau N, Davis G, Prabucki K. Searching for evidence on the validity of generalized anxiety disorder: psychopathology in children of anxious mothers. Psychiatry Res 1987;20:285–97.
[13] Fyer A, et al. Specificity in familial aggregation of phobic disorders. Arch Gen Psychiatry 1995;52:564–73.
[14] Last CG, et al. Anxiety disorders in children and their families. Arch Gen Psychiatry 1991; 48:928–34.
[15] March J, Mulle K. OCD in children and adolescents: a cognitive-behavioral treatment manual. New York: Guilford Press; 1998.
[16] Piacentini J, et al. Cognitive-behavior therapy for childhood obsessive-compulsive disorder: efficacy and predictors of treatment response. J Anxiety Disord 2002;16:207–19.
[17] Ollendick TH. Cognitive behavioral treatment of panic disorder with agoraphobia in adolescents: a multiple baseline design analysis. Behav Ther 1995;26:517–31.
[18] March J, et al. Cognitive-behavioral psychotherapy for children and adolescents with post-traumatic stress disorder following a single incident stressor. J Am Acad Child Adolesc Psychiatry 1998;37:585–93.
[19] Barrett P, Dadds M, Rapee R. Family treatment of childhood anxiety: a controlled trial. J Consult Clin Psychol 1996;64:333–42.
[20] Kendall P. Treating anxiety disorders in children: results of a randomized clinical trial. J Consult Clin Psychol 1994;62:100–10.
[21] Kendall P, et al. Therapy for youths with anxiety disorders: a second randomized clinical trial. J Consult Clin Psychol 1997;65:366–80.
[22] Rapee R. The development of generalized anxiety. In: Vasey MW, Dadds MR, editors. The developmental psychopathology of anxiety. New York: Oxford University Press; 2001. p. 481–503.
[23] Barlow DH. Anxiety and its disorders: the nature and treatment of anxiety and panic. New York: Guilford Press; 1988.
[24] Lang PJ. The application of psychophysiological methods to the study of psychotherapy and behavior modification. In: Bergin AE, Garfield SL, editors. Handbook of psychotherapy and behavior change: an empirical analysis. New York: John Wiley & Sons; 1971. p. 75–125.

[25] Rachman S, Hodgson R. Synchrony and desynchrony in fear and avoidance. Behav Res Ther 1974;12:311–8.
[26] Kagan J, Reznick J, Gibbons J. Inhibited and uninhibited types of children. Child Dev 1989;60:838–45.
[27] Kagan J, Reznick J, Snidman N. The physiology and psychology of behavioral inhibition in children. Child Dev 1987;58:59–73.
[28] Biederman J, et al. Psychiatric correlates of behavioral inhibition in young children of parents with and without psychiatric disorders. Arch Gen Psychiatry 1990;47:21–6.
[29] Biederman J, et al. A 3-year follow-up of children with and without behavioral inhibition. J Am Acad Child Adolesc Psychiatry 1993;32:814–21.
[30] Rosenbaum J, et al. Behavioral inhibition in childhood: a risk factor for anxiety disorders. Harv Rev Psychiatry 1993;1:2–16.
[31] Hayward C, et al. Linking self-reported childhood behavioral inhibition to adolescent social phobia. J Am Acad Child Adolesc Psychiatry 1998;37:1–9.
[32] Beidel D, Turner S. At risk for anxiety: I. psychopathology in the offspring of anxious parents. J Am Acad Child Adolesc Psychiatry 1997;36:918–24.
[33] Fyer A, et al. A direct interview family study of social phobia. Arch Gen Psychiatry 1993; 50:286–93.
[34] Turner S, Beidel D, Costello A. Psychopathology in the offspring of anxiety disorders patients. J Consult Clin Psychol 1987;55:229–35.
[35] Ginsburg G, Silverman W, Kurtines W. Family involvement in treating children with phobic and anxiety disorders: a look ahead. Clin Psychol Rev 1995;15:457–73.
[36] Messer S, Beidel D. Psychosocial correlates of childhood anxiety disorders. J Am Acad Child Adolesc Psychiatry 1994;33:975–83.
[37] Silverman W, Cerny J, Nelles W. The familial influence in anxiety disorders: studies on the offspring of patients with anxiety disorders: In: Lahey BB, Kazdin AE, editors. Advances in clinical child psychology. New York: 1988. p. 223–47.
[38] Ollendick TH, King N. Empirically supported treatments for children with phobic and anxiety disorders. J Clin Child Psychol 1998;27:156–67.
[39] Piacentini J, Bergman RL. Developmental issues in cognitive therapy for childhood anxiety disorders. Journal of Cognitive Psychotherapy 2001;15:165–82.
[40] Chambless D, Gillis M. Cognitive therapy of anxiety disorders. J Consult Clin Psychol 1993; 61:248–60.
[41] Velting ON, Setzer NJ, Albano AM. Update on and advances in assessment and cognitive-behavioral treatment of anxiety disorders in children and adolescents. Prof Psychol Res Pr 2004;35:42–54.
[42] Kendall P, et al. Anxiety disorders in youth: cognitive-behavioral interventions. Needham Heights (MA): Allyn and Bacon; 1992.
[43] Kendall P, Southam-Gerow M. Long-term follow-up of a cognitive behavioral therapy for anxiety disordered youth. J Consult Clin Psychol 1996;64:724–30.
[44] Kendall P, et al. Child anxiety treatment: outcomes in adolescence and impact on substance use and depression at 7.4-year follow-up. J Consult Clin Psychol 2004;72:276–87.
[45] Pina AA, et al. Exposure-based cognitive-behavioral treatment for phobic and anxiety disorders: treatment effects and maintenance for Hispanic/Latino relative to European-American youths. J Am Acad Child Adolesc Psychiatry 2003;42:1179–87.
[46] Silverman W, et al. Treating anxiety disorders in children with group cognitive-behavioral therapy: a randomized clinical trial. J Consult Clin Psychol 1999;67:995–1003.
[47] Silverman W, et al. Contingency management, self-control, and education support in the treatment of childhood phobic disorders: a randomized clinical trial. J Consult Clin Psychol 1999;67:675–87.
[48] Biederman J, et al. High risk study of young children of parents with panic disorder and agoraphobia with and without comorbid major depression. Psychiatry Res 1991;37:333–48.
[49] Gruner K, Muris P, Merckelbach H. The relationship between anxious rearing behaviours and

anxiety disorders symptomatology in normal children. J Behav Ther Exp Psychiatry 1999;30: 27–35.

[50] Chorpita B, Albano A, Barlow D. Cognitive processing in children: relation to anxiety and family influences. J Clin Child Psychol 1996;25:170–6.

[51] Dadds M, Barrett P. Family processes in child and adolescent anxiety and depression. Behav Change 1996;13:231–9.

[52] Barrett P, et al. Cognitive-behavioral treatment of anxiety disorders in children: long-term (6-year) follow-up. J Consult Clin Psychol 2001;69:135–41.

[53] Howard BL, Kendall PC. Cognitive-behavioral family therapy for anxiety-disordered children: a multiple-baseline evaluation. Cognit Ther Res 1996;20:423–43.

[54] Cobham VE, Dadds MR, Spence SH. The role of parental anxiety in the treatment of childhood anxiety. J Consult Clin Psychol 1998;66:893–905.

[55] Spence SH, Donovan C, Brechman-Toussaint M. The treatment of childhood social phobia: the effectiveness of a social skills training-based, cognitive-behavioural intervention, with and without parental involvement. J Child Psychol Psychiatry 2000;41:713–26.

[56] Nauta M, et al. Cognitive-behavioral therapy for children with anxiety disorders in a clinical setting: no additional effect of a cognitive parent training. J Am Acad Child Adolsc Psychiatry 2003;42:1270–8.

[57] Silverman W, Ginsburg G, Kurtines W. Clinical issues in treating children with anxiety and phobic disorders. Cognitive and Behavioral Practice 1995;2:93–117.

[58] Silverman W, Kurtines W. Anxiety and phobic disorders: a pragmatic approach. New York: Plenum Press; 1996.

[59] Barrett PM. Group therapy for childhood anxiety disorders. J Clin Child Psychol 1998;27: 459–68.

[60] Toren P, et al. Case series: brief parent-child group therapy for childhood anxiety disorders using a manual-based cognitive-behavioral technique. J Am Acad Child Adolesc Psychiatry 2000;39: 1309–12.

[61] Flannery-Schroeder EC, Kendall PC. Group and individual cognitive-behavioral treatments for youth with anxiety disorders: a randomized clinical trial. Cognit Ther Res 2000;24:251–78.

[62] Manassis K, et al. Group and individual cognitive-behavioral therapy for childhood anxiety disorders: a randomized trial. J Am Acad Child Adolesc Psychiatry 2002;41:1423–30.

[63] Muris P, Meesters C, van Melick M. Treatment of childhood anxiety disorders: a preliminary comparison between cognitive-behavioral group therapy and a psychological placebo intervention. J Behav Ther Exp Psychiatry 2002;33:143–58.

[64] Last C, Hansen C, Franco N. Cognitive-behavioral treatment of social phobia. J Am Acad Child Adolesc Psychiatry 1998;37:404–11.

[65] Brady E, Kendall P. Comorbidity of anxiety and depression in children and adolescents. Psychol Bull 1992;111:244–55.

[66] Strauss CC, et al. Associations between anxiety and depression in children and adolescents with anxiety disorders. J Abnorm Child Psychol 1988;16:57–68.

[67] Kendall PC, Brady EU, Verduin T. Comorbidity in childhood anxiety disorders and treatment outcome. J Am Acad Child Adolesc Psychiatry 2001;40:787–94.

[68] Rapee RM. The influence of comorbidity on treatment outcome for children and adolescents with anxiety disorders. Behav Res Ther 2003;41:105–12.

[69] Kendall PC, Chu BC. Retrospective self-reports of therapist flexibility in a manual-based treatment for youths with anxiety disorders. J Clin Child Psychol 2000;29:209–20.

[70] Jacobson NS, et al. Research-structured vs. clinically flexible versions of social learning-based marital therapy. Behav Res Ther 1989;27:173–80.

[71] Ost LG, Jerremalm A, Johansson J. Individual response patterns and the effects of different behavioral methods in the treatment of social phobia. Behav Res Ther 1981;19:1–16.

[72] RUPP Anxiety Study Group. An eight-week placebo-controlled trial of fluvoxamine for anxiety disorders in children and adolescents. N Engl J Med 2001;344:1279–85.

ELSEVIER
SAUNDERS

Child Adolesc Psychiatric Clin N Am
14 (2005) 877–908

CHILD AND
ADOLESCENT
PSYCHIATRIC CLINICS
OF NORTH AMERICA

Psychopharmacologic Treatment of Pediatric Anxiety Disorders

Shauna P. Reinblatt, MD, FRCPC*, John T. Walkup, MD

*Division of Child and Adolescent Psychiatry, Johns Hopkins University School of Medicine,
600 North Wolfe Street, CMSC 346, Baltimore, MD 21287, USA*

Anxiety disorders are among the most prevalent groups of psychiatric disorders in youth, and they affect 6% to 18% of children and adolescents [1–4]. Anxiety disorders have a significant impact on school, social, and family function [2] and are associated with an increased risk of anxiety or depressive disorders in adulthood [5]. The high prevalence and the increased risk for morbidity highlight the public health importance of treating childhood anxiety disorders. Although remarkable progress has been made in child and adolescent anxiety psychopharmacologic research, much remains to be done. Multiple treatment trials are being conducted in pediatric obsessive-compulsive disorder (OCD) [6–15], and three randomized, controlled trials are being conducted in other pediatric anxiety disorders [16–18]. Currently underway is a large randomized clinical trial, the Child/Adolescent Anxiety Multimodal Treatment Study (CAMS), which compares the efficacy of medication management with a selective serotonin reuptake inhibitor (SSRI), cognitive behavioral therapy (CBT), their combination, and pill placebo. Given the experience with other large-scale comparative treatment trials—multimodal treatment of attention deficit hyperactivity disorder (ADHD), the Treatment of Adolescent Depression Study, and the Pediatric OCD Treatment Study—CAMS likely will set the standard for treatment in childhood anxiety disorders.

This work was supported in part by National Institute of Mental Health T32 training grant MH20033.

* Corresponding author.
  E-mail address: sreinbl1@jhmi.edu (S.P. Reinblatt).

This article reviews the psychopharmacologic treatment of child and adolescent anxiety disorders and is divided into the following sections: historical background, general treatment principles, OCD, other anxiety disorders, including separation anxiety disorders (SAD), generalized anxiety disorder (GAD), and social phobia, elective mutism, and post-traumatic stress disorder (PTSD) and specific phobia. Short-term and long-term psychopharmacologic treatment strategies are reviewed, as are approaches for managing comorbidity and treatment-refractory cases. This article is organized by diagnostic categories rather than by medication classes to emphasize the clinical perspective.

Historical background

The earliest psychopharmacologic trials of childhood anxiety and mood disorders were conducted by child and adolescent psychiatrists at the Johns Hopkins Hospital in the late 1950s. In a National Institute of Mental Health–funded trial, Drs. Leon Eisenberg and Leon Cytryn compared the relative efficacy of neuroleptic agents (prochlorperazine and perphenazine) [19,20] and minor tranquilizers (meprobamate) added to psychotherapy for child and adolescent psychiatric disorders, including anxiety. Neither medication class was found to be effective [19,20] in these and subsequent trials [21]. A decade later, Rachel Gittleman-Klein and Donald Klein pioneered the antidepressant era of pediatric anxiety treatment research with the use of tricyclic antidepressants (TCAs). Building on the efficacy of imipramine for panic disorder in adults, Gittleman-Klein and Klein established the efficacy of imipramine for pediatric anxiety [22].

In the subsequent three decades, significant progress has been made in the pharmacologic treatment of pediatric anxiety disorders. Several factors support this progress, including (1) the development of standard diagnostic criteria [23], (2) operationalized, diagnostic interviews (eg, Kiddie-Schedule of Affective Disorders and Schizophrenia [24], Diagnostic Interview Schedule for Children [25], and more recently, the Anxiety Disorders Interview Schedule), and (3) several new antidepressant medications with favorable safety profile (eg, SSRIs) [26]. Currently there is good evidence for the efficacy of medication and psychotherapy for OCD and SAD, GAD, and social phobia. Preliminary evidence also exists regarding the relative efficacy of combined medication and psychotherapy in OCD.

Despite advances, significant work remains to be done. There are no comparative trials for SAD, GAD, and social phobia to answer which treatment works best for which child, although studies are underway. No large definitive trials are studying either psychotherapy or medication in pediatric PTSD. Few studies are evaluating the long-term impact of medication on outcome or side effects. No studies are evaluating the sequencing of treatment (ie, which to use first: medication or psychotherapy) and how long to treat with medication.

General treatment principles

Key to the pharmacologic treatment of pediatric anxiety disorders are a comprehensive diagnostic assessment, comprehensive treatment planning (including the selection of treatments, time course for implementation, and monitoring strategies for outcome and side effects), psychoeducation of parents and child about the disorder and the proposed treatment, and informed consent and assent for treatment. This article provides rich information that clinicians should use for details regarding assessment. Assessments should include current and past symptom inventories to establish the current symptomatology and course of illness and should include history of past treatment. Treatment planning includes not only picking a medication but also understanding the family and patient readiness for treatment and what psychosocial issues must be addressed. Psychoeducation about the anxiety disorder and the potential for risk and benefit of the proposed and alternative treatments helps ready the patient and family for treatment. Although many of these medications discussed do not have US Food and Drug Administration (FDA) indications, there may be good efficacy and safety data in this age group to support the use of a specific medication or class. Once treatment has begun, ongoing monitoring of outcome and side effects is particularly critical for optimal outcome with minimal risk. The duration of treatment should be addressed, including if and when medication should be discontinued. Although the exact minimum duration of pharmacologic treatment is not currently known, it is prudent to consider a slow tapering of medication after a period of sustained improvement.

Obsessive-compulsive disorder

OCD is characterized by obsessions or compulsions, which are respectively recurrent, intrusive, and stereotyped thoughts or behaviors that cause functional impairment. OCD is common, with a point prevalence in children and adolescents of 0.5% [6,15,27] and a lifetime rate of 1% to 3% [28,29]. OCD begins in either childhood or young adulthood, with 80% of cases beginning in childhood [30]. Of all the pediatric anxiety disorders, OCD has the strongest evidence base for pharmacologic treatment [31], more than pediatric depression or the non-OCD anxiety disorders. OCD is a heterogeneous disorder, and some subtypes of OCD [32,33] may have different treatment outcomes [34]; however, these phenotypes and their treatment implications are not yet fully understood. Although this article focuses only on the pharmacologic treatment of OCD, the benefit of psychotherapeutic treatments, such as CBT [35] and combination of medication with psychotherapy, should be acknowledged. Agents with serotonergic activity are the most helpful, although the exact mechanism of antiobsessional action of serotonergic medications remains unclear [31].

Short-term treatment of obsessive-compulsive disorder

The SSRIs are clearly effective in adult [36] and pediatric cases of OCD [7,9–13,15,27,37]. Sertraline, fluvoxamine, fluoxetine, and, more recently, paroxetine have been studied in large randomized, placebo-controlled trials of childhood OCD (Table 1) [11,12,14,27]. Three of these SSRIs have a US FDA indication for pediatric OCD, including sertraline (≥6 years) [38], fluoxetine (≥7 years) [39], and fluvoxamine (≥8 years) [38–40]. A large controlled trial of paroxetine has demonstrated efficacy, but this trial has not led to a US FDA indication for paroxetine in childhood OCD [10]. Clomipramine also has demonstrated efficacy, carries a US FDA indication, and may be particularly useful in patients who do not tolerate the SSRIs.

A meta-analysis of 13 studies of SSRIs for childhood OCD documented a combined effect size of 0.46 (moderate); there were no significant differences in effect sizes noted among the SSRIs fluoxetine, paroxetine, sertraline, or fluvoxamine [41]. Doses typically used in controlled trials can be considered the highest safe dose (as opposed to the lowest effective dose) because the medications were increased as per protocol if there were residual symptoms and minimal side effects. Despite a clinically significant treatment response to SSRIs, patients still may have residual OCD symptoms after 8 to 12 weeks of treatment. Data from longitudinal studies described later suggest that continued treatment may improve on acute phase response.

Medication treatment, although effective, may be associated with unwanted side effects. Because the SSRIs have been available for many years, the expected side effect profile is well known. More recently, reports have documented rarer and more unexpected side effects of antidepressants. Perhaps of most concern currently is the apparent increase risk for suicidal thoughts and behavior associated with SSRIs. It is important to note that no individual OCD study described seems to document a significant risk for suicidal ideation or behavior. No increase in relative risk was identified in pooled analyses of the SSRI studies of anxious youth [42]. Behavioral side effects variously labeled as activation, akathisia, disinhibition, impulsivity, and hyperactivity do appear in these reports, however. It is unclear whether one SSRI has a greater risk for such behavioral adverse events or if there is a link between such activation and suicidal ideation. Sexual side effects, although not commonly described in most large-scale clinical trials, also should be reviewed specifically in adolescents because they may impact adherence [43]. Recent reports of growth suppression associated with SSRIs suggest that ongoing monitoring of height may be advisable [44,45].

Because all SSRIs seem to be equally effective and head-to-head studies are unlikely to be conducted, the choice of SSRI should be made based on respective pharmacokinetic properties, the potential for drug-drug interactions, and side effect profiles of specific patients. When treating patients clinically, it is helpful to know what the highest safe dose is so that maximum benefit can be achieved. On the other hand, most clinicians and patients are interested in the lowest effective dose. Practically speaking, slow upward titration to reduce risk for side effects but willingness to maximize dose to improve outcome is the right course to take. Too slow upward adjustment and too low a dose put patients at risk for increased morbidity and demoralization with treatment.

Clomipramine was the first SSRI studied for pediatric OCD and the only TCA with a US FDA indication for a pediatric internalizing disorder (> 10 years) [6,7]. It has demonstrated efficacy in three small clinical trials [6,7,46]. The largest trial, which was an 8-week, multicenter, double-blind ($n = 60$) study, found clomipramine to be effective for the short-term treatment of OCD in children and adolescents aged 10 to 18 years [7]. Clomipramine has several potential side effects based on its anticholinergic and antihistaminic properties, including sedation, weight gain, increased seizure risk, and cardiovascular events, such as hypotension and arrhythmias [38]. Compared with the SSRIs, clomipramine may have more nuisance side effects but may be more useful than the SSRIs for patients who have OCD and suffer from sleep difficulties, decreased appetite, or a history of activation on the SSRIs. Clomipramine is dosed up to 200 mg/d or 3 mg/kg/d, whichever is least. Dosing outside these ranges for partially responsive or treatment-refractory patients may require monitoring of blood levels and electrocardiograms and specific documentation in a child's medical record.

Fluoxetine, at a fixed dose of 20 mg/d, was first found to be efficacious for childhood OCD ($n = 14$) in a 20-week, double-blind, placebo-controlled trial [13]. This trial was also the first to document treatment-emergent adverse behavioral changes [13]. The efficacy of fluoxetine, 20 to 60 mg/d, was later replicated in a much larger randomized, placebo-controlled trial ($n = 103$) [11]. The behavioral side effects of fluoxetine described in the previous trial were not reported in this study.

Fluvoxamine, up to 200 mg/d, was found to be effective in a large, 10-week, multicenter, randomized, placebo-controlled trial in children aged 8 to 17 years [12]. Side effects more common on active drug than on placebo included fatigue, insomnia, and gastrointestinal distress.

Sertraline, up to 200 mg/d, was found to be effective in a large, multicenter, randomized, controlled trial for children aged 6 to 17 years with OCD [27]. The incidence of insomnia, nausea, agitation, and tremor were noted to be significantly greater in the sertraline treatment group, but it was otherwise generally well tolerated. More recently, the Pediatric OCD Treatment Study compared the efficacy of sertraline, CBT, their combination, and placebo as the initial treatment for pediatric OCD [15]. Children and adolescents ($n = 112$) were followed for 12 weeks, and combined treatment with CBT and sertraline had the best rate of clinical remission. There was no evidence of treatment-emergent suicidal behavior noted in the study.

Paroxetine, up to 50 mg/d, was found to be effective in a large, 10-week, multicenter, placebo-controlled trial for children aged 7 to 17 years [10]. It is notable that one adolescent in the paroxetine group reportedly experienced suicidal thoughts versus none in the placebo group. This experience was apparently in the context of a psychosocial stressor, however. In a separate study, paroxetine efficacy was evaluated in a large, randomized, placebo-controlled discontinuation

Table 1
Acute randomized, controlled trials in pediatric obsessive-compulsive disorder

Drug	Study [reference]	Duration (wk)	Study design	N	Dose range (mg/d)
Chlomipramine	Leonard et al, 1989 [46]	10	Crossover with desipramine	48	Chlomipramine, 97–203
Chlomipramine	Flament et al, 1985 [6]	10	Crossover	19	111–171
Chlomipramine	DeVeaugh-Geiss et al, 1992 [7]	8	Multicenter; 1-year open extension phase	60	3 mg/kg daily
Fluoxetine	Riddle et al, 1992 [13]	20 (crossover at 8 wk)	Crossover	14	Fixed dose, 20
Fluoxetine	Geller et al, 2001 [11]	13	ITT analysis	103	Flexible dose, 10–60; titration schedule 10 mg × 2 wk, 20 mg × 2 wk; option to increase by 20 mg at 4 wk and 7 wk
Fluvoxamine	Riddle et al, 2001 [12]	10	Multisite; extension 1-year open label; LOCF; analysis	120	Flexible dose, 50–200
Paroxetine	Geller et al, 2003 [47]	32	Multisite two-phase Randomized, pbo-controlled, double-blind trial; 16 wk open label (phase 1) and 16 wk double-blind withdrawal from treatment (phase 2); LOCF	335	10–60
Paroxetine	Geller et al, 2004 [10]	10	LOCF	203	Flexible dose, 10–50

Mean dose (mg/d)	Findings	Common side effects
150	Chlomipramine superior to desipramine; 64% recurrence when switched to desipramine	Dry mouth, tremor, sweating, constipation, fatigue, dizziness
141	75% had at least moderate improvement irrespective of depressive symptoms	Dry mouth, tremor, constipation, sweating; one participant had a seizure
Maximum, 200	37% reduction in CY-BOCS versus 8% in pbo group; 60% "very much improved"; maintained gains during open-label phase	Dry mouth, tremor, fatigue, dizziness, constipation
Fixed dose, 20	Plasma fluoxetine levels corresponded to improvement; CY-BOCS decreased 44% versus 27% pbo; CGI improvement fluoxetine versus pbo	Insomnia, fatigue, motor activation, increased tics (preexisting in some participants); *serious AE*: 13-year-old boy with suicidal ideation after 3-wk fluoxetine, comorbid MDD, ODD and SAD (resolved after fluoxetine stopped)
25	Response: 40% reduction in CY-BOCS score with fluoxetine 49% responders versus 25% pbo ($P = 0.03$); clinician rated CGI (responder 1 or 2) fluoxetine group $P >$ pbo ($P < 0.01$); significant differences between two groups at wk 5	Same rate of discontinuation as pbo; more hyperkinesias in fluoxetine group, and diarrhea
165	Maximum improvement at wk 3; response: 25% reduction CY-BOCS, 42% fluvoxamine versus 26% pbo	Activation, hyperkinesias, somnolence and asthenia (fatigue, weakness, tiredness); asthenia and insomnia were 10% more in active treatment group than pbo
33	Response: 25% CY-BOCS; 71% participants responded; 75% OCD group; less when comorbid with ADHD, tic disorder, or ODD (56%, 53%, or 39%, respectively); double-blind relapse phase II: overall, paroxetine group relapse rate was 44% versus 35% pbo, with this 10% difference increasing with number of comorbid disorders; psychiatric comorbidity was associated with greater relapse rate	58% had one comorbid illness; 30% had at least two comorbidities
30	Entry CY-BOCS: 24.8, (moderate OCD); mean decrease in CY-BOCS scores of 9 for paroxetine group versus 5 with pbo; significant difference in mean response rates	AEs (twice as common as pbo group) included hyperkinesias and trauma (physical injuries); agitation, decreased appetite, somnolence, nausea and abdominal pain were also noted; 10% treatment group versus 3% pbo group discontinued treatment due to AEs; *serious AEs*: one child on paroxetine developed

(continued on next page)

Table 1 (*continued*)

Drug	Study [reference]	Duration (wk)	Study design	N	Dose range (mg/d)
Sertraline	March et al, 1998 [27]	12	Multisite; ITT analysis	187	Forced titration from 25 mg (children) or 50 mg (adolescents) to 200 mg maximum
Sertraline	Pediatric OCD Treatment Study Team, 2004 [15]	12	Randomized controlled trial at three centers; randomized to CBT alone, sertraline alone, sertraline and CBT, or pill pbo alone; ITT analysis	112	Flexible titration 25–200 mg over 6 wk

Abbreviations: AE, adverse event; CGI-I, Clinical Global Impression Scale-Improvement; CY-BOCS, Children's Yale-Brown Obsessive-Compulsive Scale; ITT, intent-to-treat; LOCF, last observation carried forward; ODD, oppositional defiant disorder; pbo, placebo.

trial ($n = 335$), and a high percentage of pediatric subjects responded to open treatment [47]. In perhaps the only trial that addressed the effect of comorbidity on outcome, children who have OCD and comorbid conditions had decreased response rates to open treatment and increased relapse risk after transition to placebo. The data on relapse rates on medication and placebo have not been published.

Which treatment is best for whom?

Limited data are available to help define which treatment—medication or CBT—is best for whom and how to sequence treatment. To date, one comparative treatment trial suggests that CBT or combination treatment is the best first choice; however, prominent site differences in CBT efficacy ultimately may impact on the clinician choice of first treatment (Pediatric OCD Treatment Study). In the absence of evidence, OCD treatment parameters may provide some guidance [48]. In general, such guidelines advocate the use of CBT alone as first line for most children and adolescents. As children get older and symptoms become more severe, however, there is greater support for either adding medi-

Mean dose (mg/d)	Findings	Common side effects
		suicidal ideation (without attempt) in context of psychosocial stressor and two cases of aggressive behavior in treatment group versus one case pbo group
167	Significant differences in efficacy emerged at 3 wk; response: CY-BOCS decrease of at least 25%; results: 53% response for sertraline versus 37% pbo; CGI-I: 42% rated improved or very much improved for treatment group versus 26% pbo	Agitation, insomnia, tremor, and nausea significantly more frequent in treatment group
Mean highest daily dose: combined 133 mg/d, sertraline 170 mg/d (median doses were 150 and 200 mg, respectively)	Outcome measure: CY-BOCS under 10 by blind independent evaluator; significant improvement with CBT or sertraline or combined treatment versus pbo; combined treatment was superior to CBT or sertraline alone, which did not differ; site differences may have played a role in CBT response; combined treatment may be less susceptible to site differences	Motor overactivity and activation, nausea, diarrhea, stomach ache, enuresis

cation to CBT or initiating treatment with medication. Because high-quality CBT is not universally available, beginning treatment with medication may be the default strategy in many communities.

Long-term treatment of obsessive-compulsive treatment

Three key issues exist with respect to the length of time children should stay on medication. (1) How long does it take to get maximum benefit? (2) How durable is pharmacologic treatment? (3) How long should a child stay on medication to reduce the risk for relapse with discontinuation? Few data are available to answer these questions, but the data that are available can be useful in considering a treatment duration that may be required to achieve these goals.

How long does it take to get maximum benefit?

It is clear that acute treatment of 8 to 12 weeks results in significant symptom reduction occurs, but patients are still symptomatic and may continue to meet diagnostic criteria at the end of acute treatment. Two long-term, open studies have documented continued symptomatic improvement after the acute phase, but at a much slower rate [49,50]. In these studies a total exposure of 4 to 6 months of active treatment was required to achieve maximum benefit. In both studies, maximum benefit resulted in the average patient experiencing a 40% to 50% reduction in symptoms and a level of symptom severity that may be consistent with the loss of diagnosis.

How durable is pharmacologic treatment?

Longitudinal studies to assess the durability of treatment often have significant methodologic problems, including the lack of a control condition for the duration of the study, problems with adherence that may lead to an underestimation of durability, adjunctive treatments that actually may enhance the apparent durability of medication, and ultimately how durability rates are reported (ie, intent to treat versus study completors). Despite these problems, it seems that ongoing medication treatment can be necessary for some patients who have OCD. In a long-term cross-over study of clomipramine, subjects were randomized to continue on blinded clomipramine or were transitioned to desipramine for a period of 2 months [51]. Subjects who transitioned to desipramine had reduced symptom control, which suggested that long-term treatment with clomipramine was required to maintain response. An open-label extension of the multicenter sertraline trial in childhood OCD suggested that responders to treatment who continued on medication for a period of 12 months maintained their response [49]. This evidence supports the role of SSRIs such as sertraline as being effective in pediatric OCD for up to 12 months [49,52] and is consistent with the adult literature [53]. An open-label, flexible dose study using citalopram (maximum dose, 40 mg) combined with coadministered CBT in children and adolescents who had OCD was effective for a 1-year period to decrease OCD symptoms [54].

How long should a child stay on medication to reduce the risk for relapse with discontinuation?

Given the lack of long-term discontinuation studies, it is important to note that different lengths of treatment may be associated with different relapse rates (ie, longer treatment may result in lower relapse rates) and that clinicians, children, and families may have differing views of what constitutes "too much risk" for relapse. For example, discontinuation after 6 months of treatment may have a higher rate of relapse than after 12 months of treatment. If the rate of relapse after 6 months is 30% and 20% after 12 months, however, families may want to discontinue after 6 months. Some patients may have such a severe disorder that they want to continue treatment until risk of relapse is less than 10% to 15%. Identifying the specific optimum length of treatment for childhood OCD requires a large, long-term study.

Given the lack of data, guidance is provided. Before discontinuation, (1) a patient should be stable with minimal fluctuation in symptom control; (2) psychoeducation regarding the risk of relapse and how relapse presents should be completed; (3) a plan for how to taper the medications, how to monitor for a return of symptoms, and how long a patient should be followed after he or she is off medication should be discussed; and (4) medication should be tapered slowly to minimize potential withdrawal symptoms. If possible, the patient, family, and clinician should choose the most appropriate time for discontinuing medication, such as during the summer, when there is less possible adverse impact on academic performance. It is just as important to follow a patient closely after discontinuation of treatment as it is to monitor during discontinuation. This is particularly true if the chance of relapse is high because of short duration of treatment. Multiple episodes of illness may make it more difficult to discontinue treatment successfully and may be associated with increased relapse risk. Adult OCD consensus guidelines suggest long-term treatment for persons with three to four mild/moderate relapses or two to four severe relapses with concurrent CBT [48]; the evidence is less clear for pediatric OCD [55]. A meta-analysis regarding the long-term outcome of pediatric OCD analyzed 16 studies that followed patients between 1 and 15 years [56]; the OCD overall remission rate (not fulfilling criteria for subthreshold or full OCD) was 40%, with pooled mean persistence rates of 41% for full OCD and 60% for full or subthreshold OCD. Poor prognostic factors included a poor initial treatment response and comorbid psychiatric illness.

Treatment of obsessive-compulsive disorder and co-occurring conditions

Several conditions commonly co-occur with OCD, the most common of which are other anxiety disorders, mood disorders, ADHD, tic disorders (including Tourette's disorder), and disruptive behavior disorders [47,56]. Children who have OCD and other co-occurring conditions may not be as responsive to SSRIs for OCD [41] and may be more vulnerable to relapse with SSRI discontinuation [47]. Although there is limited empirical support for using medication combinations for OCD plus co-occurring conditions, it is commonly performed in clinical practice (eg, SSRIs plus stimulants for OCD/ADHD or SSRIs plus neuroleptic agents for OCD/tics).

The treatment of co-occurring OCD and tics may require specific care because case reports suggest that tics may be worsened by SSRIs [13]. It is not uncommon in clinical care to see improvement in tic severity after successful treatment of mood and anxiety disorders with SSRIs, however. The treatment of OCD with co-occurring mood disorder is less complex because the SSRIs are effective for both; however, co-occurring depression and OCD may indicate more severe OCD that is less responsive to single drug treatment [57,58]. Monitoring for the emergence of manic symptoms is particularly important when there is a comorbid affective disorder. The treatment of OCD and ADHD with stimulants also may present a challenge because theoretical concerns exist that stimulants may increase obsessional symptoms.

Treatment-resistant obsessive-compulsive disorder

Short-term SSRI treatment of children who have OCD often leaves children with residual symptoms. Over an extended treatment period, some children experience greater improvement [49]. Some children do not receive significant benefit short-term or are left with residual and impairing symptoms even after a longer trial, however. For children who do not receive typical benefit, a re-evaluation of the diagnosis and an assessment of the adequacy of dose, duration, and compliance with the medication trial are critical. For most patients with a partial response, the addition of CBT is the first and best approach. Although some treatment guidelines suggest switching SSRIs for patients who do not respond [48], the next best step actually may be augmentation with another medication. An augmentation trial takes advantage of the benefit derived from the SSRI and limits the risks associated with discontinuing a partially effective medication.

Although augmentation strategies are commonly used, there are a limited number of augmentation strategies with demonstrated efficacy. Antipsychotic medication, particularly risperidone, has been demonstrated to be effective in augmenting SSRIs for OCD complicated by tics and schizotypy [59,60]. Other augmentation strategies are designed to enhance serotonergic functioning and include combining an SSRI with clomipramine, buspirone, lithium, or pindolol or combining two SSRIs or an SSRI plus NSRI. Clonazepam may be a useful adjunctive treatment in children and adolescents with refractory OCD; however, the potential for sedation and behavioral disinhibition are limitations to its use [61].

Combining SSRIs with low-dose clomipramine [62,63] is recommended in expert guidelines in partially responsive patients [48]. The combination of an SSRI with a TCA takes advantage of the pharmacokinetic and pharmacodynamic interactions of these medications. Although this combination can be helpful, it is important to monitor for side effects, particularly cardiovascular effects: electrocardiogram, heart rate and blood pressure monitoring, and the emergence of serotonin toxicity (ie, serotonin syndrome). A similar strategy involves combining two different SSRIs; however, the risk for drug interaction is greater because the SSRIs as a class inhibit cytochrome P-450 and combinations may result in increased blood levels of each SSRI. Other strategies include augmenting with inositol (an isomer of glucose that is also a precursor in the phosphotidylinositol cycle in the second messenger system), which has been helpful in cases of depression and OCD [64], and pindolol, a beta-blocker with 5-HT1A autoreceptor antagonist activity [65].

Intravenous clomipramine has been examined in adults and one controlled trial in adolescents [66–68]. Clomipramine undergoes nearly complete first pass metabolism to desmethylclomipramine, which has little serotonergic activity. With intravenous clomipramine the medication bypasses the liver and goes directly to the brain, which results in increased brain exposure to the serotonergically active clomipramine and the potential for increased benefit compared with orally administered clomipramine. For patients on clomipramine, adding inhibitors of cyp-450 3A4, such as fluvoxamine, also can increase the circulating levels of clomipramine versus desmethylclomipramine.

Psychosurgery, including cingulotomy and subcaudate tractotomy, has been used in adults with severe, intractable treatment-resistant adult OCD [69]. These irreversible surgical methods are not used in pediatric OCD because of the lack of data in children and the unknown effects on their developing brains [55].

Pediatric autoimmune neuropsychiatry disorders associated with streptococcal infections

Of the children and adolescents who have OCD and tics, there is a group whose symptoms seem to be secondary to group A beta-hemolytic streptococcal infections [70]. The putative mechanism is an autoimmune reaction much akin to rheumatic fever and Sydenham's chorea. Clinical characteristics of pediatric autoimmune neuropsychiatry disorders associated with streptococcal infections include tic and OCD symptoms, an episodic course, prepubertal onset, and neurologic symptoms, such as choreiform movements and the presence of documented streptococcal infection or elevated antistreptococcal antibodies [71].

Given the potential autoimmune mechanism of pediatric autoimmune neuropsychiatry disorders associated with streptococcal infections, potential treatments include anti-inflammatory, immunologic, and antibiotic prophylaxis treatments [72]. Steroids, plasmapheresis, and intravenous immunoglobulin (Ig) and antibiotics have been used in small trials. Plasma exchange and intravenous Ig were more effective than placebo intravenous IG in a small 4-week trial of patients with pediatric autoimmune neuropsychiatry disorders associated with streptococcal infections. In a trial of chronic OCD, plasma exchange was not effective and is not recommended [73]. Currently, these treatments have not been replicated, and given the potential significant risks, investigators at the National Institute of Mental Health have advised that these treatments only be considered for severely ill patients, such as part of clinical research protocols and not routine care [73a,73b].

Much as penicillin prophylaxis is used to prevent systemic infection in individuals with rheumatic heart disease, the use of penicillin prophylaxis for pediatric autoimmune neuropsychiatry disorders associated with streptococcal infections also has been explored. Tics, OCD, and other psychiatric symptoms, along with streptococcal antibody titers and throat cultures, were assessed in an 8-month placebo-controlled cross-over trial (4 months $\times$ 4 months) ($n = 37$) [74]. There was an equal number of infections in placebo and active treatment groups and no difference in OCD or tic symptoms exacerbations, which may have been caused by the failure of the antibiotic agent used as prophylaxis. More recently a comparison of azithromycin and penicillin documented improvement in short- and long-term outcome [75]. The lack of a placebo control makes it difficult to interpret the findings.

Discussion

As with cases of adult OCD, SSRIs are the cornerstones of pharmacotherapy for childhood OCD. Although the evidence may be slightly stronger for clomipramine than for the other SSRIs, its use is limited by the need for more extensive monitoring and the potential cardiac and anticholinergic side effects. All four SSRIs extensively studied (fluvoxamine, fluoxetine, sertraline, and paroxetine) seem to have similar efficacies; however, no direct comparison studies have confirmed these findings. CBT and other psychotherapeutic interventions have been less well studied but seem to have a prominent place in the therapeutic armamentarium, especially for initial treatment and in combination with medication. Although data are needed regarding the optimal long-term treatment of OCD and its comorbidities, initial studies indicate the importance of using adequate doses for adequate duration. Augmentation strategies that enhance serotonergic function are the most commonly used. Atypical neuroleptic agents are the only augmentation strategy with documented efficacy.

Non–obsessive-compulsive disorder, non–post-traumatic stress disorder anxiety disorders

The non-OCD, non-PTSD anxiety disorders (eg, SAD, social phobia, and GAD) are commonly grouped together because there is significant symptom overlap; children with one of the disorders often have symptoms of the others [1,76]. There is significant comorbidity among these anxiety disorders; up to 60% of children with one anxiety disorder have another disorder and 30% have all three [77]. This rate of comorbidity exceeds the high comorbidity seen in adults [78,79]. Finally, childhood anxiety seems to be continuous with adult anxiety disorders. For this reason, in contrast to adult anxiety studies, several pediatric psychopharmacologic studies and psychosocial treatment trials have either grouped SAD, social phobia, and GAD or targeted one of these disorders but allowed for children with more than one disorder to be included in the study [16,17,80]. In this way, studies of anxiety disorder treatment can reflect the true nature of overlap and complexity of these disorders.

The pharmacologic management of anxiety disorders in youths with antidepressant medication began with the TCAs more than 30 years ago. It was hypothesized that TCAs would be useful in children based on the efficacy of TCA treatment in adult panic patients and the common finding that adults with anxiety often suffered the onset of their symptoms during childhood [81]. The first trial documented the efficacy of imipramine on school phobia using the return to school and improved anxiety as outcomes [22]. More recently, imipramine has been effective in reducing anxiety and depression in youth who refuse to attend school [82]. Ultimately, concerns regarding the safety of TCAs and their apparently lower efficacy compared with the SSRIs have led to a shift away from using TCAs as a first-line treatment of pediatric anxiety disorders.

Over the course of the last 20 years, SSRIs have replaced the TCAs as the first line treatment for anxiety disorders in children and adolescents. The success of the SSRIs was first demonstrated in pediatric subjects who had OCD, which paved the way for studies of other anxiety disorders. Successful open trials paved the way for larger, placebo-controlled trials [80,83].

One large, multicenter, randomized, controlled trial and one smaller single site trial support the use of SSRIs in SAD, social phobia, and GAD. The Research Units of Pediatric Psychopharmacology Anxiety Study Group [79] investigated the use of fluvoxamine for SAD, social phobia, and GAD. This randomized, placebo-controlled trial enrolled children and adolescents aged 6 to 17 years ($n = 128$) who did not respond to 3 weeks of brief supportive psychoeducation. They were then randomized for 8 weeks of fluvoxamine, 50 to 300 mg/d ($n = 39$), or placebo ($n = 43$) at six participating sites across the country [84]; a fixed-flexible dose strategy was used. During the trial, subjects were assessed using various self, parent, and clinician rating scales, with the primary outcome measures being the Clinical Global Impressions scale and the Pediatric Anxiety Rating Scale [84]. The fluvoxamine group differentiated itself from the placebo group at week 2. At study endpoint, fluvoxamine was superior to placebo on the Pediatric Anxiety Rating Scale and the Clinical Global Impressions-I Scale: 76% versus 29%, respectively. Fluvoxamine was well tolerated, with few youths discontinuing use because of side effects (8% in the active treatment group versus 2% of placebo) [79]. The main side effects in the fluvoxamine group compared with the placebo group were gastrointestinal symptoms and an increase in activity level (28% versus 12%). It is noteworthy that the placebo response rate was lower than that found in many studies that examined pediatric depression, which resulted in a large effect size (1.1).

Fluoxetine was shown to be efficacious in a 12-week, randomized, controlled trial of fluoxetine, 20 mg/d, for youths aged 7 to 17 years ($n = 74$) with mixed anxiety disorders [17]. Medication was superior to placebo by week 9, and 61% of the fluoxetine group versus 35% in the placebo group were considered responders. The fluoxetine group had more gastrointestinal symptoms, headaches, and drowsiness during the first 2 weeks of the study; by study endpoint the only side effect more common on medication was headache. Although the sample was small, children with primary GAD and social phobia improved significantly better than children on placebo; the participants with SAD showed only a trend toward better response to medication than children on placebo. Similar to treatment trials in children who had OCD, more participants improved on medication than placebo, yet many had residual anxiety symptoms at the end of the study. The severity of illness at intake and a family history of anxiety disorders tended to predict a poorer response at the end of the study. No differences were noted regarding agitation or disinhibition between the placebo and treatment groups. In contrast to the Research Units of Pediatric Psychopharmacology Study, with an early separation between medication and placebo, the fluoxetine group took longer to separate from placebo and document response. The longer time to response and residual symptoms could be related to a fixed dose and the resultant inability to optimize response. Outcome with fluoxetine in clinical practice could be better than that observed in this trial if dose could be adjusted to optimized outcome.

Because of the limited sample size and large effect size of treatment, there are few predictors, moderators, or mediators. With regards to the predictors of response to SSRIs the Research Units of Pediatric Psychopharmacology Anxiety Group Study found that increased symptom severity or the presence of social phobia predicted a lessened response to pharmacotherapy [79]. The study by Birmaher and colleagues [17] found that greater symptom severity decreased medication response, as did a positive family history.

Current practice recommendations include starting medications at low doses and gradually increasing the dose according to side effects and response [2]. As evidenced by the placebo-controlled trials, the treatment effect can be seen early but may take longer. Although only two SSRIs have been studied, it is likely that the class of SSRIs is effective for these disorders. The choice of SSRI should be guided by drug factors, such as half-life, drug interactions, and side effects, and patient factors, such as family history of medication response and history of sensitivity to other SSRIs.

Safety concerns

Recent concerns have arisen around the potential for increased suicidality during treatment with SSRIs and other antidepressants, particularly in children and adolescents [85,86]. The media have focused much attention on this issue since it first emerged in 2003, when the United Kingdom's Medicines and Health Care Products Regulatory Agency published a warning regarding prescribing antidepressants to patients who are younger than age 18 years [87]. With this warning, the Medicines and Health Care Products Regulatory Agency essentially relegated the use of SSRIs to specialists in the United Kingdom.

In September 2004, the US FDA held public hearings to review the safety and efficacy of antidepressant medications in youth, with a specific focus on the risk of suicidal ideation and behavior in early treatment. Although no completed suicides occurred and no individual study demonstrated a clear increased risk of suicidality, the US FDA concluded that suicidality may be associated with antidepressant treatment in some children and adolescents. The risk of suicidal thoughts and behavior was 4% in youths treated with antidepressants compared with 2% in the placebo group [42,88]. Based on these data, the US FDA Advisory Committee recommended the following: a black box warning about the risk of suicidality for all antidepressants when used in pediatric patients [85], a medication guide for parents provided with each prescription, closer monitoring of all youth taking antidepressant medications, and a plan for antidepressants to be prescribed in unit doses [89]. In late 2004, leading up to and just after these hearings, the number of patients younger than age 18 who received antidepressant prescriptions dropped 19% in the third quarter and 16% in the fourth quarter compared with the same time periods in 2003 [90]. Although the black box warning may reduce unnecessary prescribing and improve practice standards, it also may result in unanticipated and increased barriers to pharmacologic treatment for anxious youth who might otherwise benefit from antidepressant treatment.

Other medications

Although no data support the use of antihistamines, such as diphenhydramine and hydroxyzine, they have been used for the short-term treatment of anxiety and emotional upset in pediatric patients for decades [91]. Diphenhydramine was studied by Korein and colleagues [21] and found to be sedating in "neurotic disorder" patients but not anxiolytic. More recent surveys based on number of medication prescriptions has documented that antihistamines are still used frequently in child psychiatry, particularly for agitation and anxiety [92]. These medications are generally best used only for the short-term management of anxiety or bedtime sedation [40]. In view of the paucity of data and the propensity these medications have for anticholinergic [93] side effects, including confusion, they are not first-line medications for long-term treatment of pediatric anxiety.

In summary, double-blind trials have demonstrated the use of the SSRIs fluoxetine and fluvoxamine for treating pediatric SAD, social phobia, and GAD. Although these studies included patients with mixed anxiety disorders, in the subsequent sections we review trials for each of these disorders individually.

Separation anxiety disorder and school phobia and refusal

Gittleman-Klein and Klein [22] examined imipramine and CBT in children aged 6 to 14 years for school phobia ($n = 35$). The study posited CBT as useful for the core avoidance symptoms in school phobia, whereas pharmacotherapy helps with the physical symptoms of anxiety. Improvement was seen in 81% of the imipramine/CBT group as opposed to a 47% improvement in the placebo/CBT group after 6 weeks. Despite a lower response using nonpharmacologic therapy, 41% of children still returned to school. This study played an important role in inspiring future antidepressant trials in depressed youths. A subsequent study did not replicate these findings [22,94,95]. In the later trial, youths with SAD ($n = 45$) who did not respond to 4 weeks of CBT were randomized to receive either imipramine or placebo for an additional 6 weeks of treatment. Although half of the children showed improvement, there were no group differences in the ratings overall and the treatment group showed more side effects [95]. Compared with the earlier study, these participants did not have school refusal, had a greater placebo response rate, and may have had less severe levels of baseline anxiety. The authors concluded that imipramine "need not be precluded" from pediatric anxiety treatment but that the effect of imipramine in the initial study may not occur regularly.

Another controlled study examined the role of imipramine plus CBT in teen-agers with anxiety, depression, and school refusal [82]. Attendance increased significantly for the treatment group; anxiety and depression also decreased significantly. At 1-year follow-up, most children met criteria for an anxiety disorder, although school attendance remained improved [96]. Another trial compared imipramine (50–175 mg/d) and alprazolam (0.75–4 mg/d) for treating school phobia and related anxiety [97] over a 2-month period. Although significant differences were found between the two treatment groups in this small ($n = 24$), randomized, controlled trial, the results are difficult to interpret because the analyses of covariance showed no significant improvement.

Clomipramine failed to demonstrate benefit in a group of 51 children and adolescents with school refusal [98]. Doses used in this study (40–75 mg/d) were lower than those used in the clomipramine OCD studies described earlier (doses up to 250 mg/d) [6,7,46]. The ability to review this study critically was limited by the lack of specific diagnostic information. Overall, the evidence to support the use of TCAs for separation anxiety is mixed. Although clomipramine fails to demonstrate efficacy, imipramine may be useful with more severely ill children. The results are variable, however, and diagnostic developments limit generalization of these older studies to current practice.

Although commonly used in adults, few data support the use of benzodi-azepines for separation anxiety in children and adolescents. A small 4-week, double-blind, randomized, controlled trial of clonazepam in children and ado-lescents aged 7 to 13 years ($n = 15$) [99] did not demonstrate efficacy. Although the children seemed to benefit from clonazepam up to 2 mg/d, the effect was not found to be statistically significant. The main side effects were drowsiness and disinhibition, possibly because of rapid titration.

The strongest empirical evidence supporting the efficacy of the pharmaco-logic treatment of SADs is found in the trials that also include other anxiety disorders, as discussed earlier in this article. Few trials specifically focus on SAD alone. The literature generally supports the use of SSRIs as first-line phar-macologic management of SADs in children and adolescents [17,79]. Few data are available regarding the newer atypical antidepressants, and limited data sug-gest the use of TCAs mainly as second-line treatment because of possible adverse events and less clear supporting evidence [95,97].

Generalized anxiety disorder

Historically, barbiturates were the first agents used to treat GAD (anxiety neurosis) in adults and pediatric patients because of their availability and their sedative-hypnotic properties. Benzodiazepines replaced barbiturates because they are generally safer, particularly in overdoses. Although studies have documented the safety and efficacy of benzodiazepines in adults [100–102], few studies have been conducted in the pediatric age group. The studies are small and included children with multiple co-occurring conditions [97,99,103]. A 4-week open-label trial of alprazolam, up to 3.5 mg/d, in 12 children aged 8 to 16 years with overanxious or avoidant disorder failed to demonstrate efficacy [104]. No symptoms of withdrawal were noted; side effects were mild and included dry mouth and fatigue.

In adults, benzodiazepines are used commonly to alleviate anxiety symptoms, whereas SSRIs are titrated to benefit. Benzodiazepines can be used similarly in children for short duration and with close monitoring for side effects, such as sedation [105] and disinhibition (eg, temper tantrums, aggressive behavior, and irritability) [99] and behavioral dyscontrol in adolescents [106]. To minimize side effects, benzodiazepines are titrated slowly. Children tend to metabolize benzodiazepines more rapidly than adults [107,108]; however, if coadministering a benzodiazepine and an SSRI, lower doses of the benzodiazepine may be needed because of SSRI inhibition of benzodiazepine metabolism [109]. Withdrawal symptoms can occur with rapid discontinuation, including insomnia, anxiety, gastrointestinal discomfort, headache, concentration problems, and seizures [110]. Gradually tapering a benzodiazepine by reducing the dose every 5 days by 10% of the highest dose [111] reduces the risk of withdrawal symptoms [107]. Clinicians also should keep in mind the potential for abuse, particularly when treating teenagers with a history of substance abuse.

Fortunately, non-benzodiazepine options are available to treat pediatric GAD. The literature supports the safety and efficacy of SSRIs in adults [112–114], and some open-label [80,83] and controlled studies [17,18,79] have been conducted that included children and adolescents with GAD. A double-blind, placebo-controlled trial examined the use of sertraline treatment over a 9-week period to treat children aged 5 to 17 years with GAD [18]. Sertraline up to 50 mg was superior to placebo at 4 weeks (90% versus 10% response, respectively) and was well tolerated without any significant adverse events.

There are no reports of TCAs to specifically treat pediatric GAD, despite the fact that TCAs have been studied more extensively in other childhood anxiety disorders. Given the lack of data, TCAs are not the first-line treatment of children and adolescents with GAD.

Buspirone is a partial agonist at the serotonin 5HT1A receptor [3]. Although data exist regarding its efficacy for GAD in adults, there is some controversy concerning its clinical use [115,116]. Few data are available concerning its use in children and adolescents. Similar to antidepressants, it may take up to 4 weeks for buspirone to manifest benefit [117]. Often considered to have a mild side effect profile, an open trial of buspirone in prepubertal children hospitalized with anxiety and aggression ($n = 25$) documented agitation and manic symptoms in a significant number of subjects [118]. The efficacy of the SSRIs and scant data supporting the use of buspirone argue against its use in cases of pediatric anxiety.

Panic disorder

Although children with anxiety disorders often report attacks of anxiety secondary to confronting a feared stimulus, spontaneous panic attacks and panic disorder are uncommon in children [109]. Randomized, controlled trials have found SSRIs and TCAs to be efficacious treatments for adults with panic disorder

[109]. Data from noncontrolled studies of pediatric panic disorder support the use of SSRIs. In an open-label prospective study that examined SSRIs in 12 pediatric patients who had panic disorder, 75% responded and 67% could be considered remitted [119]. A second study examined the response of several pediatric anxiety disorders to fluoxetine over a 6- to 9-week period; 5 of 16 patients had panic disorder and 3 of 5 improved with fluoxetine treatment [83]. The mean dose in children was 24 mg and 40 mg in adolescents.

The lack of large, randomized, controlled trials regarding pediatric panic disorder is likely because of the low prevalence. Adult data and open clinical trials suggest that SSRIs should be considered first-line pharmacologic treatment choice for unusual pediatric patients with panic disorder, however. SSRIs should be instituted at low doses because patients who have panic disorder may have an exacerbation of their symptoms early in their treatment (eg, sertraline, 25 mg/d, or fluoxetine, 5 mg/d). Extrapolating from adult treatment guidelines [120], an adequate SSRI trial should last at least 12 weeks. If patients have not shown any response within 5 to 8 weeks, the diagnosis should be reconsidered and adherence to treatment should be verified.

Benzodiazepines sometimes can be effective in treating adult patients who have panic disorder, but they have not been studied for chronic use and there is some risk for tolerance and dependency [120]. Few data are available that focus specifically on the use of benzodiazepines in pediatric panic disorder, which suggests that they would not be a good first-line treatment.

For adults with panic disorder, it is recommended to continue treatment for 12 to 18 months [120]. In youths with anxiety disorders, the situation is less clear, although some experts suggest considering a gradual taper off the therapeutic agent after at least 1 year of symptomatic stability while carefully monitoring for signs of relapse [121].

Social phobia

Evidence in the adult literature supports the use of pharmacologic treatments in cases of adult social phobia [120]. Several randomized studies have examined the treatment of children with social phobia and other anxiety disorders with SSRIs [17,79]. Only one trial of primary social phobia or social phobia alone has been conducted. In this large, industry-sponsored, 16-week multicenter, randomized, placebo-controlled trial, for children and adolescents (aged 8–17 years) with social anxiety disorder ($n = 322$) as their predominant psychiatric disorder, paroxetine, 10 to 50 mg/d, was found to be superior to placebo (78% versus 39%). Side effects found significantly more commonly with paroxetine than placebo included insomnia, decreased appetite, and vomiting [122].

Selective mutism

Despite the fact that behavioral approaches are often considered first-line treatment, medication is likely to play a beneficial role in the treatment of selective mutism [123]. Selective mutism, often seen as a more severe variant of social phobia, has not been studied in controlled trials [79,124]; however, case reports or open-label studies demonstrate the usefulness of antidepressant medications [124–129]. The largest open-label study investigated the use of fluoxetine (mean dose, 28 mg) in 21 children who met criteria for selective mutism over a 9-week treatment course; 76% of participants' symptoms improved, with age correlating inversely with improvement. Five of the 21 children did not improve, and 2 children developed behavioral disinhibition that caused them to discontinue the study [129]. In another small trial of fluoxetine ($n = 16$), treatment outcomes were mixed [130]. The fluoxetine group (mean maximum dose, 0.6 mg/kg/d) responded significantly better than subjects on placebo on parent rating scales but not the clinician or teacher rating scales. It is also noteworthy that many participants were still symptomatic at the end of the trial.

Specific phobias

The first-line treatments for the specific phobias in adults and children are behavioral. Because many children with specific phobias have other co-occurring anxiety disorders and some may not benefit from behavioral treatments, however, medications have been used consistently as an adjunct. Similar to other anxiety disorders, SSRIs have been used with increasing frequency. Published reports are limited to a few case reports [131–133], however, and small controlled trials in adults [134]. Paroxetine, up to 20 mg/d, was given to 11 adult participants with specific phobias over a 4-week period. This study did not include "pure" phobia patients, which suggested that medication could have been moderated by comorbid anxiety; 50% of participants on paroxetine and 17% of participants on placebo responded. In a 9-week open-label trial, fluoxetine was administered to 16 children and adolescents with mixed anxiety disorders using a flexible fixed dose titration from up to 40 mg/d in children and up to 80 mg in adolescents [83]. Four of the six children with specific phobias responded to treatment without any reported problems of side effects.

Long-term treatment of non–obsessive-compulsive disorder and non–post-traumatic stress disorder anxiety disorders

For the non-OCD, non-PTSD anxiety disorders, limited data are available on how long it takes to reach maximum benefit, how durable treatment is, and how long one should treat to reduce the risk for relapse—issues that are critical to long-term treatment decision making. In a 6-month extension of the Research Units of Pediatric Psychopharmacology Anxiety Group Study, 94% of the responders to fluvoxamine continued in remission and approximately half of the placebo nonresponders responded to open fluvoxamine treatment [135]. Of the fluvoxamine nonresponders in the acute phase, 71% showed a significant decrease in their level of anxiety when switched to fluoxetine, which suggested that a switch within the class of SSRI medications may be helpful for some nonresponders. More studies are needed to examine the long-term safety of SSRIs and address the needs of youths with treatment-resistant anxiety.

In general, once the anxiety symptoms have remitted, a medication-free trial may be attempted. The length of time for treatment is unclear; however, patients who discontinue treatment after a shorter term should be followed closely for relapse. Longer term treatments may be associated with full recovery with smaller risks for relapse. Discontinuation should occur preferably during a period of lower stress for a child, such as during summer and after a trial of CBT [121].

Treatment-resistant non–obsessive-compulsive disorder and non–post-traumatic stress disorder anxiety disorders

Although we have increasing empirical evidence regarding the efficacy of SSRIs to treat pediatric anxiety disorders, many children remain symptomatic after an initial partial response to treatment. A longer treatment period and higher dosage may be needed to optimize treatment. Given the empirical support for CBT, it is possible that combined treatment may be the best approach for partially responsive patients. Few augmentation studies have been conducted; however, augmentation strategies used in OCD may be useful in non-OCD anxiety disorders.

Comorbidities with non–obsessive-compulsive disorder and non–post-traumatic stress disorder anxiety disorders

Anxiety disorders are commonly comorbid with affective disorders [136,137], substance abuse [138,139], and ADHD [140–142]. Many children and adolescents (up to 30%) have co-occurring ADHD and anxiety disorders [140,142]. Diagnosis may be challenging because symptoms can overlap each other. The Multimodal Treatment Study of ADHD (MTA) multicenter study found that the presence of these disorders concurrently does not affect the use of stimulants to treat ADHD. The MTA group also found that behavioral management had a place in addition to pharmacology in treating ADHD and anxiety symptoms [142,143]. Combining classes of medication such as SSRIs and stimulants can be helpful when treating these coexisting disorders despite limited empirical data [144,145]. The number of children with ADHD and anxiety who require multiple medications is unknown. One open study suggested that the adjunctive use of fluoxetine may help treat anxiety in children with ADHD [146]. Recent evidence suggests that children with ADHD and anxiety disorders have a similar response rate to stimulants as children with only ADHD; the benefit of adding fluvoxamine to stimulant treatment remains unclear [147]. More research is needed to clarify definitively the effect of stimulants and SSRIs on coexisting anxiety and ADHD.

Anxiety and depressive disorders are common internalizing disorders in children and adolescence. Analyses of comorbidity have shown that depression is significantly increased with all of the anxiety disorders except OCD [137]. The coexistence of anxiety disorders with depressive disorders tends to increase with age and may be seen more with social anxiety disorders [148,149]. Because SSRIs are effective for anxiety and depression, they are likely the treatment of choice. The presence of depression in children with anxiety requires additional attention to risk for suicidality.

Different anxiety disorders have varying associations with substance abuse, although all seem to increase the risk for alcohol abuse in the teenage years [138]. Specifically, children with social anxiety disorder may be more prone to drink alcohol than youths with GAD [136,150].

Bipolar disorder is another important comorbidity to consider when treating pediatric anxiety disorders, given the risk of switching into a manic or a hypomanic state secondary to antidepressant treatment. It is important to ascertain whether a patient has a personal or family history of bipolar disorder before starting an SSRI and to monitor carefully for any emergent manic symptoms.

Post-traumatic stress disorder

PTSD occurs frequently in children and adolescents, with up to 6% of youth meeting criteria for the diagnosis [151]. Despite the relatively high prevalence, relatively few studies support the use of medication in pediatric patients who have PTSD compared with adult patients [152–154].

In adults, clonidine and propanolol have been used to treat PTSD symptoms [152], particularly nightmares and exaggerated startle. Propanolol was evaluated in 11 pediatric patients who had PTSD (mean age, 8.5 years) with agitation, hyperarousal, and a history of sexual or physical abuse [155]. This study used an "A-B-A" approach, which compares participants off medication to on medication to off medication over a 4-week period. The study found efficacy for propanolol in alleviating symptoms, particularly arousal and intrusive symptoms, in 8 of 11 children. Clonidine also may be helpful in alleviating symptoms of hyperarousal and activation in PTSD. An open-label trial reported the use of transdermal clonidine as being effective for alleviating seven patients' symptoms [156], with the main adverse events being skin irritation and rebound hypertension. Similarly, relatively low doses of oral clonidine (0.05–0.1 mg twice a day) also have been shown to diminish hyperarousal and impulsivity symptoms in children and adolescents ($n = 17$) [157,157a]. Guanfacine was reported as being helpful in a case report when used to treat nightmares of a 7-year-old patient.

SSRIs frequently are used in children with PTSD based on extrapolation from adult evidence [158]. Citalopram, 20 to 40 mg/d, was useful over 8 weeks of open treatment [159]. SSRIs also may be useful in youths with PTSD symptoms and comorbid depressive or panic symptoms [160]. Several open-label pediatric studies have been conducted using nefazodone with youths with PTSD [161]; however, because of potential liver toxicity, it is not a first-line treatment [162]. Finally, one study was conducted regarding the use of TCAs in the pediatric trauma population. Robert and colleagues [163] used low-dose imipramine to treat acute stress disorder symptoms in children with burns. In these 25 children, it seemed that imipramine was a useful treatment particularly for sleep problems.

Other classes of medications also have been described as being useful in open trials. Carbamazepine (300–1200 mg/d dose range) was found beneficial in 22 of 28 youths with PTSD symptoms in one study [164]. There is limited scientific evidence to support the use of atypical antipsychotic agents in cases of pediatric PTSD.

Summary

The pharmacologic treatment of pediatric anxiety disorders has historic roots, which coupled with recent advances over the last decade, has expanded evidence-based practice; however, much work still remains to be done. This article provides a practical overview of the current literature with an emphasis on the results of controlled and open trials, side effects, short- and long-term treatment strategies, and treatment-resistant illness. SSRIs seem to be the treatment of choice for most pervasive and impairing anxiety disorders in youth. Despite extensive experience with the TCAs, side effects and less overall efficacy data relegate the TCAs to second-line treatment. Although benzodiazepines have been evaluated extensively in adults, they are less commonly used in children because of better alternatives and the risk for dependency in this vulnerable population. As research on the treatment of pediatric anxiety disorders continues, our understanding of who responds best to what treatment, how to combine medication with psychosocial treatments, how long to treat to reduce the risk for relapse off medication, and the long-term safety of current medications will improve the outcome for children who suffer from these disorders.

References

[1] Anderson JC, Williams S, McGee R, et al. DSM-III disorders in preadolescent children: prevalence in a large sample from the general population. Arch Gen Psychiatry 1987;44(1): 69–76.

[2] Bernstein GA, Shaw K. Practice parameters for the assessment and treatment of children and adolescents with anxiety disorders. J Am Acad Child Adolesc Psychiatry 1997;36(10 Suppl): 69S–84S.

[3] Velosa JF, Riddle MA. Pharmacologic treatment of anxiety disorders in children and adolescents. Child Adolesc Psychiatr Clin N Am 2000;9(1):119–33.

[4] Costello EJ, Angold A. Epidemiology. In: March JS, editor. Anxiety disorders in children and adolescents. New York: Guilford Press; 1995. p. 109–24.

[5] Pine DS, Cohen P, Gurley D, et al. The risk for early-adulthood anxiety and depressive disorders in adolescents with anxiety and depressive disorders. Arch Gen Psychiatry 1998; 55(1):56–64.

[6] Flament MF, Rapoport JL, Berg CJ, et al. Clomipramine treatment of childhood obsessive-compulsive disorder: a double-blind controlled study. Arch Gen Psychiatry 1985;42(10): 977–83.

[7] DeVeaugh-Geiss J, Moroz G, Biederman J, et al. Clomipramine hydrochloride in childhood and adolescent obsessive-compulsive disorder: a multicenter trial. J Am Acad Child Adolesc Psychiatry 1992;31(1):45–9.

[8] Montgomery SA, McIntyre A, Osterheider M, et al. A double-blind, placebo-controlled study of fluoxetine in patients with DSM-III-R obsessive-compulsive disorder: the Lilly European OCD Study Group. Eur Neuropsychopharmacol 1993;3(2):143–52.

[9] Tollefson GD, Rampey Jr AH, Potvin JH, et al. A multicenter investigation of fixed-dose fluoxetine in the treatment of obsessive-compulsive disorder. Arch Gen Psychiatry 1994; 51(7):559–67.

[10] Geller DA, Wagner KD, Emslie G, et al. Paroxetine treatment in children and adolescents with obsessive-compulsive disorder: a randomized, multicenter, double-blind, placebo-controlled trial. J Am Acad Child Adolesc Psychiatry 2004;43(11):1387–96.

[11] Geller DA, Hoog SL, Heiligenstein JH, et al. Fluoxetine treatment for obsessive-compulsive disorder in children and adolescents: a placebo-controlled clinical trial. J Am Acad Child Adolesc Psychiatry 2001;40(7):773–9.

[12] Riddle MA, Reeve EA, Yaryura-Tobias JA, et al. Fluvoxamine for children and adolescents with obsessive-compulsive disorder: a randomized, controlled, multicenter trial. J Am Acad Child Adolesc Psychiatry 2001;40(2):222–9.

[13] Riddle MA, Scahill L, King RA, et al. Double-blind, crossover trial of fluoxetine and placebo in children and adolescents with obsessive-compulsive disorder. J Am Acad Child Adolesc Psychiatry 1992;31(6):1062–9.

[14] Riddle MA, Hardin MT, King R, et al. Fluoxetine treatment of children and adolescents with Tourette's and obsessive compulsive disorders: preliminary clinical experience. J Am Acad Child Adolesc Psychiatry 1990;29(1):45–8.

[15] Pediatric OCD Treatment Study Team. Cognitive-behavior therapy, sertraline, and their combination for children and adolescents with obsessive-compulsive disorder: the Pediatric OCD Treatment Study (POTS) randomized controlled trial. JAMA 2004;292(16):1969–76.

[16] Walkup JT, Labellarte MJ, Riddle MA, et al. Fluvoxamine for the treatment of anxiety disorders in children and adolescents. N Engl J Med 2001;344(17):1279–85.

[17] Birmaher B, Axelson DA, Monk K, et al. Fluoxetine for the treatment of childhood anxiety disorders. J Am Acad Child Adolesc Psychiatry 2003;42(4):415–23.

[18] Rynn MA, Siqueland L, Rickels K. Placebo-controlled trial of sertraline in the treatment of children with generalized anxiety disorder. Am J Psychiatry 2001;158(12):2008–14.

[19] Eisenberg L, Gilbert A, Cytryn L, et al. The effectiveness of psychotherapy alone and in conjunction with perphenazine or placebo in the treatment of neurotic and hyperkinetic children. Am J Psychiatry 1961;117:1088–93.

[20] Cytryn L, Gilbert A, Eisenberg L. The effectiveness of tranquilizing drugs plus supportive psychotherapy in treating behavior disorders of children: a double blind study of eighty outpatients. Am J Orthopsychiatry 1960;30:113–28.

[21] Korein J, Fish B, Shapiro T, et al. EEG and behavioral effects of drug therapy in children: chlorpromazine and diphenhydramine. Arch Gen Psychiatry 1971;24(6):552–63.

[22] Gittleman-Klein R, Klein D. Controlled imipramine treatment of school phobia. Arch Gen Psychiatry 1971;25:204–7.

[23] American Psychiatric Association. Diagnostic and statistical manual of mental disorders. 3rd edition. Washington (DC): American Psychiatric Association; 1980.

[24] Kaufman J, Birmaher B, Brent DA, et al. K-SADS-PL. J Am Acad Child Adolesc Psychiatry 2000;39(10):1208.

[25] Shaffer D, Fisher P, Lucas CP, et al. NIMH diagnostic interview schedule for children version IV (NIMH DISC-IV): description, differences from previous versions, and reliability of some common diagnoses. J Am Acad Child Adolesc Psychiatry 2000;39(1):28–38.

[26] Labellarte M, Ginsburg GS. Anxiety disorders. In: Martin A, Scahill L, Charney D, et al, editors. Pediatric psychopharmacology: principles and practice. New York: Oxford University Press; 2003. p. 496–510.

[27] March JS, Biederman J, Wolkow R, et al. Sertraline in children and adolescents with obsessive-compulsive disorder: a multicenter randomized controlled trial. JAMA 1998; 280(20):1752–6.

[28] Flament MF, Whitaker A, Rapoport JL, et al. Obsessive compulsive disorder in adolescence: an epidemiological study. J Am Acad Child Adolesc Psychiatry 1988;27(6):764–71.

[29] Douglass HM, Moffitt TE, Dar R, et al. Obsessive-compulsive disorder in a birth cohort of 18-year-olds: prevalence and predictors. J Am Acad Child Adolesc Psychiatry 1995;34(11): 1424–31.

[30] Pauls DL, Alsobrook JP, Goodman W, et al. A family study of obsessive-compulsive disorder. Am J Psychiatry 1995;152(1):76–84.

[31] Geller DA, Spencer T. Obsessive-compulsive disorder. In: Martin A, Seahill L, Charney D, et al, editors. Pediatric psychopharmacology: principles and practice. New York: Oxford University Press; 2003. p. 511–25.

[32] Nestadt G, Addington A, Samuels J, et al. The identification of OCD-related subgroups based on comorbidity. Biol Psychiatry 2003;53(10):914–20.

[33] Hanna GL, Piacentini J, Cantwell DP, et al. Obsessive-compulsive disorder with and without tics in a clinical sample of children and adolescents. Depress Anxiety 2002;16(2):59–63.

[34] Miguel EC, Leckman JF, Rauch S, et al. Obsessive-compulsive disorder phenotypes: implications for genetic studies. Mol Psychiatry 2005;10(3):258–75.

[35] Piacentini J. Cognitive behavioral therapy of childhood OCD. Child Adolesc Psychiatr Clin N Am 1999;8(3):599–616.

[36] Jenike MA. Pharmacologic treatment of obsessive compulsive disorders. Psychiatr Clin North Am 1992;15(4):895–919.

[37] Flament MF, Koby E, Rapoport JL, et al. Childhood obsessive-compulsive disorder: a prospective follow-up study. J Child Psychol Psychiatry 1990;31(3):363–80.

[38] Green WH. Child and adolescent clinical psychopharmacology. 3rd edition. Philadelphia: Lippincott Williams and Wilkins; 1997.

[39] Psychotropic prescribing guide (PDR). New Jersey: Thomson; 2004.

[40] Labellarte MJ, Ginsburg GS, Walkup JT, et al. The treatment of anxiety disorders in children and adolescents. Biol Psychiatry 1999;46(11):1567–78.

[41] Geller DA, Biederman J, Stewart SE, et al. Which SSRI? A meta-analysis of pharmacotherapy trials in pediatric obsessive-compulsive disorder. Am J Psychiatry 2003;160(11):1919–28.

[42] Hammad T. Review and evaluation of clinical data: relationship between psychotropic drugs and pediatric suicidality. Available at: http://www.fda.gov/ohrms/dockets/ac/04/briefing/2004-4065b1-10-TAB08-Hammads-Review.pdf. Accessed February 3, 2005.

[43] Scharko AM. Selective serotonin reuptake inhibitor-induced sexual dysfunction in adolescents: a review. J Am Acad Child Adolesc Psychiatry 2004;43(9):1071–9.

[44] Nilsson M, Joliat MJ, Miner CM, et al. Safety of subchronic treatment with fluoxetine for major depressive disorder in children and adolescents. J Child Adolesc Psychopharmacol 2004;14(3):412–7.

[45] Weintrob N, Cohen D, Klipper-Aurbach Y, et al. Decreased growth during therapy with selective serotonin reuptake inhibitors. Arch Pediatr Adolesc Med 2002;156(7):696–701.

[46] Leonard HL, Swedo SE, Rapoport JL, et al. Treatment of obsessive-compulsive disorder with clomipramine and desipramine in children and adolescents: a double-blind crossover comparison. Arch Gen Psychiatry 1989;46(12):1088–92.

[47] Geller DA, Biederman J, Stewart SE, et al. Impact of comorbidity on treatment response to paroxetine in pediatric obsessive-compulsive disorder: is the use of exclusion criteria empirically supported in randomized clinical trials? J Child Adolesc Psychopharmacol 2003; 13(Suppl 1):S19–29.

[48] March J, Franklin M, Carpenter D, et al. The expert consensus guideline series: treatment of obsessive-compulsive disorder. J Clin Psychiatry 1997;58(Suppl 4):12–27.

[49] Cook EH, Wagner KD, March JS, et al. Long-term sertraline treatment of children and adolescents with obsessive-compulsive disorder. J Am Acad Child Adolesc Psychiatry 2001; 40(10):1175–81.

[50] Walkup JT, Reeve E, Yaryuya-Tobias J, et al. Fluvoxamine for childhood OCD: long-term treatment. Presented at the 45th Annual Meeting of the American Academy of Child and Adolescent Psychiatry. Anaheim (CA), October 1998.

[51] Leonard HL, Swedo SE, Lenane MC, et al. A double-blind desipramine substitution during long-term clomipramine treatment in children and adolescents with obsessive-compulsive disorder. Arch Gen Psychiatry 1991;48(10):922–7.

[52] Wagner KD, Ambrosini P, Rynn M, et al. Efficacy of sertraline in the treatment of children and adolescents with major depressive disorder: two randomized controlled trials. JAMA 2003; 290(8):1033–41.

[53] Greist JH, Jefferson JW, Kobak KA, et al. A 1 year double-blind placebo-controlled fixed dose study of sertraline in the treatment of obsessive-compulsive disorder. Int Clin Psychopharmacol 1995;10(2):57–65.

[54] Thomsen PH. Child and adolescent obsessive-compulsive disorder treated with citalopram: findings from an open trial of 23 cases. J Child Adolesc Psychopharmacol 1997;7(3):157–66.

[55] American Academy of Child and Adolescent Psychiatry. Summary of the practice parameters for the assessment and treatment of children and adolescents with obsessive-compulsive disorder. J Am Acad Child Adolesc Psychiatry 1998;37(10):1110–6.

[56] Stewart SE, Geller DA, Jenike M, et al. Long-term outcome of pediatric obsessive-compulsive disorder: a meta-analysis and qualitative review of the literature. Acta Psychiatr Scand 2004; 110(1):4–13.

[57] Leonard HL, Swedo SE, Lenane MC, et al. A 2- to 7-year follow-up study of 54 obsessive-compulsive children and adolescents. Arch Gen Psychiatry 1993;50(6):429–39.

[58] Wewetzer C, Jans T, Muller B, et al. Long-term outcome and prognosis of obsessive-compulsive disorder with onset in childhood or adolescence. Eur Child Adolesc Psychiatry 2001;10(1):37–46.

[59] McDougle CJ, Kresch LE, Goodman WK, et al. A case-controlled study of repetitive thoughts and behavior in adults with autistic disorder and obsessive-compulsive disorder. Am J Psychiatry 1995;152(5):772–7.

[60] Jacobsen FM. Risperidone in the treatment of affective illness and obsessive-compulsive disorder. J Clin Psychiatry 1995;56(9):423–9.

[61] Leonard HL, Topol D, Bukstein O, et al. Clonazepam as an augmenting agent in the treatment of childhood-onset obsessive-compulsive disorder. J Am Acad Child Adolesc Psychiatry 1994;33(6):792–4.

[62] Figueroa Y, Rosenberg DR, Birmaher B, et al. Combination treatment with clomipramine and selective serotonin reuptake inhibitors for obsessive-compulsive disorder in children and adolescents. J Child Adolesc Psychopharmacol 1998;8(1):61–7.

[63] Simeon JG, Thatte S, Wiggins D. Treatment of adolescent obsessive-compulsive disorder with a clomipramine-fluoxetine combination. Psychopharmacol Bull 1990;26(3):285–90.

[64] Fux M, Benjamin J, Belmaker RH. Inositol versus placebo augmentation of serotonin reuptake inhibitors in the treatment of obsessive-compulsive disorder: a double-blind cross-over study. Int J Neuropsychopharmacol 1999;2(3):193–5.

[65] Dannon PN, Sasson Y, Hirschmann S, et al. Pindolol augmentation in treatment-resistant obsessive compulsive disorder: a double-blind placebo controlled trial. Eur Neuropsychopharmacol 2000;10(3):165–9.

[66] Warneke L. Intravenous chlorimipramine therapy in obsessive-compulsive disorder. Can J Psychiatry 1989;34(9):853–9.

[67] Warneke LB. Intravenous chlorimipramine in the treatment of obsessional disorder in adolescence: case report. J Clin Psychiatry 1985;46(3):100–3.

[68] Fallon BA, Campeas R, Schneier FR, et al. Open trial of intravenous clomipramine in five treatment-refractory patients with obsessive-compulsive disorder. J Neuropsychiatry Clin Neurosci 1992;4(1):70–5.

[69] Baer L, Rauch SL, Ballantine Jr HT, et al. Cingulotomy for intractable obsessive-compulsive disorder: prospective long-term follow-up of 18 patients. Arch Gen Psychiatry 1995;52(5): 384–92.

[70] Swedo SE, Leonard HL, Garvey M, et al. Pediatric autoimmune neuropsychiatric disorders associated with streptococcal infections: clinical description of the first 50 cases. Am J Psychiatry 1998;155(2):264–71.

[71] Swedo SE, Leonard HL, Garvey M, et al. Pediatric autoimmune neuropsychiatric disorders associated with streptococcal infections: clinical description of the first 50 cases. Am J Psychiatry 1998;155(2):264–71.

[72] Leonard HL, Swedo SE. Paediatric autoimmune neuropsychiatric disorders associated with streptococcal infection (PANDAS). Int J Neuropsychopharmacol 2001;4(2):191–8.

[73] Nicolson R, Swedo SE, Lenane M, et al. An open trial of plasma exchange in childhood-onset obsessive-compulsive disorder without poststreptococcal exacerbations. J Am Acad Child Adolesc Psychiatry 2000;39(10):1313–5.

[73a] National Institute of Mental Health. Pediatric autoimmune neuropsychiatric disorders associated with streptococcal infections. Available at: http://intramural.nimh.nih.gov/pdn/faqs.htm. Accessed August 9, 2005.

[73b] Snider LA, Swedo SE. Childhood-onset obsessive-compulsive disorder and tic disorders: case report and literature review. J Child Adolesc Psychopharmacol 2003;13(Suppl 1):S81–8.

[74] Garvey MA, Perlmutter SJ, Allen AJ, et al. A pilot study of penicillin prophylaxis for neuropsychiatric exacerbations triggered by streptococcal infections. Biol Psychiatry 1999;45(12): 1564–71.

[75] Snider LA, Lougee L, Slattery M, et al. Antibiotic prophylaxis with azithromycin or penicillin for childhood-onset neuropsychiatric disorders. Biol Psychiatry 2005;57(7):788–92.

[76] McGee R, Feehan M, Williams S, et al. DSM-III disorders from age 11 to age 15 years. J Am Acad Child Adolesc Psychiatry 1992;31(1):50–9.

[77] Kashani JH, Orvaschel H. A community study of anxiety in children and adolescents. Am J Psychiatry 1990;147(3):313–8.

[78] Clark DB, Smith MG, Neighbors BD, et al. Anxiety disorders in adolescence: characteristics, prevalence, and comorbidities. Clin Psychol Rev 1994;14(2):113–37.

[79] Research Units for Pediatric Psychopharmacology (RUPP) Anxiety Study Group. Fluvoxamine for the treatment of anxiety disorders in children and adolescents. N Engl J Med 2001;344:1279–85.

[80] Birmaher B, Waterman GS, Ryan N, et al. Fluoxetine for childhood anxiety disorders. J Am Acad Child Adolesc Psychiatry 1994;33(7):993–9.

[81] Mendel JG, Klein DF. Anxiety attacks with subsequent agoraphobia. Compr Psychiatry 1969; 10(3):190–5.

[82] Bernstein GA, Borchardt CM, Perwien AR, et al. Imipramine plus cognitive-behavioral therapy in the treatment of school refusal. J Am Acad Child Adolesc Psychiatry 2000;39(3): 276–83.

[83] Fairbanks JM, Pine DS, Tancer NK, et al. Open fluoxetine treatment of mixed anxiety disorders in children and adolescents. J Child Adolesc Psychopharmacol 1997;7(1):17–29.

[84] The Pediatric Anxiety Rating Scale (PARS): development and psychometric properties. J Am Acad Child Adolesc Psychiatry 2002;41(9):1061–9.

[85] Licinio J, Wong ML. Depression, antidepressants and suicidality: a critical appraisal. Nat Rev Drug Discov 2005;4(2):165–71.

[86] Gibbons RD, Hur K, Bhaumik DK, et al. The relationship between antidepressant medication use and rate of suicide. Arch Gen Psychiatry 2005;62(2):165–72.

[87] Medicines and Healthcare Products Regulatory Agency. Safety of selective serotonin reuptake inhibitor antidepressants. Available at: http://www.mhra.gov.uk/news/2004/SSRIs_061204.pdf. Accessed February 3, 2005.

[88] US Food and Drug Administration. FDA statement on recommendations of the Psychopharmacologic Drugs and Pediatric Advisory Committee. Available at: http://www.fda.gov/cder/drug/antidepressants/default. Accessed February 3, 2005.

[89] US Food and Drug Administration. FDA recommendation for black box warning. Available at: http://www.fda.gov/cder/drug/antidepressants.PL_template.pdf. Accessed February 3, 2005.

[90] Elias M. Kids' antidepressant use declines. Available at: http://www.usatoday.com/news/health/2005-01-31-antidepressant-inside_x.htm. Accessed August 9, 2005.

[91] Lader M. Clinical pharmacology of non-benzodiazepine anxiolytics. Pharmacol Biochem Behav 1988;29(4):797–8.

[92] Zito JM, Safer DJ, dosReis S, et al. Trends in the prescribing of psychotropic medications to preschoolers. JAMA 2000;283(8):1025–30.

[93] Barnett SR, Riddle MA. Anxiolytics: benzodiazepines, buspirone, and others. In: Martin A, Scahill L, Charney D, et al, editors. Pediatric psychopharmacology: principles and practice. New York: Oxford University Press; 2003. p. 341–51.

[94] Gittleman-Klein R, Klein D. School phobia: diagnostic considerations in light of imipramine effects. J Nerv Ment Dis 1973;156:199–215.

[95] Klein RG, Koplewicz HS, Kanner A. Imipramine treatment of children with separation anxiety disorder. J Am Acad Child Adolesc Psychiatry 1992;31(1):21–8.

[96] Bernstein GA, Hektner JM, Borchardt CM, et al. Treatment of school refusal: one-year follow-up. J Am Acad Child Adolesc Psychiatry 2001;40(2):206–13.

[97] Bernstein GA, Garfinkel BD, Borchardt CM. Comparative studies of pharmacotherapy for school refusal. J Am Acad Child Adolesc Psychiatry 1990;29(5):773–81.

[98] Berney T, Kolvin I, Bhate SR, et al. School phobia: a therapeutic trial with clomipramine and short-term outcome. Br J Psychiatry 1981;138:110–8.

[99] Graae F, Milner J, Rizzotto L, et al. Clonazepam in childhood anxiety disorders. J Am Acad Child Adolesc Psychiatry 1994;33(3):372–6.

[100] Rickels K, Csanalosi I, Greisman P, et al. A controlled clinical trial of alprazolam for the treatment of anxiety. Am J Psychiatry 1983;140(1):82–5.

[101] Rickels K, Case WG, Downing RW, et al. Long-term diazepam therapy and clinical outcome. JAMA 1983;250(6):767–71.

[102] Rickels K, Schweizer E, Case WG, et al. Long-term therapeutic use of benzodiazepines. I. Effects of abrupt discontinuation. Arch Gen Psychiatry 1990;47(10):899–907.

[103] Simeon JG, Ferguson HB, Knott V, et al. Clinical, cognitive, and neurophysiological effects of alprazolam in children and adolescents with overanxious and avoidant disorders. J Am Acad Child Adolesc Psychiatry 1992;31(1):29–33.

[104] Simeon JG, Ferguson HB. Alprazolam effects in children with anxiety disorders. Can J Psychiatry 1987;32(7):570–4.

[105] Riddle MA, Bernstein GA, Cook EH, et al. Anxiolytics, adrenergic agents, and naltrexone. J Am Acad Child Adolesc Psychiatry 1999;38(5):546–56.

[106] Reiter S, Kutcher SP. Disinhibition and anger outbursts in adolescents treated with clonazepam. J Clin Psychopharmacol 1991;11(4):268.

[107] Coffey B, Shader RI, Greenblatt DJ. Pharmacokinetics of benzodiazepines and psychostimulants in children. J Clin Psychopharmacol 1983;3(4):217–25.

[108] Simeon JG. Use of anxiolytics in children. Encephale 1993;19(2):71–4.

[109] Birmaher B, Ollendick TH. Childhood-onset panic disorder. In: Ollendick TH, March JS, editors. Phobic and anxiety disorders in children and adolescents: a clinician's guide to effective psychosocial and pharmacological interventions. Oxford: Oxford University Press; 2004. p. 306–33.

[110] Kutcher SP, Reiter S, Gardner DM, et al. The pharmacotherapy of anxiety disorders in children and adolescents. Psychiatr Clin North Am 1992;15(1):41–67.

[111] Kutcher SP, Reiter S, Gardner DM, Klein RG. The pharmacotherapy of anxiety disorders in children and adolescents. Psychiatr Clin North Am 1992;15(1):41–67.

[112] Pollack MH, Zaninelli R, Goddard A, et al. Paroxetine in the treatment of generalized anxiety disorder: results of a placebo-controlled, flexible-dosage trial. J Clin Psychiatry 2001;62(5):350–7.

[113] Rickels K, Pollack MH, Sheehan DV, et al. Efficacy of extended-release venlafaxine in

nondepressed outpatients with generalized anxiety disorder. Am J Psychiatry 2000;157(6): 968–74.

[114] Gelenberg AJ, Lydiard RB, Rudolph RL, et al. Efficacy of venlafaxine extended-release capsules in nondepressed outpatients with generalized anxiety disorder: a 6-month randomized controlled trial. JAMA 2000;283(23):3082–8.

[115] Rickels K. Buspirone in clinical practice. J Clin Psychiatry 1990;51(Suppl):51–4.

[116] Sheehan DV, Raj AB, Sheehan KH, et al. Is buspirone effective for panic disorder? J Clin Psychopharmacol 1990;10(1):3–11.

[117] Kutcher SP, Reiter S, Gardner DM, et al. The pharmacotherapy of anxiety disorders in children and adolescents. Psychiatr Clin North Am 1992;15(1):41–67.

[118] Pfeffer CR, Jiang H, Domeshek LJ. Buspirone treatment of psychiatrically hospitalized prepubertal children with symptoms of anxiety and moderately severe aggression. J Child Adolesc Psychopharmacol 1997;7(3):145–55.

[119] Renaud J, Birmaher B, Wassick SC, et al. Use of selective serotonin reuptake inhibitors for the treatment of childhood panic disorder: a pilot study. J Child Adolesc Psychopharmacol 1999;9(2):73–83.

[120] American Psychiatric Association. Practice guidelines for the treatment of psychiatric disorders: compendium 2000. Washington (DC): American Psychiatric Association; 2000.

[121] Pine DS. Treating children and adolescents with selective serotonin reuptake inhibitors: how long is appropriate? J Child Adolesc Psychopharmacol 2002;12(3):189–203.

[122] Wagner KD, Berard R, Stein MB, et al. A multicenter, randomized, double-blind, placebo-controlled trial of paroxetine in children and adolescents with social anxiety disorder. Arch Gen Psychiatry 2004;61(11):1153–62.

[123] Garcia AM, Freeman JB, Francis G, et al. Selective mutism. In: Ollendick TH, March JS, editors. Phobic and anxiety disorders in children and adolescents: a clinician's guide to effective psychosocial and pharmacological interventions. Oxford (UK): Oxford University Press; 2004. p. 433–55.

[124] Black B, Uhde TW. Elective mutism as a variant of social phobia. J Am Acad Child Adolesc Psychiatry 1992;31(6):1090–4.

[125] Carlson JS, Kratochwill TR, Johnston HF. Sertraline treatment of 5 children diagnosed with selective mutism: a single-case research trial. J Child Adolesc Psychopharmacol 1999;9(4): 293–306.

[126] Wright HH, Cuccaro ML, Leonhardt TV, et al. Case study: fluoxetine in the multimodal treatment of a preschool child with selective mutism. J Am Acad Child Adolesc Psychiatry 1995;34(7):857–62.

[127] Golwyn DH, Weinstock RC. Phenelzine treatment of elective mutism: a case report. J Clin Psychiatry 1990;51(9):384–5.

[128] Golwyn DH, Sevlie CP. Phenelzine treatment of selective mutism in four prepubertal children. J Child Adolesc Psychopharmacol 1999;9(2):109–13.

[129] Dummit III ES, Klein RG, Tancer NK, et al. Fluoxetine treatment of children with selective mutism: an open trial. J Am Acad Child Adolesc Psychiatry 1996;35(5):615–21.

[130] Black B, Uhde TW. Treatment of elective mutism with fluoxetine: a double-blind, placebo-controlled study. J Am Acad Child Adolesc Psychiatry 1994;33(7):1000–6.

[131] Abene MV, Hamilton JD. Resolution of fear of flying with fluoxetine treatment. J Anxiety Disord 1998;12(6):599–603.

[132] Balon R. Fluvoxamine for phobia of storms. Acta Psychiatr Scand 1999;100(3):244–5.

[133] Viswanathan R, Paradis C. Treatment of cancer phobia with fluoxetine. Am J Psychiatry 1991;148(8):1090.

[134] Benjamin J, Ben Zion IZ, Karbofsky E, et al. Double-blind placebo-controlled pilot study of paroxetine for specific phobia. Psychopharmacology (Berl) 2000;149(2):194–6.

[135] Walkup J, Labellarte M, Riddle MA, et al. Treatment of pediatric anxiety disorders: an open-label extension of the research units on pediatric psychopharmacology anxiety study. J Child Adolesc Psychopharmacol 2002;12(3):175–88.

[136] Angold A, Costello EJ. Depressive comorbidity in children and adolescents: empirical, theoretical, and methodological issues. Am J Psychiatry 1993;150(12):1779–91.

[137] Lewinsohn PM, Zinbarg R, Seeley JR, et al. Lifetime comorbidity among anxiety disorders and between anxiety disorders and other mental disorders in adolescents. J Anxiety Disord 1997;11(4):377–94.

[138] Schuckit MA, Hesselbrock V. Alcohol dependence and anxiety disorders: what is the relationship? Am J Psychiatry 1994;151(12):1723–34.

[139] Manassis K, Monga S. A therapeutic approach to children and adolescents with anxiety disorders and associated comorbid conditions. J Am Acad Child Adolesc Psychiatry 2001; 40(1):115–7.

[140] Biederman J, Newcorn J, Sprich S. Comorbidity of attention deficit hyperactivity disorder with conduct, depressive, anxiety, and other disorders. Am J Psychiatry 1991;148(5):564–77.

[141] Kendall PC, Brady EU, Verduin TL. Comorbidity in childhood anxiety disorders and treatment outcome. J Am Acad Child Adolesc Psychiatry 2001;40(7):787–94.

[142] Jensen PS, Hinshaw SP, Kraemer HC, et al. ADHD comorbidity findings from the MTA study: comparing comorbid subgroups. J Am Acad Child Adolesc Psychiatry 2001;40(2):147–58.

[143] March JS, Swanson JM, Arnold LE, et al. Anxiety as a predictor and outcome variable in the multimodal treatment study of children with ADHD (MTA). J Abnorm Child Psychol 2000; 28(6):527–41.

[144] Pliszka SR, Greenhill LL, Crismon ML, et al. The Texas Children's Medication Algorithm Project: Report of the Texas consensus conference panel on medication treatment of childhood attention-deficit/hyperactivity disorder. Part I. Attention-deficit/hyperactivity disorder. J Am Acad Child Adolesc Psychiatry 2000;39(7):908–19.

[145] Rushton JL, Whitmire JT. Pediatric stimulant and selective serotonin reuptake inhibitor prescription trends: 1992 to 1998. Arch Pediatr Adolesc Med 2001;155(5):560–5.

[146] Barrickman L, Noyes R, Kuperman S, et al. Treatment of ADHD with fluoxetine: a preliminary trial. J Am Acad Child Adolesc Psychiatry 1991;30(5):762–7.

[147] Abikoff H, McGough J, Vitiello B, et al. Sequential pharmacotherapy for children with comorbid attention-deficit/hyperactivity and anxiety disorders. J Am Acad Child Adolesc Psychiatry 2005;44(5):418–27.

[148] Manassis K, Menna R. Depression in anxious children: possible factors in comorbidity. Depress Anxiety 1999;10(1):18–24.

[149] Bernstein GA. Comorbidity and severity of anxiety and depressive disorders in a clinic sample. J Am Acad Child Adolesc Psychiatry 1991;30(1):43–50.

[150] Kaplow JB, Curran PJ, Angold A, et al. The prospective relation between dimensions of anxiety and the initiation of adolescent alcohol use. J Clin Child Psychol 2001;30(3):316–26.

[151] Giaconia RM, Reinherz HZ, Silverman AB, et al. Traumas and posttraumatic stress disorder in a community population of older adolescents. J Am Acad Child Adolesc Psychiatry 1995; 34(10):1369–80.

[152] Ursano RJ, Bell C, Eth S, et al. Practice guideline for the treatment of patients with acute stress disorder and posttraumatic stress disorder. Am J Psychiatry 2004;161(11 Suppl):3–31.

[153] The Expert Consensus Panels for PTSD. The expert consensus guideline series: treatment of posttraumatic stress disorder. J Clin Psychiatry 1999;60(Suppl 16):3–76.

[154] Cohen JA, Mannarino AP. Posttraumatic stress disorder. In: Ollendick TH, March JS, editors. Phobic and anxiety disorders in children and adolescents: a clinician's guide to effective psychosocial and pharmacological interventions. Oxford (UK): Oxford University Press; 2004. p. 405–32.

[155] Famularo R, Kinscherff R, Fenton T. Propranolol treatment for childhood posttraumatic stress disorder, acute type: a pilot study. Am J Dis Child 1988;142(11):1244–7.

[156] Harmon RJ, Riggs PD. Clonidine for posttraumatic stress disorder in preschool children. J Am Acad Child Adolesc Psychiatry 1996;35(9):1247–9.

[157] Perry BD. Neurobiological sequelae of childhood trauma: PTSD in children. In: Murburg MM, editor. Catecholamine function in posttraumatic stress disorder: emerging concepts. Washington (DC): American Psychiatric Press; 1994. p. 233–55.

[157a] Horrigan JP. Guanfacine for PTSD nightmares. J Am Acad Child Adolesc Psychiatry 1996; 35(8):975–6.

[158] Donnelly C. Post-traumatic stress disorder. In: Martin A, Scahill L, Charney D, et al, editors. Pediatric psychopharmacology: principles and practice. New York: Oxford University Press; 2003. p. 580–91.

[159] Seedat S, Stein DJ, Ziervogel C, et al. Comparison of response to a selective serotonin reuptake inhibitor in children, adolescents, and adults with posttraumatic stress disorder. J Child Adolesc Psychopharmacol 2002;12(1):37–46.

[160] Brent DA, Perper JA, Moritz G, et al. Posttraumatic stress disorder in peers of adolescent suicide victims: predisposing factors and phenomenology. J Am Acad Child Adolesc Psychiatry 1995;34(2):209–15.

[161] Domon SE, Andersen MS. Nefazodone for PTSD. J Am Acad Child Adolesc Psychiatry 2000;39(8):942–3.

[162] Schwetz BA. From the Food and Drug Administration. JAMA 2002;287(9):1103.

[163] Robert R, Blakeney PE, Villarreal C, et al. Imipramine treatment in pediatric burn patients with symptoms of acute stress disorder: a pilot study. J Am Acad Child Adolesc Psychiatry 1999;38(7):873–82.

[164] Looff D, Grimley P, Kuller F, et al. Carbamazepine for PTSD. J Am Acad Child Adolesc Psychiatry 1995;34(6):703–4.

ELSEVIER
SAUNDERS

Child Adolesc Psychiatric Clin N Am
14 (2005) 909–923

CHILD AND
ADOLESCENT
PSYCHIATRIC CLINICS
OF NORTH AMERICA

Cumulative Index 2005

Note: Page numbers of article titles are in **boldface** type.

1056-4993/05/$ – see front matter © 2005 Elsevier Inc. All rights reserved.
doi:10.1016/S1056-4993(05)00088-X

childpsych.theclinics.com

United States Postal Service
Statement of Ownership, Management, and Circulation

1. Publication Title	2. Publication Number	3. Filing Date
Child and Adolescent Psychiatric Clinics of North America	1 0 5 6 - 4 9 9 3	9/15/05

4. Issue Frequency	5. Number of Issues Published Annually	6. Annual Subscription Price
Jan, Apr, Jul, Oct	4	$175.00

7. Complete Mailing Address of Known Office of Publication (Not printer) (Street, city, county, state, and ZIP+4)

Elsevier, Inc.
6277 Sea Harbor Drive
Orlando, FL 32887-4800

Contact Person
Gwen C. Campbell

Telephone
215-239-3685

8. Complete Mailing Address of Headquarters or General Business Office of Publisher (Not printer)

Elsevier, Inc., 360 Park Avenue South, New York, NY 10010-1710

9. Full Names and Complete Mailing Addresses of Publisher, Editor, and Managing Editor (Do not leave blank)

Publisher (Name and complete mailing address)

Tim Griswold, Elsevier, Inc., 1600 John F. Kennedy Blvd. Suite 1800, Philadelphia, PA 19103-2899

Editor (Name and complete mailing address)

Sarah Barth, Elsevier, Inc., 1600 John F. Kennedy Blvd. Suite 1800, Philadelphia, PA 19103-2899

Managing Editor (Name and complete mailing address)

Heather Cullen, Elsevier, Inc., 1600 John F. Kennedy Blvd. Suite 1800, Philadelphia, PA 19103-2899

10. Owner (Do not leave blank. If the publication is owned by a corporation, give the name and address of the corporation immediately followed by the names and addresses of all stockholders owning or holding 1 percent or more of the total amount of stock. If not owned by a corporation, give the names and addresses of the individual owners. If owned by a partnership or other unincorporated firm, give its name and address as well as those of each individual owner. If the publication is published by a nonprofit organization, give its name and address.)

Full Name	Complete Mailing Address
Wholly owned subsidiary of	4520 East-West Highway
Reed/Elsevier, US holdings	Bethesda, MD 20814

11. Known Bondholders, Mortgages, and Other Security Holders Owning or Holding 1 Percent or More of Total Amount of Bonds, Mortgages, or Other Securities. If none, check box   ▶ ☐ None

Full Name	Complete Mailing Address
N/A	

12. Tax Status (For completion by nonprofit organizations authorized to mail at nonprofit rates) (Check one)
The purpose, function, and nonprofit status of this organization and the exempt status for federal income tax purposes:
☐ Has Not Changed During Preceding 12 Months
☐ Has Changed During Preceding 12 Months (Publisher must submit explanation of change with this statement)

(See Instructions on Reverse)

PS Form 3526, October 1999

13. Publication Title				14. Issue Date for Circulation Data Below
Child and Adolescent Psychiatric Clinics of North America				July 2005

15.	Extent and Nature of Circulation	Average No. Copies Each Issue During Preceding 12 Months	No. Copies of Single Issue Published Nearest to Filing Date
a.	Total Number of Copies (Net press run)	2050	1900
b. Paid and/or Requested Circulation	(1) Paid/Requested Outside-County Mail Subscriptions Stated on Form 3541. (Include advertiser's proof and exchange copies)	1170	1112
	(2) Paid In-County Subscriptions Stated on Form 3541 (Include advertiser's proof and exchange copies)		
	(3) Sales Through Dealers and Carriers, Street Vendors, Counter Sales, and Other Non-USPS Paid Distribution	101	108
	(4) Other Classes Mailed Through the USPS		
c.	Total Paid and/or Requested Circulation [Sum of 15b. (1), (2), (3), and (4)] ▶	1271	1220
d. Free Distribution by Mail (Samples, complimentary, and other free)	(1) Outside-County as Stated on Form 3541	72	88
	(2) In-County as Stated on Form 3541		
	(3) Other Classes Mailed Through the USPS		
e.	Free Distribution Outside the Mail (Carriers or other means)		
f.	Total Free Distribution (Sum of 15d. and 15e.) ▶	72	88
g.	Total Distribution (Sum of 15c. and 15f.) ▶	1343	1308
h.	Copies not Distributed	707	592
i.	Total (Sum of 15g and h.) ▶	2050	1900
j.	Percent Paid and/or Requested Circulation (15c. divided by 15g. times 100)	95%	93%

16. Publication of Statement of Ownership
☐ Publication required. Will be printed in the **October 2005** issue of this publication.
☐ Publication not required.

17. Signature and Title of Editor, Publisher, Business Manager, or Owner

Janet V. Zimmerman — Manager of Subscription Services

Date 9/15/05

I certify that all information furnished on this form is true and complete. I understand that anyone who furnishes false or misleading information on this form or who omits material or information requested on the form may be subject to criminal sanctions (including fines and imprisonment) and/or civil sanctions (including civil penalties).

Instructions to Publishers

1. Complete and file one copy of this form with your postmaster annually on or before October 1. Keep a copy of the completed form for your records.

2. In cases where the stockholder or security holder is a trustee, include in items 10 and 11 the name of the person or corporation for whom the trustee is acting. Also include the names and addresses of individuals who are stockholders who own or hold 1 percent or more of the total amount of bonds, mortgages, or other securities of the publishing corporation. In item 11, if none, check the box. Use blank sheets if more space is required.

3. Be sure to furnish all circulation information called for in item 15. Free circulation must be shown in items 15d, e, and f.

4. Item 15h., Copies not Distributed, must include (1) newsstand copies originally stated on Form 3541, and returned to the publisher, (2) estimated returns from news agents, and (3), copies for office use, leftovers, spoiled, and all other copies not distributed.

5. If the publication had Periodicals authorization as a general or requester publication, this Statement of Ownership, Management, and Circulation must be published; it must be printed in any issue in October or, if the publication is not published during October, the first issue printed after October.

6. In item 16, indicate the date of the issue in which this Statement of Ownership will be published.

7. Item 17 must be signed.

Failure to file or publish a statement of ownership may lead to suspension of Periodicals authorization.

PS Form 3526, October 1999 (Reverse)

Changing Your Address?

Make sure your subscription changes too! When you notify us of your new address, you can help make our job easier by including an exact copy of your Clinics label number with your old address (see illustration below.) This number identifies you to our computer system and will speed the processing of your address change. Please be sure this label number accompanies your old address and your corrected address—you can send an old Clinics label with your number on it or just copy it exactly and send it to the address listed below.

We appreciate your help in our attempt to give you continuous coverage. Thank you.

W. B. Saunders Company

SHIPPING AND RECEIVING DEPTS.
151 BENIGNO BLVD.
BELLMAWR, N.J. 08031

> SECOND CLASS POSTAGE
> **PAID AT BELLMAWR, N.J.**

This is your copy of the

_____ **CLINICS OF NORTH AMERICA**

00503570 DOE—J32400   101   NH   8102

JOHN C DOE MD
324 SAMSON ST
BERLIN   NH   03570

XP-D11494

JAN ISSUE

Your Clinics Label Number
Copy it exactly or send your label along with your address to:
W.B. Saunders Company, Customer Service
Orlando, FL 32887-4800
Call Toll Free 1-800-654-2452

Please allow four to six weeks for delivery of new subscriptions and for processing address changes.